THE HISTORICAL TRAUMA PROGRAMME

For Self-help or to Support Individual Therapy

A guidebook of hope and recovery for people who experienced childhood abuse, neglect, or abandonment

ISBN: 978-1-917293-43-3

IMPORTANT NOTE: There are two versions of this Guidebook, one designed to be used for *self-help or to support individual therapy* and the other to support *group therapy*. Please check the titles carefully to ensure you have the version that is right for you.

Free audio version
The Historical Trauma Programme should not discriminate against anyone who needs help. If you have a learning difficulty such as dyslexia or struggle with reading due to current psychological problems, please be aware that a free audio version of the Guidebook is available. You can download the audio version from the HTP website at www.htpcommunity.org. Alternatively, you can access the audio version on YouTube - when on YouTube, search using the words @HistoricalTraumaProgramme. *While the audio version can be very helpful it will be essential to use it alongside the print version for completing questionnaires, reviewing charts, journaling, etc.*

The HTP Community Website
The HTP website can be found at www.htpcommunity.org. The website allows you to connect with others, share your views, ask questions, make contact, and access further information.

People who experienced childhood harm describe their experiences in this Guidebook. All names have been changed, and certain identifying features have been altered in some cases to protect their identities. Also, sometimes clients use expletives (swear words) when describing their experiences. We decided to stick with their words as much as possible, so you will occasionally encounter some spicy language.

This programme is not intended to be a substitute for certified clinical treatment where this is necessary. Persons with a condition requiring professional attention should consult a qualified medical practitioner or therapist.

DEDICATION

This Guidebook is dedicated to the hundreds of people who experienced childhood harm and courageously told us their stories, shared their insights, and supported the development of this text.

CONTENTS

ACKNOWLEDGEMENTS

The author wishes to express gratitude to the many clinicians who supported the Historical Trauma Programme (HTP). First and foremost is Dr Liz Murphy, who was there right at the beginning and provided essential practical and emotional assistance. Special thanks are due to clinicians who have facilitated HTP programmes and therapy groups, including Dr Katie Williams, Fi Connington, Dr Liz Murphy, Dr Agnieszka Dixon, Analee Beesley, Dr Chelsey Church, John Woolner, Dr Christina Rowe, Dr Sam Yong, Simone Harding, Richard Ashrowan, Leslie Brooks, Nicky Taylor, Dr George Capone, Dr Liz Parry, Lottie Costello, and Dr Jennifer Martin. The author is also grateful to the many clinicians who provided individual therapy supporting clients using the HTP Guidebook, including Dr Vicky Brooks, Alex Briely, John Harris, Sarah Milton, Alex Drake, Amy Goodwin, Toney Courtney, Melissa Willis, Leslie Whyte, Laura Scott-Lowe, Antonia Nash, Dr Candy Hayward, Dr Sam Bampton, Charlotte Harrison, Jasmine Randal, Lottie Costello, Nahory Mancilla-Hernandez, Ashley Colledge, Amethyst Wheeler, Lydia Jevon, Ceinwen John, Leslie Brooks, Howard Winfield, Rosie Orchard, Jack Erasmus, Gemma Doyle, Paula Morgan, Cassie Sails, Esme Huggons, Clare Crook, Hannah Parkinson, and Lottie Costello. A debt of gratitude is also due to Professor Nick Sarra for his sage clinical supervision and Dr Hamilton Fairfax who provided support and encouragement.

While the HTP draws on a broad range of models and research findings, a handful of clinicians were especially influential. There is Judith Herman, whose insights concerning the process of recovery have proven incredibly useful; Steven Porges, who gave us such helpful language to describe how childhood trauma shapes the way the autonomic nervous system develops and operates; Christine Courtois and Julian Ford, who's research, writing and coordination has had such a positive impact on the field of childhood trauma; Bessel Van Der Kolk, who has done so much to illuminate the role of the body in respect to understanding and intervening (Van Der Kolk also needs to be recognised for how he has helped psychiatrists, psychologists, and psychotherapists talk to one another); and, Jeffrey E. Young, who has done so much to illuminate the substantial role that traumatic core beliefs (schemas) play in trauma and recovery.

INTRODUCTION

"I think there's a part of me that wants to deal with what happened and another part of me that tries to push it all away. Is that normal?"
- Charlie

There are two groups of people who know *a lot* about childhood abuse, neglect and abandonment. The first group are those individuals who were harmed in childhood. No one has a more direct and experiential understanding of childhood trauma than those who encountered it, and this is a point that needs to be acknowledged. Apart from anything else, these individuals are 'experts by experience'. The second group of people are the mental health clinicians and researchers who specialise in the field of childhood trauma. A great deal has been learned over the past 50 years. Specialists now have a better understanding concerning the prevalence of childhood trauma, the impact of abuse and neglect on development, and the ideas and strategies that can really help. This is good news and cause for those who experienced harm to feel optimistic that progress can be made. Although it's an oversimplification, we might say that specialists *know about* childhood trauma, whereas those who were harmed *know it*. Both forms of knowing are essential, and when combined, we have a powerful mix of ingredients that can support recovery. A unique feature of The Historical Trauma Programme (HTP) is the extent to which it represents a genuine partnership between those who experienced trauma and clinicians.

The Historical Trauma Programme was designed as a scientifically-based model for those who experienced childhood harm and continue to struggle with psychological problems today. Over several years, the HTP Guidebook has been used by hundreds of clients working closely with dozens of NHS clinicians within individual and group therapy. In this way, the Guidebook developed as *a close collaboration* between clients and clinicians. Clients worked with the earlier versions of the Guidebook, attended sessions, continually shared their stories, and told us what was helpful and less useful. The Guidebook was rewritten many times to include the 'voices' and feedback of those we worked with. Over time, the Guidebook came to represent what are seen as the best ideas and strategies from the field of trauma studies *and* the real-life insights and experiences provided by numerous clients. As confidence in the value of the Guidebook grew, it made sense to make it available to the general public. This version of the

Guidebook is designed for self-help or to support individual therapy, and there is a separate version designed to support group therapy.

If you experienced abuse or neglect in childhood, it might sound like a cliché to suggest that 'you are not alone'. And yet, there are credible reasons to see this as true. The challenges of identifying historical trauma and the role of secrecy make relying on statistics difficult. However, we know that there are currently 57,000 children identified as requiring protection from all types of abuse in the UK, and due to the likelihood of significant under-reporting, the NSPCC estimates this figure as approximately eight times higher – about 456,000 children.[1] Taking population size into account, rates of child abuse and neglect appear similar in America, where around 3.2 million children are annually subjected to an investigation.[2]

However, the statistics do not convey what the experience is like, and each individual's history is unique. Childhood harm may have taken the form of physical, emotional or sexual abuse, neglect or abandonment. Or, there may have occurred a mix of these experiences. Those who caused harm may have been a parent or step-parent, another family member, a teacher, a child-minder, school peers or others. Harm can occur in the family home, in foster care or residential settings, in school, within clubs, athletic or religious organisations, or in other places. Also, the effects of trauma during childhood and in later life can vary. In other words, there is no 'single story' about who a person is that experienced harm in childhood. They are male and female, people of every age, people of every ethnicity, belief, gender or sexual orientation, people who are very successful in life and those who have had serious social difficulties. If someone were to walk past an individual who experienced childhood harm in the street or meet them at a social event, they can't be told apart from the rest of society.

While such individuals are unique, the consequences of childhood trauma are not random. In general, people who were harmed as children experience difficulties in getting essential needs met. If we look closer, we see that there are important *themes* that most people who experience childhood harm can identify with. These themes also help us appreciate the significant challenges posed by childhood harm *and* point us in the general direction of recovery.

Five themes which pull such individuals together as a group are: first, whereas childhood should have been characterised by enduring safety and love, these individuals had **experiences of threat and fear**. Second, childhood trauma (in whatever form) compromises a **child's developing self**. How people come to think and feel about themselves is *normally* affected by trauma in a significant manner. Third, such individuals are more likely to experience a range of **distressing psychological problems** in adulthood, including emotional and attentional issues, post-traumatic reactions, psychosomatic issues (trauma expressed as a medical problem), and so on. For many, this can also include further trauma as an adult, referred to as retraumatisation. Fourth, the effects of trauma often compromise the individual's **quality of relationships** and **general life development**. Fifth, **the role of silence** is often a complicated issue. Many children will have found it nearly impossible to talk about what was happening during childhood, or perhaps they did try to talk about it but did not get the help they needed. As clinicians, we often find that we are speaking with individuals in their 30s, 40s, 50s or even later in life, and they are only now really discussing and exploring past experiences.

If all of this sounds gloomy, there are at least a couple of points of optimism. As mentioned above, there are good reasons for clinicians and people who experienced childhood harm to feel that progress can be made. And the political and cultural landscape is changing. While research in this area is lacking, more and more people appear to be able to think and talk about what happened to them and seek help.[3]

There are some good books and lots of online resources available for adults who experienced childhood trauma, so what's different about the HTP? First, you will note (possibly with some alarm) that the HTP is a *big* programme. The Guidebook contains 21 chapters, each focusing on an essential theme and related practices. And, you will be encouraged take your time, engaging in an unhurried but sustained pace (more about this later). While the HTP is admittedly 'a big ask', there is a reason for this. Childhood trauma is cunning, has deep roots, as well as multiple and complex impacts on wellness – impacts which are emotional, cognitive (effecting how we think), body-based, and which affect our sense of self and relationships. It's for this reason that the HTP asks you to go slowly and work with historical trauma in a comprehensive way. Here's an analogy which may help. Lionel Messi is a wonderful football player, but if you put him up against any premier team, things are going to go wrong. Childhood trauma is likewise a challenging opponent, so it's important to approach it with care and have lots of resources on your side. The HTP is not for everyone, and some might need a recovery model with a more narrow focus that asks for less of an investment in time.

Second, the HTP will emphasise the need for continued safety and stability. As boring as safety may sound, if you really engage with what happened to you and your recovery, things are going to get *emotional*. We have seen this happen repeatedly among the clients who have worked with us. The HTP proceeds at a careful and gradual pace, but it will get fairly intense in terms of what you will be asked to remember and think about.

Third (and as mentioned), through continuous feedback, hundreds of clients have taught us clinicians what is helpful about the HTP and what needs development. We have been deeply touched by the generosity and tolerance clients have shown and their willingness to help us get the Guidebook right. Also, you will find the 'voices' of numerous clients throughout the Guidebook. This not only acts to complement research and ideas from trauma studies, but it can also be really helpful. On countless occasions, people we work with have told us how the words of a client found in the Guidebook have been comforting, inspiring, or helpful.

Fourth, while certainly not exclusive to the HTP, our model is firmly based on the principles of 'mental health recovery'. Childhood trauma is *not* seen as a 'mental illness' that an individual must simply live with. The programme attends to post-traumatic symptoms (the painful stuff) but is also greatly interested in post-traumatic growth.[4] An individual should not merely aim for some state of 'stability' but should be supported to develop their unique abilities and create the life they want. People who experienced childhood harm are seen as active and capable participants. The principles of hope, empowerment, learning, personal identity, creativity and meaning are essential for recovery.

General overview of the programme

Where do the ideas and strategies which make up the HTP come from? Or, what's it all about? There are three ways of answering this question. 1. There are several available books which can support those who experienced childhood harm, and most can be helpful. However, many available books are based in a particular model of helping or they focus more narrowly on specific topics. The HTP is highly 'integrative'. This means that the HTP is not tied to one model of trauma or psychological therapy. Rather, the HTP relies on the most useful ideas and practices from a wide range of theoretical models – psychodynamic, attachment psychology, humanistic and existential, cognitive behavioural, body-based approaches, compassion-based approaches, neuropsychology, and more.

The HTP covers a broad range of significant issues or needs related to childhood harm. If you have read other books on trauma, the HTP can support your confidence and help consolidate your recovery. However, because of the breadth of topics covered, the HTP can be a good place to start. 2. The HTP is informed by what we see as the most valid and useful medical and psychological research. 3. As mentioned, the HTP guidebook has been used with hundreds of clients over several years in individual and group psychotherapy. Clients describe their experiences and often share their personal insights, which you will find throughout the Guidebook.

The ethos and structure of the programme owe a debt to the ground-breaking work of Judith Herman.[5] It was Herman who really understood the need to feel in control and the importance of relationships to recovery. In Herman's words, "The core experiences of psychological trauma are disempowerment and disconnection from others. Recovery, therefore, is based upon the empowerment of the survivor and the creation of new connections."[6] Historical traumas involve circumstances where a child experienced a profound lack of control. This sense of lacking a healthy sense of control is often carried into adult experiences and relationships. Clients can share with us this sense that past traumatic events exert control over their minds (thoughts), their body-based reactions and related emotions, and even at times their choices or behaviours. Consistent with Herman's view, The HTP seeks to empower you to develop a healthy sense of control and find connections with others. There are many essential ways you will find here of working with your mind (thoughts), body-based distress and emotions, and the behaviours (choices) you will decide to make for yourself.

This programme contains 21 chapters which you will work through. You will be introduced to what we believe are the most helpful ideas and strategies for understanding and overcoming the effects of child abuse or neglect. The insights you will find here come from a broad understanding of research into complex trauma, our clinical experiences and numerous exchanges with people we have supported over the years.

The initial pages of the *Guidebook* provide opportunities to establish any necessary safety and stability. The words of the British philosopher A. C. Grayling perhaps capture why safety and stability are so important: "It is often the case that truth is as painful as it is liberating."[7] While this Guidebook will not aim to tell you what is 'true', your work with it can help you build on previous insights or find 'personal truths'. If you are like many who engage with this programme, such insights or personal truths can be, as Grayling suggests, painful as well as liberating. This is why a focus on stability can be so important.

Part I then allows you to explore the nature and impact of historical trauma. You will not only learn a lot about how historical trauma tends to affect people in general, but you will be looking at this in a very personal way. *Part II* can be the most challenging because you will be asked to explore what happened to you as a child in ways which can stir up memories and some difficult feelings, but this is quite a necessary part of the process. Remembering and reflecting on what happened provides opportunities for insight and new ways of thinking, not only about the past but about your relationship with yourself, others, and life. We then added a chapter right in the middle of the programme that encourages reflection on what recovery or personal development looks like for you. *Part III* focuses more on recovery, and you will be offered many ideas and strategies to help you overcome the impact of past trauma, develop your sense of self, get your needs met better, and shape relationships and life in ways important to you.

The structure of the programme described above reflects ideas developed by Herman,[5] who pointed out that successfully recovering from childhood trauma involves *three successive stages*: 1. Establishing safety and stability, 2. 'Processing' or being able to reflect on and make sense of the past (Herman has called this remembering and morning), and 3. Engaging in life and relationships in new ways which are less constrained by past harm (Herman has referred to this as reconnection and integration).

Clinicians and researchers interested in childhood trauma have, over many years, developed specialist language. These professionals use words like *somatisation*, *trauma bond*, *traumatic re-enactment*, *dissociation*, and so on. This sort of language can be useful but comes with a risk. More than anything, the people who use this programme should feel empowered and encouraged by what they find here – they should not feel confused and frustrated. Our view is this: It *is* sometimes important to use specialist terminology because many of these terms have some lovely explanatory power that can support moments of insight. And, if you come across a term or concept which seems important, you may want to go and learn more about it elsewhere (the internet is an amazing resource). But we will always do our best to explain such terminology in a clear and meaningful way.

On the subject of language, it's been a challenge to know how to refer to people engaging with this programme. Language is important, especially when it relates to an individual's identity. For several years we used the term *survivors*, which is quite a common descriptor. Many individuals connected with this word, but others felt uncomfortable (or even annoyed) with it for various reasons. The term *victim* doesn't work well. As children, many people truly *were* victims because they lacked the power to respond to what was happening to them. However, as adults, the word victim is associated with a sense of powerlessness or helplessness, which is really not useful.

Eventually, we asked the eight members of one of our therapy groups what language might work best. After some discussion, the group settled on the descriptor *people who experienced childhood harm*. It's inclusive and captures any or all relevant childhood experiences, e.g. every form of abuse, emotional or physical neglect, abandonment or vicarious trauma. Occasionally we may use the very similar descriptors of *childhood trauma* or *childhood adverse experiences*.

We also want to mention a few points about the programme's general perspective. The first point is nicely illustrated by some words which were apparently falsely attributed to Ben Franklin: "Tell me and I forget. Teach me and I remember. Involve me and I learn." Wherever this idea came from (some say it's a Chinese philosopher named Xun Kuang), it represents our view about what makes the programme effective. We do not see people who use this programme as 'students' or passive recipients of the information being taught. Whether you use the Guidebook as self-help or alongside individual therapy, the programme's success depends on you being actively involved with these materials. It might sound corny, but you will have 'a relationship' with this Guidebook. In ways which may be surprising, this Guidebook is about you. You won't make a connection with everything you find here, but you will identify with many ideas and certain experiences of others who have used the programme. If you are like most, you will see yourself in these pages. There can be a strange sense of recognition.

Second, your expertise as someone who experienced childhood harm is as valid as all the research and theory in this Guidebook. The programme seeks to empower you to get important needs met and develop your life as you wish. With this in mind, the programme *will never tell you* how to think, feel, or cope. Instead, you will be provided with numerous opportunities to *reflect* on your experiences and experiment with certain tools for change. You can decide what is most useful in the context of your life.

Third, we believe there are a couple of values that are important and which you will often find in the 'subtext' of the Guidebook: *hope* and *patience*. Hope, because however entrenched the effects of past trauma may seem, if you can create reasonable safety and stability and think about your past, there are opportunities for change – change in terms of developing insight or change within your life. However, a counterbalance to the value of hope is the need for patience concerning recovery and patience with yourself. Childhood trauma *normally* has deep roots, and the effects of trauma do not want to heal easily or quickly. We appreciate the challenge you are facing, and we are not fond of any model that offers simplistic or quick-fix solutions. This programme itself requires patience in that it is designed to go at a careful and thoughtful pace. We hope you will make progress within the course of this programme, but in certain respects, you are likely to be working with your recovery for many years to come or for the rest of your life. Hope and patience are twin values which can work together for you.

Is the programme a good fit for you?

The programme is for adult men and women and is likely to be appropriate if:

1. You experienced **physical, emotional or sexual abuse, neglect or abandonment** in childhood, i.e. between birth and 18. If you're not sure how you think or feel about these terms, this is quite common. We will explore them in further detail in chapter 1.

2. **You experience psychological problems related to childhood events**. You may experience intrusive and unwanted thoughts or memories of what happened, or you might feel you have to push such memories away. You may sometimes have bad dreams, you might feel the need to avoid situations or people in your life which remind you of the past, or you may have painful psychological symptoms which seem connected to

childhood harm, e.g. depression, anxiety, sleeping problems, compulsive behaviours, eating difficulties, being mistrustful or 'hyper-vigilant' to possible threats, etc...

3. You will likely recognise that abuse or neglect was detrimental to your **sense of self**. This may be recognised in difficulties with self-worth, self-confidence or self-image. Related to impaired self-development, you may recognise that it's been difficult (at least at times in your life) to build or maintain healthy, intimate or stable **relationships**. As a result, you may see a pattern (past or present) where you either feel **cut off** from others or find yourself in painful relationships in which you do not get your needs met.

4. To benefit, there is another essential ingredient: **readiness to engage with the programme.** This programme asks quite a bit of you. You will need to consider the impact of childhood events on your development, think about upsetting events from your past, work at building insight and engage with specific exercises. So you have to be in the right 'place' to commit the time and resources to do this work. The section entitled *Preparing for a Safe and Productive Experience* will help you explore in more detail whether now is the right time to engage with this programme.

Will the HTP help and are there risks?

All models of helping have their *strengths* and *limitations*, and we will describe both as openly as possible regarding the HTP. We will also mention a particular risk concerning the HTP. This may help you decide if the HTP is right for you at this time in your life. Based on feedback received and our clinical experiences, the HTP can help in the following ways:

- You will learn **a lot** about childhood harm, both in a general and highly personal manner. Knowledge can provide a sense of control and hope, and at the end of this programme, you may feel like something of an expert on childhood trauma. You should be able to think and talk about childhood trauma with increased confidence.
- Through increased insight, you may develop a stronger sense of self. This can mean developing thoughts and feelings that are less self-critical or shame-based. Self-compassion, self-care, and confidence may also increase.
- You may see improvements in your current relationships or develop healthier relationships.
- As children try and adapt to traumatic circumstances, their autonomic nervous system understandably becomes more sensitive to possible threats. As adults, they often have an overly sensitive nervous system as a result. Within our therapy groups it's not unusual for

us to see clients in a state of fear or emotional shut-down. Brains and bodies got 'shaped' through experience to overreact in situations where basic safety is present. The HTP can help you make progress with this common issue.

- You may develop ways of coping which are more likely to get 'deeper' needs met. Reductions in 'retraumatisation' can occur.
- You may feel more confident developing your life in ways that provide increased meaning and self-expression.
- You may see an eventual reduction in painful psychological symptoms such as depression, anxiety, sleep difficulties, or intrusive memories. However, it's not unusual for increases in psychological symptoms to occur before things improve.

The specific reasons a person wants to engage with the HTP are personal. However, there are a couple of goals that are common (perhaps even universal) for almost everyone who comes to this programme. 1. There is a need to explore what happened and find words to explain it to yourself and, to whatever extent possible, to others. This is a process of remembering – of making sense of what happened and the impact on your development. 2. Your body and mind need to learn that the threats that existed in the past are over so that you can be present in the moment, play, be productive, and commune with others in ways that are as meaningful and fulfilling as possible.[8] The HTP is designed to help with both of these tasks.

However, there are areas of recovery for which the HTP may not be adequate for some people. And the HTP might not even be the right model for you at this time. Certain post-traumatic symptoms related to childhood harm are an example, i.e. intrusive thoughts or images, nightmares, or 'flashbacks'. While the Guidebook contains what is hopefully helpful information in this area, it's not unusual for people to complete the Guidebook and find that post-traumatic symptoms continue to be a problem. They may need additional specialist therapy such as Eye Movement Desensitization and Reprocessing (EMDR) or CBT for PTSD. Or, if post-traumatic symptoms are very disturbing for you now, it's probably best to engage with specialist therapy *before* working with the HTP.

We spend time at the front end of the programme helping you identify instability and ways of responding if it should occur. Nevertheless, for a minority of people, there can be a risk that using the HTP results in instability which is more significant or worrying. If this occurs, they may need to continue their work with the HTP or other models with a therapist. And, for those who currently experience *significant* emotional instability or risk as a primary problem, it's advisable to get specialist therapy for this issue. We have seen many examples of people who made really good progress with the HTP, but they needed to better manage significant emotional instability or risk *before* doing the HTP work.

It's not unusual for a reader to find a certain chapter and topic really helpful, but it may not feel sufficient – the individual feels a need to go further with that topic. In a sense, this is good news and can be seen as more an opportunity than a problem. Part of what the HTP aims to do is stimulate hope and enthusiasm for your recovery, and if you are left wanting more following your work here, that's great. At the end of the book, you will find a *recommended reading* section for almost all of the topics we cover.

References

1. Child Protection Register and Plan Statistics for all UK Nations, 2015
2. US Department of Health and Human Services Report, 2014
3. Saner, E. *Women and men are speaking out about abuse – is this the end of the patriachy?* The Guardian. October 30th, 2017.
4. Calhoun, L. G. & Tedeschi, R. G. (2013). *Post-traumatic Growth in Clinical Practice*. London: Routledge.
5. Herman, J. (1992). *Trauma and Recovery: The Aftermath of Violence – From Domestic Abuse to Political Terror*. NY: Basic Books.
6. Herman, J. (2002). *Recovery from Trauma*. Wiley online library. https://doi.org/10.1046/j.1440-1819.1998.0520s5S145.x.
7. Grayling, A.C. (2023). *Philosophy and Life: Exploring the Great Questions of How to Live. London*: Penguin Books.
8. Van Der Kolk, B. (2015). *The body keeps the score: Mind, brain and body in the transformation of trauma*. London: Penguin Books.

PREPARING FOR A SAFE AND PRODUCTIVE EXPERIENCE

If you buy a new power tool or food processor, you will probably skip the 'safety information' and go straight to the description of how to use your new appliance. We do need to spend time considering safety and stability, but this *really is* an important consideration in the context of childhood trauma. It's essential that people who experienced childhood harm are reasonably safe and stable *before* they start working at understanding and 'processing' past issues.[1] And, even if they feel reasonably stable before starting this work, it's common to experience some challenges to stability along the way. Stretching and warming up your muscles before a workout can prevent an injury. In the same way, being prepared to spot and respond to instability is the best means of protecting yourself if it occurs.

Aside from stability simply being a good thing, there is another reason why it's important. Even with the support of therapy, about 20% of people drop out of the work they are doing.[2] A common reason why people disengage from therapy or personal development work is because they begin to lose confidence in their stability in response to exploring their past experiences. You're much less likely to benefit from therapy or personal development programmes if you drop out,[3] and considering safety and stability at the outset increases the chances that you will make it right through to the end.

Should you use the programme as self-help or alongside therapy?

We use the word self-help because it is the most common term to convey that you are using a resource without professional help. However, the word self-help has a solitary feel which we imagine conveys the wrong idea. Childhood trauma was interpersonal because it involved other people. Recovering from childhood trauma is also interpersonal because it requires other people – people you should feel reasonably safe with. For some, a therapist will be a necessary other person. Where therapy is not essential, individuals tend to require others they can trust to talk with about the work they are doing with the HTP Guidebook. This person might be a friend, partner, family member, people in a face-to-face or online community support group, or others.

Talking with others about the work you are doing with the Guidebook is not always a popular idea among people who were harmed by others. Many have difficulties with trust and some are fiercely self-reliant (or try to be). This helps to explain why childhood trauma is often kept a secret for many years. Below we help you think about whether to do the programme as self-help or alongside individual therapy, but whatever decision you make, it's important not to do the HTP in an isolated fashion.

While it is possible to use the programme as self-help, this is advisable for people who feel relatively stable, have support, and can already think about their past without becoming significantly distressed.

If you are experiencing any of the following, we advise that you do not use this programme as self-help. Instead, seeking help from a qualified therapist or mental health clinician will be advisable. Tic what applies.

___ You are experiencing significant vulnerability or instability due to current life events.
___ You are self-harming or having suicidal thoughts/impulses.
___ You are social isolated or there is no one you feel safe enough to talk about the work you are doing with the HTP.
___ You are hallucinating, experiencing significant paranoia, or delusional thinking.
___ You are experiencing post-traumatic stress symptoms which you feel you have little control over, e.g. disturbing thoughts/images, very high levels of anxiety, significant social avoidance, frequent nightmares.
___ You can't think about the past without feeling very disturbed or that you are losing control.
___ Your current relationships are unstable and painful in ways that will make it difficult to work on your past trauma.
___ You are struggling with addiction or substance misuse, or you are in the early stages of recovery from addiction or substance misuse.

If you need professional therapy before or while doing this programme, you may want to speak to a family doctor/GP or other medical clinician for advice. Ask a therapist any questions you need to before you decide to work with them. Ensure they are properly registered or certified for the country you live in, have training and experience in working with childhood trauma, and seem trustworthy.

If you feel you can use the Guidebook as self-help (without therapy), we still advise that you have someone you can talk to about the work you are doing, and how you are managing. This person (or people) should be someone you can trust, who will listen, keep what you say confidential, take you seriously, and care about how you are coping.

Exercise 1: If using the HTP as self-help, indicate below who you can speak with while doing this programme.

Suggestions on how to best use the Guidebook

The Guidebook has been rewritten many times in an attempt to include only what seems most essential to recovery. However, we appreciate that the Guidebook can seem very 'big', and some might wonder if they can fit it into their lives. If the Guidebook seems big, this reflects the fact that childhood trauma is normally experienced as a *big problem*. Our modern world is often about speed, and there is nothing necessarily wrong with that. If a two-minute YouTube video can sort out your problem, that's great. But childhood trauma is a different sort of problem – childhood trauma has deep roots and will not 'go willingly'. This program is, therefore, designed to go at a fairly unhurried pace, and that's how we suggest you relate to it. Many people we work with cope by rushing like mad (as if being chased) or coming to a dead stop and collapsing. These are ways of coping with experiences of threat that are based in the nervous system, which we will look at later. You will be encouraged to work with the Guidebook in a *gentle* but *sustained* manner, giving yourself time to integrate what you discover in the context of your lived experiences.

The chapters are not that long – they range from 8 to about 20 pages. You might imagine you could read through the book in a few weeks. However, we strongly recommend you do not approach things this way for a couple of reasons. First, the ideas and exercises you encounter here will stir up memories, feelings, and thoughts. After reading and doing exercises, it's helpful to just get on with life and give yourself time to reflect on or integrate what you are encountering. Anna experienced childhood physical and emotional abuse, and she described her experience this way:

> **"I could relate to most of the ideas without much trouble, and so I often just wanted to go straight onto the next chapter. But I realised that I needed to slow down because after finishing a chapter, I would keep thinking about what I read and seeing how these ideas related to my life and how I saw myself."**

You will encounter many important ideas while reading the Guidebook, but this is a rather superficial form of learning. The most powerful way to understand these ideas is to see how they actually work in the context of your life and relationships. You will read about, for example, the impact of trauma on your body and nervous system, retraumatisation and traumatic core beliefs, but you will get a more powerful understanding of these ideas in relation to your lived experience. So the programme requires reading and doing exercises *plus* time to go and live your life. And some exercises are not done sitting at a table – they are done in response to life events, which can develop spontaneously.

Doing a chapter over the course of a week is often a good pace for many, which means spending something like five or six months to work your way through the entire programme. This might seem like a long time, but consider this: you have struggled with past events and related psychological problems for most of your life. What's another five or six months in the greater scheme of things? The Guidebook only feels 'big' or overwhelming if you imagine you have to do it in a few weeks. If you are using the Guidebook while seeing a therapist, working with one chapter between each session can often create a useful rhythm, although it may be helpful for you and your therapist to work out together what the right pace may be.

The Guidebook is yours to use, develop and keep for the rest of your life. You can underline, highlight, make notes in the page margins, do the exercises, draw pictures, etc... At the moment, this Guidebook is identical to every other copy. When you finish, there will be a lot of *you* between these pages.

The content of each chapter is designed to build on the chapters which came before it, so it's helpful to read the chapters in order. Certain earlier chapters offer opportunities for developing insight into the nature of childhood trauma. This work helps prepare you for later chapters, which focus more explicitly on remembering or 'processing' historical trauma, and still later chapters, which focus explicitly on recovery.

Within this Guidebook, you will encounter exercises encouraging you to reflect on your experience (past or present) and to express your thoughts and feelings. Many exercises offer an opportunity for writing, some are checklists, and others are questionnaires. There is evidence that expressing yourself through writing can be helpful with respect to resolving past trauma[4] and for general health.[5] This makes sense. As we explore later, children who experience trauma often cope by not consciously absorbing what is happening to them. They 'split off' or deny their own experiences. To survive, children often deny parts of who they are. Reflecting and exploring through writing can be a powerful way to integrate aspects of your experience and to get in touch with parts of you that had to be denied.

However, exercises involving writing may feel intimidating for many who have had negative school experiences, have a learning difficulty such as dyslexia, or have problems with concentration. These issues are common for adults who have experienced childhood harm. If you struggle in any of these ways, we have a few pieces of advice: 1. *Don't worry* about getting anything 'right or wrong' or 'failing'. Only you have the 'correct answer' because you are reflecting on your own experience. 2. Writing is not the only way to respond to these exercises. Some will find it more beneficial to make drawings, write poetry, paint or use other art media. If the amount of space offered in the Guidebook is not sufficient, use more paper and place this work in the book. 3. If there are certain words you just can't write because it feels too distressing, perhaps use initials or some code. If putting something down on paper still feels impossible, see if you can talk it through with someone you trust or your clinician (if you are in therapy). 4. If it helps, there is a free audio version of the Guidebook you can download from the HTP Website or find on YouTube (see final section of book for further information). If you use the audio version you will still require the Guidebook to complete exercises.

Some people using this programme can feel unsure about how much of their work should be shared with others. Doing this programme can give some people the confidence to talk more about what happened, and many have found it helpful to share the Guidebook and work they are doing with others they trust. There is a truism which suggests that 'talking helps', and for many who experienced childhood harm, there is evidence that this is accurate.[6] If you can share your work in the Guidebook with someone you trust, we suggest you do that. Some people we have worked with have had powerful and therapeutic experiences by reading the Guidebook with someone they trust or sharing their guidebook work. Others may talk to someone they trust about their work, but they want privacy concerning the writing they are doing in the Guidebook. You should feel in control, so do what's right for you.

If the reading or an exercise elicits disturbing emotions or impulses, don't force yourself to do it. If you're in therapy, tell your clinician what happened so they can give you more support. Otherwise, as you progress in the programme, you may develop more confidence, making it possible to circle back to certain sections or exercises you felt the need to avoid earlier.

Creating the necessary time and space

You will need some protected time and space to focus on the reading and exercises. Below you have a chance to think about when and where you will read the Guidebook. Consider when you are less likely to encounter interruptions. And see if there is a way to make that time pleasant. First thing in the morning with a hot drink can work well for many people, or later on works better for others. The only time we find it doesn't work well is right before bed. You're usually tired, and the work can sometimes stir up memories and feelings, affecting your sleep.

Exercise 1: Time and space for reading the Guidebook

Below, describe what you see as the best time and place for you to work with the Guidebook.

Motivation – more complex than you might think

There was a quote from Charlie at the outset of the book, which we will repeat here: "I think there's a part of me that wants to deal with what happened and another part of me that tries to push it all away. Is that normal?"

If by 'normal' we mean common, then yes, Charlie's experience is very normal. Pretty much everyone we know who has approached this programme has experienced 'mixed feelings'. There is a part of them that wants to get to grips with their past experience, to spend time remembering and making sense of what happened and the way it impacted their development, to work at making changes in how they think and cope, and to (hopefully) feel better about themselves and life. One of the biggest motivating factors for some is that they are just so fed up living with the impact of their past experiences on their daily lives.

However, there is also another part of people who experienced childhood harm that can resist or avoid doing this work, and there can be many *genuine* reasons for this. For example, learning about the effects of past trauma can be upsetting, remembering what happened can feel worrying, contemplating letting go of unhealthy ways of coping may not be something you want to do, and doing this work might affect your relationships in some way. Just thinking about your needs can be something many feel uncomfortable with.

Sometimes the issue of motivation is looked at in quite a punitive way. As in, "hey, that person just isn't motivated," suggesting laziness. But, in the context of this programme, it makes no sense to think of motivation in a punitive way – we need to consider it *psychologically*. In other words, it's understandable that a part of you wants to face this, and a part of you wants to avoid it.

For many, it isn't whether they do this programme (or use another model); it's about *when* they do it. Here is a question to consider: at this point in your life, is the part of you wanting to get to grips with your past and its impact on your life bigger than the part that doesn't want to deal with it? What is your gut response? If you want to go for it, that's great. If not, that's okay too. This programme (or other models) will be here when you're ready. We knew one individual who left the Guidebook on a bookshelf in her kitchen for almost a year. She told us she'd glance at it most days when making meals or doing the dishes, wondering when to start. So, it took a while for her motivation to tip over and for her to get going, but when she did, she had a safe and helpful experience.

Considering difficult life issues or distractions

The exercise below helps you consider your current stability and any distractions in your life. Have a look at the potential issues below that can interfere with security or stability and tick any that currently apply to you. If you tick certain issues, this doesn't necessarily mean you can't or shouldn't do this programme. But you may need to sort some things out first.

Exercise 2: Identifying difficult issues or distractions

___ I'm having medical or physical health problems which are so significant it's hard to focus on much else

___ I'm having to deal with significant financial, legal or debt problems right now

___ My housing or living circumstances are precarious or insecure, and I have to focus on that right now

___ I'm having a serious relationship problem now that I have to focus on

___ I'm grieving or dealing with a significant loss right now

___ There is a major challenge like school, work, or a personal project which makes it difficult to give time to the past or mental health issues

___ There are people in my life whose problems are so bad that it's very difficult to focus on my problems and needs

___ Alcohol, drug use or other compulsive issues are a big enough problem that they would get in the way of this work

___ I have anxiety which is so bad that I'm not sure I can face much of anything

___ I'm so depressed I'm not sure I can focus on anything

Any other distractions? ____

We are not suggesting that your life needs to be completely sorted and that you should have perfect stability before you start this programme. However, if you ticked any of the above issues or identified other significant issues not in the checklist, we suggest you consider two options. First, if a life challenge is worrying or distracting, it may be important to delay the programme until you can sort it out or get through it. Second, perhaps you can start the programme now, but you need the support of a qualified therapist to ensure you will have the stability and support to complete the work safely.

Recognising 'destabilisation' during the programme

Virtually everyone who does personal development work or therapy concerning childhood trauma will encounter difficult feelings, thoughts and memories. This programme will ask you to fully appreciate how childhood experiences have impacted your well-being, sense of self, relationships and life development. You will be looking at patterns by which you have coped as an adult and how childhood pain has continued in adulthood (something called retraumatisation). Later, you will be asked to recall and explore childhood experiences and memories, something you may have needed to push away to a greater or lesser extent. All of this is important for developing personal insight, understanding your needs better, and developing a life less constrained by the past. But, it can be upsetting, and feelings like anger, anxiety, fear and sadness are *normal* (any time we use the word normal, we mean common).

Amanda was a biology and chemistry teacher who was physically and emotionally abused by a stepmother and neglected by her father. An intelligent individual with a scientific and analytical mind, she found the HTP work emotionally challenging and put it like this:

> **"The Guidebook can be upsetting and at times I feel like I'm coming apart. But, maybe that's how it works. Maybe you have to take something apart in order to understand it... and that allows you to put it back together in a new way... in a better way."**

We really liked Amanda's description because it captures the perils and opportunities of working with past trauma. The most common peril is probably destabilisation, the sort of experience you can have when things are being pulled apart. So, what does destabilisation mean? As you use this programme, any difficult reactions you experience will hopefully be temporary and manageable. In other words, you will be able to largely manage these reactions and get back to your life when you need to. This is *not* what is meant by destabilisation. Destabilisation means experiencing feelings, thoughts, memories or impulses that are distressing, difficult to put aside, and threatening to interfere with your ability to cope.

We take the view that 'forewarned is forearmed'. If you can spot destabilisation if it begins to happen, you will be more able to respond or get help. To support you in recognising destabilisation, we will describe the four most common ways it occurs and the *Window of Tolerance*, another helpful way to explain destabilisation. We will then provide ideas about how you might respond so you can re-establish the stability necessary for your continued recovery.

Emotional destabilisation

It's common for people who experienced childhood harm to cope by *pushing the past away*. By engaging with this programme, you will explore your past and its effect on your life, so you should not be surprised if things get... emotional. Such emotional reactions will hopefully be manageable, and you can set them aside and get back to life when you need to. Emotional destabilisation is occurring if you are experiencing powerful emotional reactions that feel overwhelming and which you are struggling to soothe or put aside.

Destabilisation in coping

You can probably identify with the idea that at times you cope in healthier ways but at other times can be vulnerable to coping in ways which undermine your personal development. Everyone is different, but difficulties in coping might mean over-reliance on alcohol or drugs, an increase in obsessive-compulsive behaviours, difficulties with food, isolating oneself from others, etc. Any impulses concerning suicide, deliberate self-harming or other risky behaviours are definite signs of destabilisation concerning coping and should be taken seriously. If you encounter material in this Guidebook that elicits painful feelings or memories leading to deterioration in your ability to cope, this is an expression of destabilisation.

Destabilisation concerning intrusive memories or a 'flashback'

Many parts of this Guidebook can cause you to recall events from your childhood, and you will be specifically asked to recall memories when you get into the middle of the programme. It's normal to experience some difficult memories while doing this work, but ideally, you can put them aside so you can get back to your life and relationships. The goal is remembering, not reliving. However, there is a possibility that exploring past events can cause you to experience painful *intrusive memories*. While less common, it's possible that some could experience a *flashback*.

The difference between an intrusive memory and a 'flashback' is probably one of degree. An intrusive memory occurs if events from your past intrude into your consciousness in a distressing way that you are struggling to control or set aside. Intrusive memories can be distressing, but people can still largely stay connected to the reality around them. With a flashback, the images, emotions and physical sensations are so powerful that someone can lose touch with reality, and it might seem like something bad is actually happening again. It's hard to know what is real. If you are struggling with painful intrusive memories which feel hard to manage or have a flashback, these are signs of destabilisation.

Shame response as destabilisation

Shame is a complex and challenging issue for many people who have experienced childhood harm, which is why we will explore this area in depth in Chapter 15. However, we mention it here briefly because just thinking about your past or how you have coped can elicit a shame response, and we want you to be aware of this from the outset. By shame, we are talking about experiencing painful feelings of self-blame, 'badness' or a sense of inadequacy. Many people we work with can be self-punitive concerning past experiences and the problems they have, which makes them vulnerable to experiencing shame. Just reading this Guidebook and recalling past experiences can trigger a shame response for some, which could be destabilising. In the next section, we will offer a suggestion as to how you can manage if you experience shame in relation to your recovery work.

The window of tolerance

Developed by Danial Seagal,[7] the window of tolerance is a further way to appreciate if you are losing stability. Humans can flip into states of fight, flight or freeze when we encounter (or imagine we encounter) a threat. Fighting or fleeing is consistent with a state of *hyperarousal,* a reaction characterised by emotions such as fear or anger. Alternatively, we can also cope with threats through freezing. This is a state of *hypoarousal,* characterised by emotional numbing, shutting down or becoming immobilised. Between hyperarousal (intense emotions) and hypoarousal (numb emotions) is *The Window of Tolerance*, a place where you are focused on the present and experiencing more moderate levels of emotion. Please read through Table 1 and see what you can identify with.

Table 1

Hyperarousal **FIGHT OR FLIGHT** **Anxiety/panic, hyperactivity, anger, defensive, racing thoughts, intrusive imagery, tension, shaking, hypervigilance (scanning for danger)**
Window of Tolerance **Grounded, present moment awareness, accessing reason, feel safe, emotions tolerable, open and curious, listening and responding in a flexible way**
Hypoarousal **FREEZE** **Emotionally shutdown, disconnected, can't access thoughts, can't defend, numb, physically immobilised, dissociating, loss of energy**

Why might those who experienced childhood trauma be more likely to flip into distressing states of hyperarousal or hypoarousal? One answer is that as children, they learned that hyperarousal or hypoarousal was an effective way of protecting themselves. A child may decide that being very alert and watching anxiously for any dangers (hyperarousal) will help them avoid harm. However, hyperarousal is more likely a means of coping if a child imagines there is a way of escaping danger. If a child is overwhelmed by threat and believes that escape isn't possible, they can learn that shutting down emotionally or becoming numb (hypoarousal) is a good means of feeling less pain. So, people who experienced childhood harm often cope today through hyperarousal or hypoarousal simply because *they learned to do it as a child.*

However, as you navigate this programme and life situations, *spending as much time as possible within the window of tolerance will be helpful.* Being 'kicked out' of the window of tolerance and into states of hyperarousal or hypoarousal can be seen as an expression of destabilization. If you can identify when you are being kicked out of the window of tolerance, this may help you respond in a way that helps you regain stability.

Responding to destabilisation

A state of destabilization can feel complex and is always specific to the context and the individual. So, there is no particular skill that is always appropriate or helpful in respect to regaining stabilization. Several skills to support stabilization are woven throughout the programme. However, we thought it was important to offer certain skills at the front end of the Guidebook, just in case you need them.

Finding the right balance between exposing yourself to the work in this Guidebook and retaining stability is important. In other words, you want to get *close enough* to memories and ideas to develop useful insight but not *so close* that you get overwhelmed.

Distraction or permission to avoid certain material

If there is a particular section of reading or an exercise you don't feel ready to do, that's okay. We have seen many people return to exercises later in their recovery when they feel ready, which is fine. If you sense that destabilisation is occurring, you can also take a break and *distract yourself.* Leave it alone for a while and immerse yourselves in life, relationships or projects. You can then return to the work you are doing when you feel ready. Distraction or temporary avoidance, when necessary, can be a good response if you are destabilised by emotions, intrusive images, or struggling with coping.

Grounding

Grounding can be useful if you struggle with disturbing memories, intrusive images, or emotions that threaten to overwhelm you. It can also be especially helpful if you are having a flashback. As mentioned, intrusive memories can be a feature of a flashback, but the images, the emotions and the physical sensations are so powerful that a person can lose touch with reality, and it might seem like something bad is actually happening again. A grounding exercise is anything that can keep you connected to reality. If you are 'grounded', you are connected to the immediate world around you. You can feel yourself sitting in a chair, and you can hear and see what is happening around you. There are different grounding exercises, and we offer three below. One of these may have more appeal to you than the others.

1. 5-4-3-2-1 grounding
- Look around and name five things that you can see.
- Now, focus your attention on four things that you can feel.
- Next, name three things that you can hear around you.
- Next, focus attention on two things that you can smell around you right now.
- Lastly, find some food which is handy. Focus on what you can taste.

2. You can focus strongly on the objects in your immediate surrounding. Say to yourself, "I'm safe and I'm here in my ________________." Then closely observe the objects around you and describe them, e.g. "This is my kitchen, those are our dinner plates, this is the table we eat at, etc… .

3. You can get back to reality by reminding yourself of who you are. "My name is____________, I'm ____ years old. I live at _____________." The friends and family in my life are ___________________, etc… Keep listing everything about yourself and life which seems important. If you get to the end and everything still feels unreal, start going through the list again.

Some find it helpful to write out the text of the grounding exercise and then keep this with them at all times. If they get triggered and begin to experience intrusive memories or a flashback, they can access the grounding exercise quickly and with greater confidence.

Responding to a shame response

As mentioned, a shame response involves feelings of inadequacy, self-blame, or a sense of 'badness'. It's possible that just reading this book and doing the exercises can trigger feelings of shame. In chapter 15, we will examine shame in detail and explore how it is fundamentally an unhelpful emotion in the context of childhood trauma. For the moment, we ask you to trust us on this point.

If you begin to punish yourself for your past or how you have coped while engaging with this programme, we encourage you to do a couple of things. First, reassure yourself that shame is a very common response for people who experience childhood harm. Second, see if you can get hold of the idea that shame is not helpful for developing insight or recovery. Imagine that shame is this road you can go down. Literally, imagine a road sign labelled *shame*, and this road you can go down is made of self-blame and a sense of badness. And, if you come across that road while doing this programme, don't go down it. Here's why you shouldn't. At every turn, we want to look at what happened and how you have coped *psychologically*, not from any perspective of self-blame, self-punishment or shame. Recovery certainly includes taking responsibility for your behaviour, but trauma-based shame (as we will explore) does not help in this respect.

Also, if you feel shame concerning decisions you made or how you have coped, try to see it with self-compassion, keeping in mind that your past experiences will have set you up for problems later on. In other words, there are reasons why you may have acted or coped as you did. This is a point we will reinforce several times during the programme. So, if a shame response begins to push you towards destabilisation, please try to care for and reassure yourself. Or seek reassurance from others you trust if you can.

Safe place imagery

If you have flipped into a fight or flight response (hyperarousal) as a response to a *genuine* threat, hyperarousal is the right response, and you need to get safe. However, if you are experiencing fear or anger which is trauma-based and out of proportion to any real threats, it makes sense to calm the state of hyperarousal itself.

Creating and accessing a 'safe place' through imagery might seem silly or pointless, but there is an interesting reason why it can help calm a state of hyperarousal. The structures in your brain responsible for firing up a hyperarousal response (sympathetic nervous system) will respond either to an actual threat in front of you, a traumatic memory which has been triggered or calming imagery (such as a safe place). The sympathetic nervous system can't really distinguish events 'out there' from events in your mind, or actual memories from images you create. So imaging a safe place can calm a state of hyperarousal, just like traumatic images, worry or facing a threat in life can activate hyperarousal.

If you are facing a genuine and immediate threat and experiencing fear or anger, you probably need to *do something* to keep yourself or others safe. But if the fear or anger is being driven by past trauma rather than the present situation or is out of proportion to any immediate threat, accessing a 'safe place' can calm the hyperarousal reaction and get you back into the window of tolerance.

Exercise 3: Creating a safe place

Imagine a place where you can feel safe and with pleasant emotions attached. This can be a real place you know, an imaginary place you create or a mix of the two. Others we have worked with have created desert islands, a warm submarine, a cosy shelter with a fire in a snowstorm, being held by a special Being or protective animal, a forest setting, and so on. However, this is *very personal imagery*, so create it as you need to. Try the imagery out, spending at least a few minutes there. Does it work for you? If it does, then that's your safe place. Briefly describe your safe place below.

Accessing a 'safe place' won't be necessary if you are managing Guidebook material without difficulties. However, if a particular section of reading or an exercise seems challenging, you can access your safe place to settle your physiology *before* doing the work. And, if a section of the Guidebook or an exercise winds you up into a state of hyperarousal, you can access your safe place *after*wards to help you get back into your window of tolerance. If having or using a safe place seems silly, perhaps suspend judgement for a bit and see how it works in practice.

Controlled breathing

When you get triggered into a state of hyperarousal, a lot is going on physically that you have little or no control over. If we said, *hey, why don't you stop producing adrenalin, cortisol, and glucose and stop perspiring, you'd say, uhm, I don't think so*. But breathing is a feature of a stress response which you can have voluntary control over. Alcohol, many street drugs, and most psychoactive medications act on your brain in ways that slow breathing. But you can act directly to slow your breathing. And, when you slow your breathing, you start a feedback loop which results in the physical reactions you don't have control over reducing as well.

Exercise 4: Controlled breathing

Find a room where you can be alone and uninterrupted. Sit in a chair in a way which is comfortable but also allows your back to be fairly straight (not slumped). Place the palm of one hand on your chest and the palm of your other hand over your stomach area. Your hands will be like a very inexpensive piece of biofeedback equipment because they will help you know what is happening with your breathing. Close your eyes and pay attention to your breathing, noticing what is happening with your hands as you do. Do this for at least a few minutes or as long as you think it useful. When finished, answer the question below.

What did you notice about your breathing, hands, and body? Was there something interesting about doing this?

When you are triggered and get kicked into hyperarousal, you will begin pumping more oxygen into your system. More oxygen means being able to run, fight or respond to an emergency. More oxygen also means more fear and/or anger. However, if there is no good reason to run, fight or respond, you want to reduce the amount of oxygen in your system. Do you know why some people breathe into a bag for a while to prevent a panic attack from occurring? If you breathe in and out of a bag, you are recycling your own carbon dioxide, the net result being less oxygen. You can use a bag in emergencies, but you don't need it if you just want to reduce fear or anger. You can manage by consciously slowing and deepening your breathing. We will describe two types of breathing: Scared/angry breathing and calm breathing. Your hands gave you some feedback about what was happening with your breathing. What you experienced may have been scared/angry breathing or calm breathing, or perhaps it transitioned from one to the other.

Scared/angry breathing feels like this:

1. The breaths come quickly and there is little or no gap between breaths.
2. The breaths seem shallow – not deep.
3. You are working not only to pull air in, but also to push it out.
4. You may notice that both upper and lower hands are moving.

Calm breathing feels like this:

1. The breaths come more slowly and there is a gap between the breaths.
2. The breaths are deeper.

3. Your diaphragm muscle (which you had your lower hand over) works to pull air in, but then just relaxes to let air out.

4. You should notice little or no movement in your upper hand, and much more movement in your lower hand.

Even though the breaths are deeper with calm breathing, the breaths come more slowly and there are gaps between the breaths, so the result is less oxygen. Reduced oxygen means a less subjective experience of fear or anger. It's really hard to have lower oxygen levels and still feel scared or angry!

Now, please re-read the points above related to scared and calm breathing and do the exercise again, i.e. place your hands on your body, close your eyes, and pay attention to your breathing. This time, see if you can create calm breathing for yourself. Let your hands tell you how you are doing, and pay attention to the pace and depth of your breathing. When finished, answer the question below.

What did you notice? How did it go?

Practising calm breathing in the privacy of your own home can be helpful. But it misses the point in many circumstances because much of the time you get kicked into hyperarousal when you are out in the world. You can think of practising calm breathing in the privacy of your home as practice for doing it when you are out in the world.

You may be in a store, at work, at school, walking the dog or somewhere else. When feelings of fear or anger and the physical sensations that go with them come over you, pay attention to your breathing. If you're in a public place, you probably won't put your hands on your chest and stomach! But you can still pay attention to the intake and release of your breath. If it's scared breathing happening in the absence of any serious threat, see if you can take control and shift it into calm breathing. By really focusing on breathing, you are not only reducing oxygen levels, but also distracting yourself from whatever perception of threat was inducing fear. It's like a 'get two for the price of one deal'.

Realising you can have direct control over hyperarousal states can increase confidence and hope. Also, many apps are available to help you slow and deepen your breathing. You can find them quickly using search terms such as 'breathing' or 'breath pacer'. They can be very supportive of this practice.

Some thoughts on managing hypoarousal

In a state of hypoarousal, you may realise you are emotionally numb, disconnected from life or others, or switched off. Your body may be slumped and seem immobilised. If hypoarousal is occurring as a response to *genuine threats* which feel overwhelming, then this is serious and you need to get help so you can stay safe.

However, if there are no genuine threats you are facing, hypoarousal may be a pattern of coping you just developed as a child. It may have helped you cope all those years ago, but today it may prevent you from accessing feelings or connecting with life or others. Perhaps you can't think clearly, act to get needs met or focus on personal development. Below are a few ideas for shifting away from hypoarousal and moving into the window of tolerance.

In hypoarousal, you may be immobilised or disconnected. Your breathing has slowed and you can find you are sighing. Just *moving* your body will get breathing, related sensations, and some emotions flowing again. Walking, stretching, or any form of exercise can get physical sensations going. Hypoarousal also means disconnecting from the world 'out there', and you may feel 'hypnotised' by inner thoughts or images. *Staying in the moment and reconnecting* to the world and other people can shift you out of hypoarousal and into the window of tolerance. Just doing what is needed in the moment can help, whether it means washing the dishes, communicating with someone, etc…

Using support from someone you trust

While every person who experienced childhood harm is unique, a common issue for many is that they have difficulties trusting others. In response to childhood experiences, they may have concluded that they should not show vulnerability, rely on others or ask for help. If you are managing the Guidebook on your own without encountering destabilisation, that's fine. However, it can sometimes help to work with guidebook materials with someone you trust. We have known several clients over the years who have used this Guidebook alongside a partner, friend or family member. Jean experienced physical and emotional abuse within her family and sometimes would approach the Guidebook with her partner Jim.

> **"There are parts of the Guidebook I don't mind dealing with on my own, but there are other sections I want to do with Jim. We sit on the couch just before dinner and sometimes I read or he reads if I ask him to. If something upsets me, I'll stop and talk about it. Jim doesn't say too much but it helps with him just being there."**

Others using this programme may not actually read the Guidebook with someone else, but having someone they trust who they can talk to about what they are learning or experiencing can help fend off destabilisation.

Seeing a therapist

The tools mentioned above and further skills you will encounter as you navigate the Guidebook may be sufficient for responding to destabilisation if it occurs. However, if you feel that you are just not managing destabilisation at any point during your work with this programme, there are a couple of choices. One way forward is to delay this work until you feel it's a better time in your life. Or, you can consider continuing your work with the support of a qualified and experienced therapist. If you need help from a therapist to do this work, this is not an indication that you are failing or inadequate for the task. It's just how childhood trauma operates for you.

Alright. You have read about how the programme works. You have been introduced to ideas about how to best use the Guidebook. You have been thoughtful about your motivation, when and where to do this work, and stability and safety. Let's go.

References

1. Herman, J. L. (1992). *Trauma and recovery: The aftermath of violence – From domestic to political terror*. New York: Basic Books.
2. Swift, J.K., Greenburg, R.P. (2012). Premature discontinuation in adult psychotherapy: A meta-analysis. *Journal of Consulting and Clinical Psychology*. 80 (4), 547–559.
3. Orlinsky, D. E., Grawe, K. & Parks, B. K. (1994). Process and outcome in psychotherapy. In S. L. Garfield & A. E. Bergin (Eds.) *Handbook of Psychotherapy and Behaviour Change, 4th ed.* (pp. 270–376). New York: Wiley.
4. Pennebaker, J.W. (2012). *Opening Up: The Healing Power of Expressing Emotions*. New York: Guilford Press.
5. Pennebaker, J.W., Kiecolt-Glaser, J.K., & Glasser, R. Disclosures of traumas and immune function: Health implications for psychotherapy. *Journal of Consulting and Clinical Psychology*. 56 (2), 239-245.
6. Lambert, M. J. (2013). The efficacy and effectiveness of psychotherapy. In A. Bergin and S. Garfield (Eds) *Handbook of psychotherapy and behaviour change, 6th Ed.* New Jersey: Wiley & Sons.
7. Siegel, D. J. (2012). *The Developing Mind: How Relationships and the Brain Interact to shape who we are. Second ed.* New York: The Guilford Press.

PART I

THE NATURE OF HISTORICAL TRAUMA

Part I offers an opportunity to explore the nature and impact of childhood harm on your development. The entire programme has been designed to build in a progressive manner. Learning about trauma, making connections and building insight comes first, and in many ways this is what part one is about. The connections you make may feel exciting and provide hope. However, feeling upset, angry or low in mood are common reactions to this information. As you work with the material in Part I, we will remind you to see your problems and how you have coped *psychologically* rather than through the lens of punitive self-blame.

Chapter 1

Are there Words that Can Describe Historical Trauma?

"I've been diagnosed with a few things over the years. It's been helpful in some ways. I don't know – I've probably just been looking for someone who can understand me."
Sam

Finding the most helpful language to describe your experience is an important aspect of recovering from childhood trauma. This means having the confidence to explain what happened, how you were affected, and the sense you are making of it. It means being able to use language that is meaningful and healing. This language can be spoken, written, or even translated into something creative. Are there words which can *entirely* capture and explain the experience of childhood trauma? Perhaps not. However, discovering and using language within yourself, and to whatever extent possible, with people you trust, can be a part of recovery. It's possible you have already made some good progress in this respect, and hopefully this chapter will help you build on this work. However, for many it can feel like a beginning – a bit like they have stepped off a plane in a foreign country. Either response is fine.

The first part of the chapter will provide generic descriptions of different forms of abuse, as well as neglect, abandonment and vicarious trauma. For some readers, this is straightforward; for others, it can feel challenging. The second part of the chapter looks at how professionals have tried to make sense of trauma and associated psychological problems. You will have an opportunity to explore whether the efforts of professionals are useful to you.

Here's the chapter headline: finding the right language to describe your experience to yourself and others can be an important feature of healing. Generic descriptions may help. The efforts of mental health professionals may help. The words of others we have worked with over the years found in the Guidebook may help. However, all of this information is simply an opportunity to reflect and find the best language for *your* recovery. The information in this chapter may help you find your voice. But this will be a unique voice – it will be your voice.

Generic descriptions of childhood harm

Some people who experienced childhood harm are quite clear in their minds about how to describe what happened to them, and they are confident in using words like *abuse*, *neglect* or *abandonment*. For others, whether they should describe it this way can feel confusing. Some may wonder if it is right to use this language. There can be many reasons why people feel unsure if they should use words like abuse, neglect or abandonment. Some of these reasons are listed below. Place a tick next to or highlight any of the following experiences you can identify with.

- ❖ In order to cope, some put a lot of effort into *not* thinking about what happened as a child
- ❖ Some got told that what was happening to them was *not* abuse, neglect or abandonment. Someone you knew may have minimised what occurred.
- ❖ For some, the events happened a long time ago, and memories can feel uncertain
- ❖ For some, there wasn't a good basis of comparison, so what occurred just seemed 'normal'
- ❖ Some just don't want to see what happened as abuse, neglect or abandonment because it would feel awful to think of it that way
- ❖ For some, it feels like they are being 'disloyal' by seeing what happened as abuse, neglect or abandonment. They may feel a need to protect someone who harmed them
- ❖ Some can still feel frightened of the person who harmed them. Using words like abuse, neglect, or abandonment can feel scary, even though this may not seem rational.
- ❖ Some imagine they 'deserved what happened', so it can't be abuse, neglect or abandonment

The purpose of this section is not to tell you how to think about or describe what happened, but merely to give you an opportunity to explore it. Also, after reading this section, some may feel confident in the language they want to use to describe childhood events. However, others may still feel unsure about the language they wish to use. If that's the case, let's not worry about it now – you will have many further opportunities to decide on the best way to describe your experiences.

Some people using this programme will have experienced multiple forms of abuse, neglect *and* abandonment. Others may have principally experienced just one form of harm. How many forms you experienced is not necessarily relevant regarding the amount of harm done. For example, we have worked with people who were not directly abused but experienced neglect, which can be very harmful.

Below are some descriptions of various forms of historical trauma. Following this section, you will have an opportunity to reflect on how this information relates to your experiences.

Physical abuse

Children on the receiving end of physical abuse may have been hit, slapped, kicked, burned, had objects thrown at them, hair pulled, etc. Being locked up or exposed to hunger, cold, or other painful circumstances is also physical abuse. The abuser is normally bigger and stronger, and the child will have been frightened and in pain. The child's development will lack the experience of physical safety. Physical abuse represents an attack on the child's body, but it can also profoundly affect the child's sense of self. Physical abuse of a child can impart a message that *you're the sort of person who deserves to be physically harmed.*

Emotional abuse

Whereas physical abuse represents an attack on a child's body, emotional abuse attacks the child's sense of self. The abuser will have spoken or shouted at the child in a humiliating, frightening or demeaning manner. Infants do not come into this world with a developed sense of self. I learn who I am through the quality of my relationships with important others. If my caregivers, siblings, or peers attack or demean me through words, this will damage my sense of who I am. Because there is no attack or interference with a child's body, some might not recognise emotional abuse *as abuse*. This should not be the case, as there is evidence that emotional abuse can be as (or more) damaging to a child's development than other forms of abuse.[1]

Sexual Abuse

Sexual abuse occurs when an adult or another child (who is often older or has more power) has sexual contact with a child for the perpetrator's gratification. It is normal for children to want physical contact and non-sexual physical intimacy from others. However, prepubescent children are not usually interested in or understand adult forms of sexuality, and they are in no way psychologically equipped for such experiences. For a perpetrator to have sexual contact with a child is abusive and damaging to that child's sense of self and experience of safety in the world. While exceptions can occur, perpetrators are often known to the child and may be parents, family members, teachers, neighbours, older children or others. Sexual abuse comes in many forms, such as fondling, oral sex, intercourse, exposure to the child, sexualised touching, etc… Even if physical contact does not occur, it is still sexual abuse if the perpetrator exposes the child to adult forms of sexuality, e.g. pornography, getting them to observe sexual behaviour, or an adult 'exposing' themselves to a child for gratification.

'Grooming' a child gradually into sexual activity is common. As a result, some children may believe that what they are doing is 'normal' or that they are willingly participating (though this does not reduce the eventual damage it does). In some cases, a child can have apparently positive experiences coinciding with sexual abuse, such as receiving attention or gifts. This is often a feature of 'grooming' and manipulation and can make sexual abuse especially confusing. It's common for those experiencing sexual abuse to keep what happened a secret for many years. This can happen because the abuser threatened them, because the individual felt ashamed or worried that someone would blame them, or because they tried to protect someone. The issues of secrecy, shame and breaches of trust are common to all forms of abuse but can be especially difficult in instances of sexual abuse.

Neglect

Physical, emotional and sexual abuse represents harm *actively* done to a child. Neglect results from an absence of care, time or affection. Infants and children naturally depend on carers for many years to provide for their physical and emotional needs. Neglect occurs when a child's physical and emotional needs are not met. Meeting **physical needs** includes providing food and feeding, ensuring the child is clean and well-clothed, caring for illness or injury, and providing a warm, safe and ordered home. Providing for **emotional needs** means giving the child time, encouragement, affection and love. It also means providing protection from others who might harm the child. Neglect can occur for many reasons. Some careers are physically or mentally unwell. Other carers may have serious drug or alcohol problems. Some carers had children at a time when their own developmental needs were not met, and they just were not ready to be parents. Some careers are simply too ego-centric to prioritise a child's needs. Experiences of abandonment or loss can overlap with the experience of neglect. For example, when a career leaves the family suddenly or dies. Or, some children can never sustain friendships because their families move around a lot. Neglect often overlaps with physical, emotional or sexual abuse. Children who are neglected are more likely to find themselves in situations or with people where abuse occurs. For example, if a child's needs for love and affection are ignored, they may be more vulnerable to sexual abuse. Trauma occurs when a child has experiences which are frightening or distressing. In this respect, neglecting a child's needs can be traumatising. For example, it can be scary to be left alone or not know if you will have warmth or food. A four-year-old will attempt to use a stove to cook a meal if she gets hungry enough, often with ill-fated results.

Abandonment

Abandonment is related to neglect and often coincides with abusive experiences. Children who were abandoned will have lost relationships with people who were important to them. This can happen through a divorce, a death or simply by getting left. Some children are part of families that constantly move, resulting in numerous peer relationships being severed.

Vicarious Trauma

The above descriptions of trauma involve a child being directly harmed. Many people imagine it shouldn't be traumatising if you see or hear someone else being abused. This is not the case. Children can be traumatised by *witnessing* others being harmed. This can occur when a child watches a parent or sibling being physically, emotionally or sexually abused. This is called vicarious trauma, and the negative impact can be serious.

Reading through the descriptions of the six forms of childhood harm can help some individuals use language with more confidence. However, at this stage in personal development or the programme, it's common for some individuals to still feel uncertain about the language they wish to use. That's fine, and there will be many further opportunities to reflect on language as you go along.

There is no correct way to use language. Some will want to say *I experienced childhood physical abuse*, or *I experienced periods of abandonment until the age of 10*, etc.... There are many variations. Some find using modifiers helpful, such as *I experienced* ***serious*** *emotional neglect,* ***moderate*** *physical abuse and* ***milder*** *vicarious trauma in childhood.* You are the final authority on the language which feels closest to your experience.

Exercise 1: Your thoughts and feelings on generic descriptions of childhood harm

The generic descriptions of childhood harm explored here include physical abuse, emotional abuse, sexual abuse, neglect, abandonment and vicarious trauma. Which terms describe your experience as a child? Do you feel confident using these terms for yourself, or do you feel unsure if these terms apply to your experiences?

Do professionals have a name for what ails you?

When people struggle with mental health problems, it's common for them to turn to professionals to explain what's going on. A clinician may then provide a diagnosis. So, is there a mental health diagnosis for people who experienced childhood trauma and struggle with related psychological problems? The short answer is that we now have a diagnosis which can be useful for some individuals, and this may include yourself. However, there is a complicated story behind professionals' attempts to develop a useful diagnosis, and we think it's worth telling.

Adults who experienced childhood trauma have been turning up in clinics since the earliest developments within psychiatry, psychology and psychotherapy. So, you might think that getting mental health clinicians to agree on a diagnosis would not be that difficult. In fact, agreeing on a diagnosis has been fraught with false starts and professional quarrelling. And the rancour continues today in some respects. If this sounds disheartening, hang in there. There are actually some quite useful diagnostic ideas that have finally come from all the years of debate. We will offer a fairly brief explanation of the history, but for those who want more detail, Bessel Van Der Kolk's *The Body Keeps the Score* is very useful in this respect.[2]

Some might suggest that discussing diagnosis in a book such as this is improper – that diagnosis should only be considered in a consulting room between a qualified clinician and a patient. While a consultation with a qualified clinician may certainly be important for some, we see this as an outdated view. Consistent with the values of the recovery movement, people suffering from mental health issues should have access to any information which may be helpful. At any rate, the purpose of this discussion is not to diagnose the reader or necessarily for the reader to self-diagnose. Whether you find diagnostic ideas helpful or less helpful is a personal experience. Some people we work with can feel anxious about exploring diagnostic ideas. They might think, *what if I don't meet all the diagnostic criteria? Will that invalidate my experience?* This is not something to worry about. Adults who experience childhood harm *are unique* and will vary in how diagnostic criteria apply to them. Some even find non-diagnostic or generic language most helpful. However, some people who have experienced childhood harm can find diagnostic ideas useful and even supportive. More importantly, your experience and the language you wish to use to describe it are the highest points of authority on the subject. The section below simply provides information and an opportunity for reflection; you can use what is most helpful and toss out what isn't.

More than 120 years ago, clinicians such as Sigmund Freud, Jean-Martin Charcot, and Pierre Janet were making the connection between abuse (especially sexual abuse) and the problems their patients were experiencing. They used the term *hysteria,* and what they often saw at the time was what we now call *somatisation* (more about somatisation later in the Guidebook). In European society, abuse was rarely discussed in the early 1900s. Often unable to recall or talk about the abuse they had experienced, many of these patients expressed their traumas within and through their bodies, e.g. frozen or shaking limbs, difficulties with movement or immobilisation, etc. Freud and his colleagues likely made a significant breakthrough by understanding that repressed memories of abuse could be expressed through the physical problems they saw in their clinics. This discovery pointed these clinicians toward what became *the talking cure* (what we now call psychotherapy). The idea was that if patients could recall and talk about their abuse, the medical problems they expressed through their bodies would diminish or disappear. However, it's possible that Freud got nervous concerning the societal implications of this insight. How would polite Viennese society react if a well-known doctor was suggesting that many adults were suffering due to repressed memories of childhood abuse, especially sexual abuse? Freud shifted his emphasis away from abuse and towards what he suggested were universal developmental intrapsychic structures and family bonds.

The experience of World War I made it clear to many clinicians that young men were suffering, and the term *shell-shock* was coined by British psychologist Charles Samuel Meyers as an attempt to describe such experiences.[3] However, the military and society were not ready to acknowledge that the primary cause of psychological and physical problems was traumatic war experiences. Instead, such reactions were thought to result from 'a lack of moral fibre' or some other character defect. Not surprisingly, similar psychological problems were seen in veterans of World War II, but despite changing the description to *combat stress reaction*, the response was similar. As with Freud 50 years earlier, society and many professionals had difficulty appreciating the true impact of traumatic experiences. And then came…Vietnam.

What was fundamentally different about Vietnam was that the images and film footage of what soldiers experienced came straight into our living rooms through TV, magazines and newspapers. Society and clinicians were obligated to rethink trauma. Explaining trauma reactions on the basis of 'a lack of moral fibre' was absurd. Blaming the traumatised for their psychological problems no longer made sense. In 1980 a group of Vietnam veterans and New York psychoanalysts Shatan and Lifton successfully lobbied the US Congress, leading to the acceptance of a new diagnosis: *Post-Traumatic Stress Disorder (PTSD)*.[4] This diagnosis resulted in a substantial amount of money which supported research and the development of therapies to help those who suffered. Furthermore, the diagnosis of PTSD *legitimise*d the psychological difficulties of not only soldiers but anyone who experienced a devastating trauma. These were patients who had genuine problems that were understandable, and they needed help. It was recognised that the principal cause of PTSD symptoms was trauma itself – not some character flaw.

The symptoms of PTSD were seen to fall into three different categories:

1. *Re-experiencing*: Intrusive and unwanted memories (thoughts or images) of the event(s) can force themselves into a person's mind, and it can be difficult to put the memories away. If the re-experiencing comes with powerful physical sensations and emotions and the person loses contact with the present moment or isn't sure what is real, this is termed a flashback. Nightmares are like re-experiencing when asleep, often in symbolic form.
2. *Sense of threat*. Following a traumatic incident or incidents, the individual loses their sense of safety in the world. They can be hyper-alert to danger and feel anxious or fearful. They can be 'jumpy', easily startled and have problems concentrating or sleeping.
3. *Avoidance*: A person may need to avoid places or people associated with the traumatic event(s), and their life experiences become narrow. They may also need to avoid inner experiences like fear or memories, so they might use drink or drugs or stay hyper-busy. They may feel numb or detached from their bodies.

The acceptance of PTSD in 1980 was an important step for clinicians and anyone who experienced trauma, but it raised a perplexing question. Imagine two people. The first felt loved and safe during childhood and had close bonds with caregivers. As an adult, they formed good relationships that mirrored the close relationships of childhood. And then, they experienced a serious traumatic event, perhaps a car accident or a physical assault. Despite the support in their lives, they develop all of the PTSD symptoms indicated above, which persist for several months. Understandably, the experience is devastating for them and seriously impacts their happiness and lives. Imagine a second person. They experienced trauma too, but it took the form of abuse, emotional neglect and/or abandonment, and it occurred during childhood. People who were meant to care for them were involved in the harm that occurred or failed to protect them. It wasn't a single event. Rather, it involved multiple events. They lacked a sense of fundamental and enduring safety. As an adult, they can identify with some or all of the three core symptoms of PTSD, although how much they suffer from these symptoms may vary at different times in their life. So, is PTSD for someone who experienced a single episode of trauma as an adult the same as PTSD associated with multiple events which occurred during childhood and involved people the child had (or was meant to have had) an intimate and important relationship with?

This is the question that has caused so much controversy, and to try and answer it, we need to point out that there are two different classification systems of mental health diagnosis. *The Diagnostic and Statistical Manual of Mental Disorders* (DSM), which is primarily used in The United States, but may be used in other countries. And the even less attractive sounding *The International Classification of Diseases* (ICD), which is used mainly in Europe and countries like Australia, but may be used elsewhere. The word 'diseases' turns up in the ICD because the manual covers physical *and* mental health problems. If this sounds complicated, please hang in there. We will limit our discussion to information that is most important and meaningful to anyone who has experienced childhood trauma.

ICD 11 (used in Europe) was released in 2018, and this edition contained a new diagnosis: *Complex Post-Traumatic Stress Disorder (C-PTSD)*. ICD had concluded that the experience of a single traumatic event in adulthood could be captured well by the diagnosis of PTSD and the three core symptoms described above, but the experience of ongoing trauma *was* different, and it required its own diagnosis. The word 'complex' captured the experience of multiple traumatic events that were ongoing over time and often occurred within relationships which were meant to be intimate or important. So, this clearly includes childhood physical, emotional or sexual abuse, emotional or physical neglect, or abandonment.

The experience of C-PTSD was seen to include the three core experiences of PTSD mentioned above, but there were three additional problems.

4. *Emotional and attentional difficulties*: A person may struggle with emotional stability and their ability to concentrate or attend. Emotions like fear, anger or shame can feel overwhelming. Other times, a person might struggle because they feel emotionally numb or 'cut off' from emotions.
5. *Problems with self-concept*: A person may struggle with negative thoughts or feelings about oneself. Issues with self-confidence or self-worth can be present. Shame or self-denigration may be problematic.
6. *Difficulties in relationships*: The person may struggle to establish intimate, trusting, enduring or safe relationships.

Chart 1 below illustrates the problems often associated with PTSD and C-PTSD, as indicated in ICD-11. You can see the three core problems for PTSD, typical for individuals who experience a single traumatising event as an adult. With C-PTSD, you will note the three additional problems which can exist for a number of people who experienced ongoing harm associated with childhood abuse, neglect or abandonment.

Chart 1

PTSD	C-PTSD
Re-experiencing	Re-experiencing
Sense of threat	Sense of threat
Avoidance	Avoidance
	Enduring emotional and attentional difficulties
	Problems with self-concept
	Difficulties in relationships

While the experience of PTSD and C-PTSD clearly overlap, there is substantial evidence that they are different and can be discriminated. In a 2017 review, the distinction between ICD-11 PTSD and C-PTSD was supported in nine out of ten studies.[5] Why might multiple events of harm occurring in childhood produce enduring emotional and attentional problems, self-concept issues and difficulties in forming stable and trusting relationships? The key here is to consider *when the harm* occurred and *the context* of the harm. When a traumatic experience occurs in adulthood, the individual will likely have a reasonably formed ego or sense of self. And, the traumatic event may involve people with whom the adult does not have an ongoing intimate or important relationship, as occurs in a sudden traffic accident, fire or mugging. The three extra difficulties seen in C-PTSD are more likely to develop as a consequence of ongoing childhood trauma for a couple of reasons. First, the traumatic events happened when the child did not have a well-formed and stable sense of self to help manage the events. Second, the ongoing harm is often caused by people who the child is meant to have an important or intimate relationship to, such as parents, partners of parents, family members or family friends, teachers, childhood friends, childminders, classmates, members of a religious group or other organisations, etc... And, the child may not have been protected from the harm by people who should have played this role. Therefore, ongoing abuse, neglect or abandonment in childhood can have a greater impact on a child's developing sense of self, capacity to trust in human relationships, and ability to regulate emotions (the three extra features of C-PTSD).

The psychological problems resulting from a single traumatic incident occurring in adulthood can be serious, and we should not underestimate the extent to which it can impact a person's well-being. However, many adults will recover in about three to six months, especially if they have good relationship support. If the problems persist for more than 3 months, that's when clinicians may start using the diagnosis of PTSD, and the individual may need specialist therapy and perhaps psychoactive medication to support their recovery.

The problems associated with childhood trauma (and C-PTSD) are normally more complex and enduring. It's common for us to meet with adult clients who appreciate that the childhood harm they experienced has had a deep and enduring impact on their sense of self, their emotional lives, their relationships, their sense of safety in the world, or their capacity to cope and get needs met. Perhaps at times in their lives things have gone better, which will often occur if they find a safe and stable relationship. But at other times, the effects of what happened in childhood can catch up to them, perhaps when there are losses or significant setbacks. The view that childhood trauma can be harder and take longer to recover from should not be disheartening. Individuals can make progress at any stage in their life. It's worth restating an idea mentioned previously – patience is required, but hope is possible.

Recall that C-PTSD is a feature of the ICD classification system, used mainly in Europe. So, what happened in America with the DSM system? DSM 5, the most current edition, came out in 2013, and only the diagnosis of PTSD appears there. In other words, no significant distinction is made between the impact of trauma on an adult and how ongoing childhood abuse, neglect or abandonment might be experienced. The problem of getting diagnostic recognition of the unique impacts of childhood harm has not been due to a lack of professional effort. As far back as the early 1990s, American trauma pioneers such as Judith Herman and Bessel Van Der Kolk have been arguing for criteria which can better capture the unique features of childhood harm. Much of the debate came to a head when Bessel Van Der Kolk and colleagues presented research and a proposal in 2009 for a new diagnosis called *Developmental Trauma Disorder (DTD)*. This diagnosis was specifically designed to capture the unique consequences of ongoing childhood harm. Specifically, it highlighted: A. Emotional and body-based dysregulation; B. Problems focusing attention or coping with stresses; C. Problems with personal identity and forming and coping within relationships; D. At least one feature of PTSD; and E. An impact on life development, e.g. difficulties with school, work, health, legal issues, etc…

You will note that DTD overlaps quite a bit with C-PTSD, adopted by ICD in 2018. But, the diagnosis of DTD was rejected by the American DSM system, which we see as an unhelpful development. At any rate, if you are an American discussing childhood trauma and related psychological problems with a clinician, you may receive a diagnosis of PTSD. This is just how it works at the moment, but perhaps things will change in the future.

At the end of this section, you will have an opportunity to reflect on the topic of diagnosis, but we want to add two final points. First, concerning diagnosing those with childhood trauma, there is a controversy concerning the PTSD symptom of re-experiencing (having intrusive and unwanted thoughts or dreams of past trauma). We find that this is harder to predict for those who experienced childhood trauma. For certain people who experienced childhood harm, this can be a real problem. They may experience intrusive childhood memories (thoughts, images or dreams) that are disturbing to them. However, others may experience the impact of childhood harm in certain ways, but memories may be repressed, or the events happened when they were very young, so they don't have good access to them. Or, re-experiencing may be a problem at one point in life, and then it will calm down. So, as a diagnostic criterion, re-experiencing can vary from one individual to another.

Second, despite how clunky mental health diagnosis can be for those who experienced childhood trauma, there is something which can be said for trying to get it as right as possible. Given our current physical and mental health services, if you don't get a diagnosis that captures childhood trauma, you may receive an inadequate or misleading diagnosis. For some, the diagnosis is simply wrong. For many, the diagnosis may be technically correct but fails to capture the role of childhood trauma. This may have the effect of minimising the impact of the harm and the challenges of recovery. Either in childhood or as an adult, a wide range of mental and physical health diagnoses are often given to people who experienced childhood trauma.

Childhood trauma frequently disrupts an individual's capacity to pay attention or remain still, so a diagnosis of *Attention Deficit Hyperactivity Disorder (ADHD)* may be given. The experience of threat and a lack of enduring safety is a key component of childhood harm, so the individual's brain and body get 'shaped' to see and experience danger (lots more about this in chapter 4). As a result, the individual may be diagnosed with various *anxiety disorders*, including social phobia, agoraphobia, panic disorder, OCD, etc. Childhood trauma commonly damages the individual's self-concept and the ability to experience intimacy and get core needs met, all of which can intersect with depressed mood. So, the individual may be diagnosed with a *depressive disorder*, e.g. clinical depression, manic depression, or dysthymia (a persistent low-level depression). If coping with past trauma means you just don't have access to feelings or associated body sensations, and you can't find the words to describe what's happening, you might get diagnosed with *Alexithymia*. For some, the impact of childhood trauma gets expressed through difficulties with empathy and impulsive or criminal behaviour. Of those who end up in prison, 24% spent time in care, 29% experienced abuse, and 41% witnessed violence in their homes.[6] Some of these individuals will be diagnosed with *oppositional-defiant disorder* (in childhood) or *antisocial personality disorder* (as an adult). For a minority of individuals, childhood trauma can result in a very insecure sense of self, fears of abandonment, highly unstable emotions, and self-injurious or high-risk behaviours. If this is the case, a person may receive a diagnosis of *Borderline Personality Disorder (BPD)* in the USA or *Emotionally Unstable Personality Disorder (EUPD)* in Europe (these are different terms for essentially the same mental health issue). A minority of people who experienced childhood harm will meet the criteria for BPD or EUPD. However, of those diagnosed with BPD or EUPD, about 81% experienced significant childhood trauma, most often before age seven.[7] As we discuss in more detail later, the effects of childhood trauma are commonly experienced or expressed through the body. Sometimes referred to as 'unexplained medical symptoms', psychosomatic problems, or somatising, trauma can also be expressed through a wide range of very real physical symptoms.[8] Such problems can include chronic muscular pain, headaches or migraines, fibromyalgia, irritable bowel syndrome or other digestive complaints, shaking or other confusing bodily experiences, etc…

Again, if you have been diagnosed with any of the above, these diagnoses are not necessarily 'wrong', and perhaps the diagnosis has been helpful in some manner. But, the diagnosis often fails to appreciate the full story. What do all of the above mental health diagnoses have in common? Well, if you look carefully at the criteria, none mention childhood abuse, neglect or abandonment. By giving an individual who experienced childhood trauma a diagnosis like an anxiety disorder, depression, ADHD, or chronic pain, we might be 'missing the forest for the trees'. These diagnoses focus on symptoms rather than capturing the underlying problem. This can be of limited use or in some cases unhelpful, because if what you see are symptoms, then what you will 'treat' are… symptoms. If you want to know why the car won't start, you can stare at the paintwork all day without learning a lot; at some point, you're going to have to open the bonnet (UK) or the hood (USA). The HTP is one way of doing just this.

So why is it that an individual who experienced childhood trauma may receive a diagnosis representing the symptomatic expression of the problem rather than the problem itself? The answer to this is likely complex and may vary from case to case. Sometimes it's because clinicians are anxious with respect to asking about childhood experiences in a direct and empathic way. *Between birth and 18, did you ever experience physical, emotional or sexual abuse, neglect or periods of abandonment?* The question is not complicated, but asking it might feel complicated. Some clinicians worry they may upset, insult or make their patients worse. This is unfortunate because patients rarely respond in this way (whether or not they experienced childhood trauma). Many patients are relieved and grateful that a clinician finally asked them. Some clinicians can worry that if they hear about significant trauma, they may be unable to refer to services that can provide what is needed. This can be an issue depending on where you live, your finances or health care coverage.

However, some individuals will go for many years without a diagnosis which captures childhood trauma because they find it difficult or impossible to talk about what happened to them when they were young. We will discuss the role of silence further in chapter 9, but there can be understandable reasons why an individual doesn't talk about their childhood experiences for many years, even with clinicians. It can be easier to talk about panic attacks or fear of social experiences than a mother who was physically abusive. It might seem simpler to talk about problems with concentration, depression or stomach pain than the uncle who was sexually abusive.

In a way, the problem Freud had more than 120 years ago is still around. He saw or correctly intuited that many patients presenting with a wide range of medical and psychological problems had been abused as children, but he got scared concerning the consequences for society and perhaps for his career. However, it's no longer 1900. More and more, people who experienced childhood trauma can recall and think about what happened. They are able to connect past events with present symptomatic expressions of what happened. They are ready to explore the best language to start explaining it to themselves and others.

Considering what language may be best for you

Some will finish this chapter and feel they can use language concerning the childhood harm they experienced with a fair degree of confidence. For others, the ideas they have come across here may feel new and disorienting. Perhaps something seems a bit clearer and they are getting a sense of the language that might be best for them, but they need more time for reflection. That's understandable. Not surprisingly, much of what you will encounter in the Guidebook offers opportunities to delve much deeper into the very features that make up a diagnosis like C-PTSD, such as your experience of emotions, relationships, self-concept, coping, core PTSD issues, and more. So, there are many further opportunities to refine how you want to use language to make sense of the past and your recovery.

Some readers may feel that generic or non-diagnostic language is perfectly adequate. With respect to exercise 1, they might feel it's sufficient to think or say something like, *I experienced childhood* abuse, *I experienced childhood physical abuse,* or *I experienced childhood neglect* or *abandonment*. Perhaps more general language works best, like *I experienced childhood trauma* or *I experienced childhood harm*. It's quite personal.

Some readers, however, might also identify with the diagnostic language we have explored here, and they may find diagnostic terms supportive or useful. Recognising your experience in a diagnostic term can feel affirming for some. We've had people say things like, *wow, I didn't know there was a word for this stuff I go through*. Knowing diagnostic terminology can also help some people search online for further information, find further reading materials, locate support groups, etc.... Despite the American DSM system not recognising *Complex Post-traumatic Stress Disorder (C-PTSD),* it's still the most internationally recognised diagnosis which can capture the impacts of childhood harm. The American psychologist Judith Herman was actually advocating for the use of C-PTSD in the early 1990s and the term C-PTSD is found all over American-based websites. So, no matter where you live, if you find this term helpful, there is no reason not to use it. *Developmental Trauma Disorder* (DTD) has the advantage of being created specifically with respect to the impacts of childhood trauma, the criteria are very good, and the term itself is probably the best choice of language. But, for now, it's not a part of ICD or DSM, so it's just less recognisable in common speech, has less presence online than C-PTSD, and is less recognisable if you are speaking with clinicians.

At the end of the day, it's the professionals who are fundamentally dependent on those who experienced childhood trauma to help them research and create diagnostic language. So, in a sense, you and those with similar experiences are the highest authority on the subject. And, this is your recovery. Finding the language that works best for you is what matters.

Exercise 2: Diagnostic language and childhood harm

Does generic language feel sufficient in helping you describe your experience of childhood harm? Or, do diagnoses like C-PTSD and / or DTD feel useful as well? What's your view?

References

1. Vachon, D. D., Kreuger, R. F., Rogosch, F. A. & Cicchetti, D. (2015). Assessment of the harmful psychiatric and behavioural effects of different forms of child maltreatment. *Jama Psychiatry, 72 (11), 1135-1142.*
2. Van Der kolk, B. (2015). *The body keeps the score: Mind, brain and body in the transformation of trauma*. London: Penguin Books.
3. Jones, E., Fear, N. & Wessely, S. (2007). Shell shock and mild traumatic brain injury: A historical review. American Journal of Psychiatry, 164:1641–1645.
4. Van Der kolk, B. (2015). *The body keeps the score: Mind, brain and body in the transformation of trauma*. London: Penguin Books.
5. Maercker, A., Brewin, C. R., Bryant, R. A. , Cloitre, M., Reed, G.M., van Ommeren, M., et al. Proposals for mental disorders specifically associated with stress in the International Classification of Diseases-11. *Lancet* 2013; 381: 1683–5.
6. Williams, K., Papadopoulou, V. & and Booth, N. (2012). Prisoners' childhood and family backgrounds: Results from the Surveying Prisoner Crime Reduction (SPCR) longitudinal cohort study of prisoners. *Ministry of Justice Research Series*. http://www.justice.gov.uk/publications/research-and-analysis/moj
7. Herman, J. L., Perry, J. C. & Van Der Kolk, B. (1989). Childhood trauma in borderline personality disorder. *American Journal of Psychiatry*, 146: 490-495.
8. Roelofs, K. & Spinhoven, P. (2007). Trauma and medically unexplained symptoms: Towards an integration of cognitive and neuro-biological accounts. *Clinical Psychology Review*, 27 (7): 798-820.

Chapter 2

Human Needs and the 'Self'

"I've always had this sense that something is missing. It's like a hole or an emptiness.
I can't describe it, really."
Tom

In this chapter, we will be exploring the impact of childhood trauma with respect to the core human needs that we all share – what can be called universal human needs. And, we will look at one of these needs in more detail – the need for a positive or secure sense of self. The discussion will be much more than 'academic' because you will have opportunities to explore your personal experience and development with respect to these ideas.

Universal human needs and the effects of complex trauma

In the mid-20th century, a psychologist named Abraham H. Maslow was creating a revolution in our thinking about the connection between universal human needs, psychological problems and personal development.[1] Up to this point, psychological difficulties had often been seen as an 'illness', and those who suffered mental illness were in some way quite different from other members of the public. Maslow's view was that human beings didn't fall from the sky last week. We evolved over millions of years, and in particular, we evolved to have needs unique to our species. A flower evolved to need nutrient soil, the right temperature and the right amount of water and sunshine. If these needs are met, the flower will grow. Maslow believed that *all* human beings evolved to have five 'core' needs and that meeting these needs was essential if an individual is going to develop in a healthy and flourishing manner. People with mental health problems are seen to be *just like everyone else* because they have the same core needs. However, their developmental experiences impacted them in such a way that needs, to a greater or lesser extent, didn't get met. Psychological problems can then be seen as an expression of unmet needs. You may be familiar with Maslow's *hierarchy of needs triangle* depicted below because it features in pretty much any course in the human sciences, business, art, etc.... It's a model with a great deal of explanatory power in many areas, including the experience of historical trauma and personal development.

Diagram 1: Maslow's Hierarchy of Needs

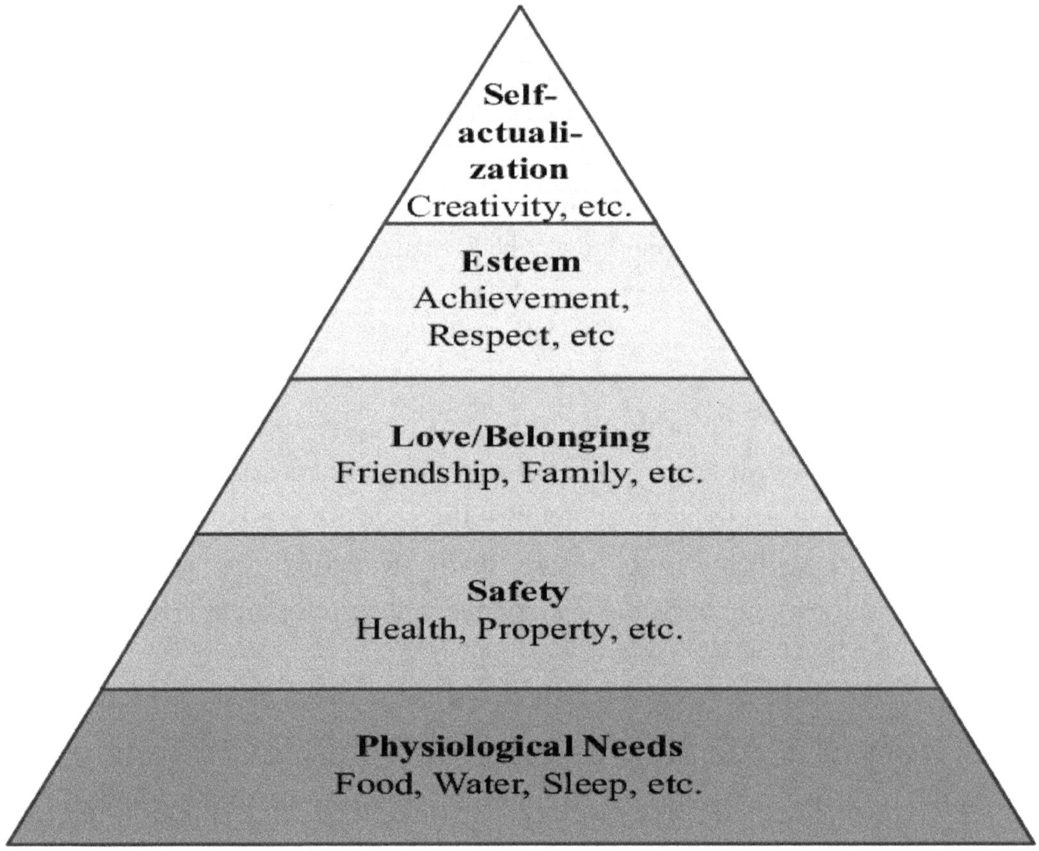

One of the appealing features of Maslow's model is its simplicity. The first layer of needs to be met are *physiological* (needs for shelter, food and water, and warmth). We then look to have needs for physical and emotional *safety* met. You must experience basic safety in order to be able to play, form intimate relationships, be creative or work productively. When I can be reasonably sure I am physically and emotionally safe from harm, my need for *love, affection, or belonging arises*. When this area of need is met, I can focus on a need for *self-esteem* (self-worth, self-love, self-expression). Having the need for self-esteem met in a basic way provides a secure place from which I can develop and express my natural abilities to the fullest extent possible (this is *self-actualising*). Some people challenge the idea that needs exist in a hierarchy, i.e. that more primary needs must be met before 'higher' needs become important. The idea that core human needs exist is less challenged, though some people want to argue about how many core needs exist and how to describe them. Maslow's model of universal human needs is not the only way of looking at this area. Perhaps you have a view on these issues.

Human beings evolved in such a way that infants and young children are dependent on caregivers for a very long time. This has to do with the fact that we have large brains compared to the rest of the animal kingdom. We have to be born at a period of gestation when our brains are quite underdeveloped. Otherwise, the process of birth would be impossible. A new-born deer can be on its feet within minutes, but it will take us about a year for our brains to coordinate our balance so that we can stagger around. Much of our brain development must take place over many years after we are born. Meanwhile, we are very dependent on our caregivers to meet our needs.

But how does Maslow's view of core human needs help us understand the impact of childhood trauma?

1. As an infant and child, you depended on adult caregivers for needs such as safety, love and belonging, positive self-esteem and self-expression. Abuse, neglect and abandonment compromise our ability to get these needs met. As a result, those who experienced childhood harm often come into their teen and adult years continuing to feel unsafe, unloved, and struggling with self-esteem or self-expression. Maslow's hierarchy of needs is progressive. This means that lower needs have to be reasonably met before a person feels the confidence to work on getting higher-level needs met. For example, if all your energy is going into staying emotionally or physically safe, it's difficult to focus on needs for self-esteem or self-expression.

2. Maslow tells us that there is a close connection between unmet core needs and painful psychological symptoms. Below we will explore common psychological symptoms of complex trauma, but we need to see that these symptoms are closely tied to unmet needs. Psychological symptoms such as depression and anxiety are important to consider, but they are *symptoms*, an expression of the *problem*. If we are going to get closer to the underlying problem, we need to see how your needs didn't get met in childhood and in what way they continue to be unmet today.

Some models of therapy can focus almost exclusively on painful psychological symptoms like depression, anxiety or PTSD symptoms. This is important, but it is not adequate for the purposes of this programme. Overcoming the effects of childhood trauma is not *just* about reducing such symptoms. It's about taking control back and developing yourself, relationships and life so that you can be as free as possible from the effects of past abuse. A feature of this goal is *getting your needs met better*. We trust that by getting these needs met better, psychological symptoms can be helped as well. If this feels like a big project, we agree.

Exercise 1: Exploring needs

In chapter 12 you will have an opportunity to explore your needs in more detail with a view to deciding how you want to develop yourself and your life. For the moment, can you identify with Maslow's point of view? Do you have some sense of the core needs which were unmet for you during childhood?

'The self' and the messages you received

One of the core needs Maslow highlighted was a positive, confident sense of self. As mentioned in chapter 1, a problem with self-concept is a core diagnostic difficulty for complex post-traumatic stress disorder (C-PTSD), so we felt this area deserved further attention. We will look at how the self can develop through the 'messages' a child receives. And, we will explore what is known as 'the adapted self', which can be quite a powerful idea for understanding what went wrong and what recovery might look like.

The language we use suggests there is something to this idea of the 'self'. We use words such as *self-worth*, *self-concept*, *self-image*, *self-confidence*, *self-knowledge*, and so on. But what is actually meant by 'the self'? The self is not a part of me like the hair on my head or my nose. The self is better thought of as something I experience. The 'self' is experienced typically through *the pattern* by which I commonly see myself, talk to myself, feel about myself or experience myself in relation to others. If I look in the mirror and have thoughts and feelings about what I see, this is an experience of the self. If someone criticises or compliments me, the thoughts or feelings elicited are an expression of the self. Self-concept or self-image are perhaps useful words to use. We can even talk about a 'bodily-felt sense of self'.[2] The sensations I experience through my body also contribute to my sense of self. If I typically have pleasant and calm or unpleasant and agitated bodily sensations, this too is an experience of who I am.

While we are born with a unique biological temperament, we are not born with a self-concept. A newborn infant cannot even see themselves as separate from the rest of the world. As we grow up, how we think and feel about ourselves depends on the *quality of relationships* we have and our experience of the world. As a child, you were exposed to thousands of 'messages' from others, including parents, siblings, other children, and teachers. These 'messages' come through everything said to us, done to us, or, in the case of neglect, what we did *not* receive. Dramatically different messages are illustrated below:

A five-year-old draws a picture of the family cat and shows it to a parent.

- *The child's parent looks carefully at the drawing and responds: "Wow, that's a really good drawing."*
- *The child's parent scowls and responds irritably: "That doesn't look anything like a cat."*
- *The parent tunes out the child and carries on drinking and watching TV.*

A five-year-old spills a glass of juice over the kitchen table and appears surprised and upset.

- *The parent says, "It was an accident," and then teaches the child how to clean up and properly hold a glass.*
- *The child's parent responds in anger: "You useless (add harsh expletive here) moron!*

A five-year-old has not had enough experience of others or the world to have a well-defined sense of self. They will absorb the above 'messages' from their parent in a manner which *informs* their sense of self. In the first example (child drawing a cat), the message received will be *I'm a good artist, I'm a lousy artist,* or *my drawings aren't worth looking at.* In the second example (spilled juice), the message received will be *it's okay to make mistakes because you can learn from them* or *I'm a useless (expletive) moron.* If messages such as these are repeated on hundreds or thousands of occasions, the child will almost certainly come to develop ways of thinking and feeling about themselves which are consistent with the messages. And the messages we hear are not just ideas or images I absorb; they also come with emotions attached and remembered. *I am good at drawing* comes with pleasant feelings of confidence. *I am a useless moron* comes with feelings of shame or fear.

Clinicians have a fancy term for explaining this phenomenon. We say that a child 'introjects' the messages they hear. It's a simple idea, actually. All it means is that if I hear a message like *you are useless* often enough, I come to believe it. I absorb or introject the message and associated feelings into my sense of self. Years later, if I make a mistake, even a small one, I may feel quite angry at myself or ashamed, and I will see or talk to myself in terms of *being useless*. The people who sent those hurtful messages years ago might not be around anymore. **They don't need to be**. Those messages have become a part of who I am, and I can see myself and talk to myself in ways consistent with the hurtful messages I heard many years ago. My experience of abuse or neglect is kept alive through how I typically think and feel about myself today.

What was *said* to me as a child is not the only way I can receive 'messages' from others. The experience of being physically abused, sexually abused or neglected can also send messages. For example, physical abuse tends to impart the message that 'you are bad' or 'you are the sort of person who deserves to be hit'. Emotional neglect or being ignored sends a message like, 'you are not worth spending time with'. As we will explore in a later chapter, people who are abused or neglected in childhood are *more* likely to be abused or neglected within adult relationships, something called retraumatisation. This makes sense. If I absorb the idea that I am bad and am the sort of person who deserves to be hit, I am more likely to accept being in an adult relationship with someone who induces bad feelings or hits me.

Some may have experienced severe and sustained abuse through multiple childhood relationships, so they will have received very few positive 'messages' to counteract the abusive ones. However, others will have received 'mixed-messages', many harmful to their developing self-image, but others which were supportive. There may have been an abusive person you encountered, but this was counter-balanced by someone who supported your sense of self. Our developing sense of self is often not simple in this respect. Samuel, an individual who experienced severe emotional neglect, expressed this issue well:

> **"I was the black sheep of the family. Everyone either ignored me or shouted at me. But in year five there was this teacher who liked me and really encouraged me. That meant a lot."**

Exercise 2: Exploring the 'messages' you received

Below you will find opposing messages which exist at either end of a spectrum. Place an X somewhere along the line between these two messages to indicate where your overall *childhood experience* lies. Keep in mind that there may have been many people that sent you messages, some positive and others negative. And, messages were sent not just by what was *said* to you, but how you *got treated*. There's no 'correct answer' – trust in your 'gut feeling' about where along the line to place an X.

You're socially
acceptable or likable ---You're not wanted

You're competent   You're likely to fail
or capable -- or get things wrong

You deserve
affection and time --- No one is interested in you

You're basically a
good person --- You're bad

You have some
special talent -- You're no good at anything

You can cope and
sort things out --- You'll make a mess of things

You're physically
attractive -- You're physically unattractive

You deserve to be   You deserve to be
treated with care and sensitivity -- hurt or punished

People will stick
with you -- You will get left or abandoned

Someone cares enough to
have expectations and
boundaries for you --- Do whatever you want

Completing the above exercise will hopefully help clarify which sorts of harmful messages were most pronounced for you during childhood. Let's see if we can take this a step further and also consider how these messages got 'introjected' – in other words, have you absorbed these messages into your sense of self? Are the messages you received in childhood still alive through your daily experience? Do you continue to relate to yourself in ways which are consistent with the harmful treatment you experienced as a child?

To help you explore this, let's consider Alan. Alan was a 40-year-old man who experienced emotional and physical abuse from his father and did not get protected by his mother, a woman with serious mental health issues. Remarkably, Alan completed university and became manager of an IT department that looked after the computer systems of a large organisation. Recently, Alan made a few relatively minor mistakes at work and had become so distraught that he had taken sick leave, convinced that he was incapable of doing his job. To keep busy at home, he had drilled a hole in a ceiling for a new light, and the hole had been too large.

> **"So now I've got a hole in my ceiling and I can't even put the light in. I'm just useless. If I can't even drill a hole that's the right size, how in the world can I manage a department? Seriously – I feel like a waste of space."**

I'm just useless... I feel like a waste of space. For Alan, this language will feel very much like his own words. But, these words clearly reflect the abusive messages imparted to him by his father throughout childhood. The highly punitive way Alan punishes himself for minor mistakes today expresses all the harmful messages he experienced in childhood. Alan had introjected these messages, and they have become a feature of his self-concept. Your experience won't be quite the same as Alan's, but perhaps you can identify with Alan in a manner which helps you explore the messages you received in childhood, and how these messages are still alive for you today.

Below you have an opportunity to summarise *in your own words* what you think are the most problematic 'messages' you received (reviewing where you placed X's on the lines above may help). Also, can you continue to talk to yourself today in ways which reflect the experiences of harm you experienced in childhood?

The adapted self

We will explain what the adapted self means in a moment, but let's begin by clarifying what a child needs as they are developing. What a child needs reflects Maslow's hierarchy of needs, but let's put it in terms specific to child development. A child needs to receive: 1. care for basic needs (feeding, warmth, sleep); 2. physical and emotional safety; 3. affection, acceptance and a sense of belonging; and 4. recognition ('I see and value you'). For these needs to be met, there must be at least one adult who is emotionally attuned to the child, i.e. can correctly understand and respond to the child's needs in an enduring manner. Emotional attunement is critical in every respect because it underlies an adult's ability to respond to any of the child's needs.

To understand the adapted self, we need to appreciate that the needs indicated above are so important that a child will do pretty much anything to try and get them met. If necessary, a child will adjust their behaviour, bury or ignore their feelings, or pretend to be something they are not. If a child experiences abuse, neglect or abandonment, they will *adapt* their emotions and behaviours to try and get safety, affection or love, or a sense of belonging or recognition. So, *the adapted self is who the child becomes to try to get these needs met.* If a child has to adapt their emotions and behaviours on a regular basis, these emotions and behaviours begin to seem 'normal', or *just who you are*.

Because children are small and vulnerable, they tend to be very sensitive to the expectations or demands of carers. Of course, any caring parent will set healthy boundaries and expectations for their child, such as regular bedtimes, brushing teeth, or keeping things tidy. However, children need to grow up in circumstances where they are confident they will be safe, loved and valued *no matter what*. Unfortunately, in circumstances of abuse or neglect, children frequently experience what have been called *conditions of worth*.[2] Conditions of worth are conditions a child imagines they must meet to gain others' acceptance, inclusion or approval. Sometimes it's not just conditions of worth – it's *conditions of safety*.

Tom never knew his father and experienced neglect and emotional abuse from his mother. When he came out as a gay man in his teens, he experienced bullying and rejection, exacerbating his earlier experiences. He often seemed emotionally numb and barely able to describe what he was feeling.

> **"It just wasn't a good idea to have emotions when I was little. My mom would get pissed off or ignore me if I was upset or scared. It's like I just wasn't supposed to ever get upset or need anything."**

Tom was experiencing conditions of worth such as 'don't have or express emotions' and 'don't be needy'. Children like Tom will adapt to circumstances of neglect and abuse by learning to ignore or suppress their emotions or by not asking for anything. Recall how we said that 'the self' is the pattern of how I learn to think about or see myself. In order to adapt to circumstances of neglect and emotional abuse, Tom was learning to see himself as someone who should not express emotions or needs. This is exactly what the adapted self means – it's the self you become as you try to adapt to abuse, neglect or conditions of worth. As mentioned, if you spend much of your childhood adapting to difficult situations, the adapted self just begins to feel like the person you are. The adapted self becomes how you typically feel, think or behave, and it can seem 'normal'.

Exercise 3: Conditions of worth or safety (basis for the adapted self)
The variety of conditions of worth or safety children can experience is quite broad and will be unique to your experience. Some of them are below, but others exist which may not be listed. Underline, tick or highlight any of the below that you can identify from childhood. *You can be safe or get some attention or acceptance if you*

… don't express anger
… don't cry
… don't think about yourself – focus on pleasing others
… are quiet or don't 'bother people'
… don't ask for anything or express your needs
… don't show weakness or vulnerability
… don't disagree or question what you are told
… don't ever fail or make mistakes
… fight and win
… don't express what you really think
… do what you're told
… don't question what you are told

Indicate any other conditions of worth or safety you experienced below

____

____

So, the adapted self is who a person becomes as a response to conditions of worth or safety. Many years later, these ideas can exist as a deeply ingrained part of a person's sense of self. Here's the big problem. As this adapted self develops, you will need to *deny* very real parts of yourself. We mentioned Tom a moment ago. As a response to emotional abuse and neglect, Tom's adapted self includes ideas such as *don't express emotions like anger* and *don't ask for help*. So, Tom learned to deny or ignore feelings like anger, and he is in the habit of never letting others see when he needs help. Psychologists sometimes say Tom has 'split off' these feelings or needs.

When a child has to deny or 'split-off' parts of who they really are, they live in a state of contradiction. They have feelings and needs that they imagine are not safe to experience or express. So, these feelings and needs have to be buried or ignored. Tom came to therapy because his wife was threatening to leave him, and he was distraught. His wife was frustrated with him because he was so 'closed-off', distant and depressed. This makes sense. Tom's adapted self required not allowing himself to have feelings like anger or to ask for help. At 35, the adapted self is still operating, but now it is a real problem for his marriage… and happiness.

The adapted self can take many forms depending on what characteristics had to be denied in order to get some safety or recognition. Juliet's mother was a heroin addict who provided little care for Juliet or her two younger siblings. Juliet told us:

> **"I had to dress my younger brother and sister and get us food from around the house a lot. I was changing diapers from the age of 6. It was just normal, I guess. It was like this role I had."**

Don't think about yourself and serve others was a condition of worth and safety for Juliet. It gave her a role, but she had to deny the part of herself that can be assertive or receive care. As an adult, she is submissive, unable to express herself, depressed and has relied on eating disordered behaviour for many years.

John was physically and emotionally abused by an alcoholic father. His father modelled and taught aggression, and John got the idea that if he was going to receive any respect, attention or affection, he would need to be a fighter.

> **"I was often in trouble for fighting and I got thrown out of school at 15. The odd thing is, I'm not really an aggressive person. I mean, I don't really want to hurt people. I don't even like conflict, really."**

When we knew John, he was largely illiterate and was learning to read and write through adult education. He'd done time in prison a few times for theft. He had plenty of acquaintances but no close relationships. Conditions of worth or safety for John were *you better fight and dominate people if you want respect or importance.* John became a fighter, but he denied or 'split-off' the sensitive and caring parts of himself and a willingness to be vulnerable in relationships.

Children often deny or 'split-off' parts of themselves because the alternative would mean losing a relationship to the person who is supposed to care for you – the person you are meant to bond with. Van der Kolk captures this idea vividly. "For many children it is safer to hate themselves than to risk their relationship to their caregivers by expressing anger or running away… they survive by denying, ignoring, and splitting off large chunks of reality. They forget the abuse; they suppress their rage or despair; they numb their physical sensations. If you were abused as a child, you are likely to have a childlike part living inside you that is frozen in time, still holding fast to this kind of self-loathing and denial."[3]

In a moment we are going to consider the 'unadapted self', or those aspects of you that might have developed if you had felt safe and cared for. But before we move on, an important point needs to be made. It's not correct to simply say that the adapted self is 'bad' or unhealthy and the unadapted self is 'good'. It's not this 'black and white'. We need to keep in mind that the adapted self developed in order to protect the child – to allow the child to try and get some limited needs met for emotional and physical safety, love, recognition, and a sense of belonging. The remnants of the adapted self which developed in childhood will still be a part of who you are today. The adaptive self may cause you worry or stress and prevent you from getting certain needs met, but there can also be positive aspects. Maggy is a hairdresser who experienced emotional abuse from both parents, and a feature of her adapted self is that she is extremely sensitive to others.

> **"When I am cutting hair I am totally focused on my customer and I want it to be just right for them. I worry a lot and if there is even a hint of unhappiness, I can feel really upset and sometimes I won't sleep. It's stressful, but I'm really good at what I do and I've got loads of customers who won't let anyone else touch their hair."**

Recovery for Maggy will need to involve seeing how the adapted self undermines her need for safety and self-esteem. However, qualities such as sensitivity and care were also a product of her childhood experiences. She won't lose those qualities – they are too much a part of who she is. So, while it's necessary to work on the unhelpful remnants of the adapted self which are alive today, it's also important to *respect* and *honour* those positive aspects of the adapted self that made you who you are today.

When speaking with people who experienced childhood harm, it's common for them to spontaneously say such things as *I feel like I don't know who I am.* Or, *I feel like I'm trying to find myself.* In the context of our discussion, these statements take on a particular meaning. If a person spends much of their childhood adapting to abuse or neglect, they become something *they have to be* in order to try and get some safety or recognition (the adapted self). But who are they really? Who are they when they can let go of the defensiveness? Who might they be if they could reclaim the parts of themselves they had to deny or bury? As adults, reclaiming lost parts of yourself is a way of understanding who you really are.

Everyone who encounters adverse childhood experiences is unique, so who they are underneath the adapted self will also be unique. However, it's possible to consider what can be called the *unadapted self.* An individual's personality comprises all the patterns by which they typically think, feel and behave in relation to themselves and others. Personality will always be the result of the unique biological temperament you were born with (nature) and your experiences, especially relationship experiences (nurture). Most parents with two or more children intuitively understand what biological temperament is. They know that aspects of their children's personality were 'baked-in' at birth – in other words, aspects of their child's personality are simply the product of biological temperament. Aspects of biological temperament can include qualities such as as how sensitive, how cautious or adventurous, or how introverted or social a person is.

We can understand the *unadapted self* in the following way. Let's say that throughout childhood there was at least one person who had been consistently attuned to your emotions and needs, and then provided dependable care, affection, and protection from harm. If we combine these experiences of nurture with the biological temperament you were born with, we can perhaps get some inkling of the unadapted self. Put simply, the unadapted self is who a person becomes when they do not have to adapt to significant childhood experiences of threat or conditions of worth. If you find the term unadapted self a bit cold, you can use terms like your *natural* or *original self.*

But what is your unadapted self? As mentioned above, the unadapted self will be unique because you are a unique individual. However, there are certain general features of the unadapted self which are more likely for those who received enduring care and protection in childhood. These include:

Having access to feelings, body sensations and needs

You may have experienced conditions of worth or safety such as *if you want to be safe or accepted, you had better focus on the needs of others*. Accessing or developing the unadapted self often means being able to attend to all of your emotions, including anger, fear and sadness. It means being able to pay attention to body sensations and being able to access your core needs.

Self-expression, agency and industry

Conditions of worth such as *be quiet, don't talk, don't act spontaneously, etc...* can crush self-expression and self-confidence. Accessing the unadapted self can mean developing self-confidence, self-expression, finding your voice, and getting hold of a stronger sense of self-agency. It might not have been safe as a child to be playful, spontaneous or creative, so these characteristics may need to be discovered or developed.

Intimacy and self-protection

If a child lives with threatening circumstances, they learn that getting close to people is dangerous, so the adapted self keeps people at a distance or may be aggressive or resistant. It can mean never allowing yourself to be trusting or vulnerable, leading to loneliness and isolation. The unadapted self does include protecting yourself when necessary but also means allowing yourself to be open and vulnerable with the right people so that you can experience intimacy. It means learning when to put your guard up and when it's safe to lower it.

Capacity for self-compassion and self-care

If conditions of worth or safety include ideas such as *think about and care for others, ignore your own needs, etc...* a person's capacity for self-compassion and self-care can get compromised. Accessing or developing the unadapted self can mean developing skills for self-compassion and self-care. This is certainly easier *said than done*, and there is a whole chapter on this area later on.

Exercise 4: Getting a sense of your unadapted self

As you were trying to adapt to abuse or neglect in childhood, you probably had to deny or bury parts of yourself. The parts of you that got buried can include:

1. Being able to access and express certain emotions like anger or sadness. Being able to know what you need
2. Self-expression, spontaneity, playfulness.
3. Being able to protect yourself when necessary, but also being able to allow for openness, trust and closeness.
4. Being able to access self-compassion and self-care.

Discovering your unadapted or natural self means seeing and acknowledging what got lost or denied in childhood. If you can do this, it can point you in the general direction of what personal development looks like for you. Below is an opportunity for reflection. Considering the four points above, are you getting some sense of what you need to be working on concerning self-development?

References

1. Maslow, A. H. (1943). A Theory of Human Motivation. *Psychological Review*, 50, 370-396.
2. Rogers, C. (1959). *'A Theory of Therapy, Personality, and Interpersonal Relationships, as Developed in the Client- Centered Framework'*. In Koch. S. (ed) (1959). New York: McGraw-Hill.
3. Van Der kolk, B. (2015). *The body keeps the score: Mind, brain and body in the transformation of trauma*. London: Penguin Books.

Chapter 3

Common Psychological Problems

"They don't really make plasters [Band-Aids] for this stuff."
Mary Ann

The painful part of the experience

Childhood traumatic events have negative impacts on a child, and these impacts tend to endure into the adult years – they do not simply disappear when an individual turns eighteen. *Psychological symptoms* can be thought of as the painful ways in which past trauma expresses itself today. As we shall see, the pain of past trauma can express itself through our emotional states, memories, thoughts, and our bodies. How symptoms express themselves within your life will be quite personal, but people who experience childhood harm often share similar experiences.

We have worked with many people who can feel anxious about exploring this topic. Your experience of this material will be unique, but Terry's reaction is not unusual. Terry was emotionally and physically abused by his mother, and at the start of a group therapy session he reflected on this chapter.

> **"I was worried about reading this chapter because... well, what if I find out its all worse than I thought. I've spent most of my life trying to believe I'm normal – trying to make people think I'm normal too. Reading this stuff, I'm like... yup that's me... yup, that's me too. It made me sad... and sort of angry. But, I also thought, okay, so maybe this is what happens if you don't feel safe when you're growing up."**

So, it's possible that reading about psychological symptoms will stir up some difficult feelings. However, recognising and acknowledging the impact of childhood harm can be important. As mentioned previously, Judith Herman suggests that 'remembering and morning' is a necessary part of recovery from childhood trauma.[1] Herman is saying that being in touch with what happened and how it affected you will naturally evoke difficult emotions – sadness often being part of the experience.

If recognising the impact of childhood harm is upsetting, there are a couple of reasons this work can be helpful. First, the psychological symptoms you will explore here are *common* reactions to childhood harm. So, if you find yourself identifying with these issues – you are not alone. Terry understood this when he said, "But, I also thought, okay, so this is what happens if you don't feel safe when you're growing up." A lot of people who experience childhood harm go through their adulthood years thinking 'I'm the problem'. This chapter may help you appreciate that there is a more realistic way to look at things: it's not that *you* are the problem. Rather, you *have* problems. *The problem* is the childhood harm you experienced and its psychological impacts. So, understanding the common psychological symptoms associated with childhood harm can help *normalise* the difficulties you have. In other words, you may appreciate that it's normal (as in common) for people to experience a range of psychological symptoms as a consequence of childhood trauma.

Second, understanding the unique impacts of childhood harm may help you feel a bit clearer about what you want to work on. Part III of the book will offer plenty of opportunities to focus on recovery or change. The issues you discover here will likely form a part of what recovery means for you. Recovering from trauma requires having some clarity about what you are recovering from. Painful psychological symptoms are only part of the story, but it's not something to overlook.

The adverse childhood experiences study

Does child abuse or neglect have negative impacts on mental and physical health? The answer, as it turns out, is *yes it does*. There are numerous studies supporting the link between historical trauma and a range of problems in later life, but the most comprehensive study ever conducted is the Adverse Childhood Experiences Study. Over 25 years, more than 17,000 people in the San Diego area were studied with a view to understanding the connection between childhood trauma and difficulties in later life. If you want to understand the detail of this study, there is a website indicated at the end of the chapter you can access.[2] Individuals who participated in the study filled out a 10 question survey which allowed them to understand how many Adverse Childhood Experiences they encountered. Adverse child experiences (or ACEs) essentially refer to forms of childhood traumatic events. If you go to the site, you can complete the same survey and discover how many ACEs you experienced. There are individual differences, but, on average, the more ACEs (answering 'yes' to any question) an individual experiences, the greater the negative impact.

A visit to the website provides much more detail, but some of the headlines from the ACE study are as follows: 1. Adverse childhood experiences were more common than expected, as seen by the fact that only one-third of respondents reported no ACEs. 2. The more ACEs a child experiences, the more likely they are to experience learning, emotional or behavioural difficulties at school. 3. Higher ACE scores coincide with increased rates of depression, higher incidents of suicide attempts, alcohol and drug abuse, problems functioning at work and financial difficulties, and increased risk of further traumatisation in adult relationships.

The point of mentioning the ACE study is not to depress or demotivate anybody. In fact, the message is quite the opposite. If you intuitively recognise that your childhood adverse experiences have put you at risk for psychological, relationship or health problems, that's an important connection to make. You can begin to appreciate that your childhood experiences have set you up for such problems. The challenge now is to move in directions in which your childhood experiences have less impact on your well-being, health and happiness.

Below is a description of common psychological symptoms related to childhood trauma. Please note that the difficulty of shame is such a complex consequence of childhood trauma, it deserves its own chapter and will be discussed later in the Guidebook.

Anxiety difficulties

It makes sense that people with abuse histories are more likely to struggle with anxiety problems. We learn through our experience whether the world is safe or filled with physical or emotional threats. If a child lives with fear because they are anticipating that physical, emotional or sexual abuse is likely to occur, fear can become ingrained into their personality – it becomes a way of just going through life. Imagine two people. One has never had anything but pleasant driving experiences. Through no fault of their own, the other has been involved in five car accidents in which they were terrified and sustained physical injuries. These two drivers will think and feel very differently about driving. With childhood abuse, it was not a car accident that hurt you – it was another person or people. So, many who experienced childhood harm tend to feel anxiety and mistrust toward others.

Fear or anxiety can be experienced in several ways. It's normally felt in our bodies as an automatic reaction to thoughts or events – a pounding heart, racing thoughts, quick and shallow breathing, sweating or feeling hot, and so on. Another natural response to anxiety is to feel a need to **avoid** anything associated with the anxiety. You might want to avoid places such as shops, public transportation or events. But it's not really places you want to avoid – it's people. Places are just where other people tend to be. People who are anxious also tend to spend time scanning for danger or being on the lookout for threats.

We call this **hypervigilance**. Hypervigilance makes it difficult to relax and enjoy others and our surroundings. Finally, those who experienced childhood harm tend to quickly imagine that they are in danger or that something bad will occur. How they **interpret events may be biased** towards imagining a threat, often in situations where they are likely to be safe. How anxiety is experienced can vary. Some might struggle with panic attacks, some can have specific phobias, some worry a lot, and some might develop obsessive-compulsive ways of coping.

Human beings evolved to feel fear. It's a feeling meant to help us because it gets us to focus our attention in ways that will keep us or others safe. The problem for many people who experience childhood harm is that they may feel anxiety in situations where there is little or no danger. As a child, it made sense to feel scared as the threats were real. Perhaps there continue to be genuine threats in your life now, which may be something you need to pay attention to. However, for many, the legitimate fear they felt in childhood gets transferred onto many social situations today in ways which are not realistic. A good analogy is to a smoke alarm. If a smoke alarm is working properly, it will sound an alarm if there is a fire. If a smoke alarm is set in a manner that is too sensitive, it will sound an alarm when someone is cooking dinner. There is nothing fundamentally wrong with the smoke alarm; its settings are just overly sensitive. As Van Der Kolk has written, the challenge is in "repairing faulty alarm systems and restoring the emotional brain to its ordinary job of being a quiet background presence that takes care of the housekeeping of the body, ensuring you eat, sleep, connect with intimate partners, protect your children, and defend against danger."[3]

Exercise 1: Can you relate to the above description of anxiety difficulties? In what manner?

Intrusive memories, flashbacks and nightmares

You probably don't remember the experience of eating your lunch on June 17th, 2015. This is because the experience of eating lunch on that day wasn't likely to have been especially important. Memory is selective. Our brains evolved to store memories which are important to our survival and to forget less important memories. Events in which we felt seriously threatened or terrified – memories of abuse – are more likely to be strongly encoded in our memories. We may forget a memory for periods of time, but it can get triggered by a particular event. We can refer to this as an unwanted or *intrusive memory*. What triggers a memory of trauma can vary between people. It might be something you see on TV or hear on the radio. It might be hearing about someone from your past. But it's not just the memory that intrudes into your mind – some old emotions and physical sensations come with it. So the memory can feel distressing. It's common for some to feel afraid of the memories and try to avoid situations that might trigger them. As one person we worked with said, 'I never listen to the news'.

A *flashback* is a term which describes an intrusive memory which is so powerful it carries a lot of the original emotional charge. When people experience a flashback, they can momentarily lose contact with what's real. They might imagine that something bad is happening to them *right now* even though no immediate threat exists. The past invades the present moment. Flashbacks are scary.

Nightmares can be thought of as another way past trauma intrudes into our lives. We might be successful to some extent in suppressing traumatic memories during our waking lives, but they can then express themselves within frightening dreams. The dreams may be very strange because the content of the trauma is presented symbolically. An important point is this: If you struggle with intrusive memories, flashbacks or nightmares, this is a normal and understandable consequence of a traumatic past. We will work with these sorts of problems later in the programme.

Exercise 2: Are intrusive thoughts, flashbacks, or nightmares difficult for you? How so?

Anger

Anger is a natural and understandable reaction when we perceive that we have been mistreated or believe a situation is unjust. Anger can also be an immediate emotion which comes out in us when we feel threatened. Those who experience abuse or neglect were mistreated and have genuine reasons to feel that what happened to them was unfair or wrong.

We find two things about anger that seem relevant for many people who experienced childhood harm. Anger is (1) a common reaction, but (2) it's often a *complicated* feeling. Some could never feel angry at the person who was hurting them when they were younger. Perhaps being angry then would have been pointless or incurred even more danger. When you are not safe to express anger, either as a child or as an adult, the anger must express itself somehow. This can explain why anger can get directed inward at the self, perhaps through self-punitive statements, deliberate self-harm, or reckless behaviours. If anger is self-directed, it can also be experienced as depression or can express itself through body-based difficulties referred to as somatisation (more about somatisation in a moment).

As adults, some can feel anger which is quite generalised – they might carry around anger or feel 'angry at the world'. They sense that the anger they feel towards daily events is 'out of proportion', but it's hard to stop it. Angry fantasies may take up space in their minds. Their anger might be 'right beneath the surface', and it doesn't take much to set it off. Some may cope with powerful feelings of anger by occasionally 'dumping' it onto others, and they may feel regret about this. People can feel worn out by their anger.

Exercise 3: Can you identify with the above description of anger? If so, in what manner?

Depression

It is not unusual for people who experienced childhood to experience depression at various times in their lives. Depressive states can be characterised by dark moods, feelings of hopelessness, sadness, despair, a lack of interest, alienation or pointlessness. And, as psychologist Dorothy Rowe has convincingly pointed out, a key component of depression is *feeling cut-off* – feeling like you are in a bubble which separates you from others and life.[4] Depression can be mixed with anxiety (anxious depression) or with anger and frustration (angry depression). But why are people who experienced abuse or neglect more vulnerable to depressive states? The answer to this question can be found in a simple idea: our historical experiences deeply inform how we tend to see ourselves, others and life.

Consider an individual who *did not* experience childhood abuse or neglect. As they were growing up, they were loved, valued, protected, encouraged, and had good opportunities to play and learn. Their childhood experiences taught them that they have value, that relationships are safe and worthwhile and that life holds interesting opportunities. As a consequence, they tend to look at themselves, others and life in positive and hopeful ways. When life presents these individuals with hardships (which it will), a perspective of hope, positivity and trust insulates them from depression or despair.

The learning experiences of people who experienced childhood harm tend to be different. What happened in childhood may have taught them that they are inadequate, that others cannot be trusted, and that existence is a bad place where you are likely to get hurt or disappointed. Understandably, a dark or pessimistic perspective may develop. This perspective can be the source of vulnerability to depressive states, especially when life doesn't go well.

However, there is no single cause for depression. A minority of people have a genetic predisposition to depression, which is true for a small number of people who experienced childhood harm. A psychoanalytic explanation for depression is that it results from not being able to access and express feelings of anger, and many who experienced abuse or neglect certainly have genuine reasons to feel anger. Another explanation for depression may relate to something a psychologist named Rollo May said. He described apathy as *the last great defence*.[5] What he meant was that by not caring about my development, other people, or life, I can protect myself from hurt, disappointment, or abandonment. The defence mechanism works like this: *I can't get hurt by something I don't care about. So, I'm not going to care or hope for something*. A lot of people we work with were truly hurt and let down by life and other people, so it's understandable that they might not hope or want for much. Experiencing apathy (or indifference) is a way of protecting ourselves from further disappointment or hurt, but it's also a recipe for depression.

Exercise 4: Can you relate to the above description of depression, now or in the past?

Somatisation

Somatisation may or may not be a problem for you. However, somatisation or psychosomatic problems are more common for people who experience trauma.[6] Somatisation occurs when psychological problems or past trauma gets expressed directly through our bodies. Examples of how psychological problems *might* express themselves physically can include gastrointestinal disturbance (e.g. IBS), chronic back or neck pain, muscular tension or spasms, migraine headaches, high blood pressure, chronic pain conditions, odd sensations such as trembling or shaking, frozen joints or limbs, loss of physiological feeling, etc. Physical expressions of unresolved past trauma can be very confusing, not only for people who experience them but also for medical physicians. Sometimes when a physician can't determine a physical causation for a physical problem, they might refer to the issue as a 'medically unexplained symptom'. If such problems are very pronounced or more chronic, the term Functional Neurological Disorder (FND) might be used.

The exact mechanism whereby psychological or emotional problems are experienced as physiological issues is not entirely understood, but there are some fairly obvious clues. Muscle tension is likely one culprit. As Van Der Kolk suggests, "when people are chronically angry or scared, constant muscle tension ultimately leads to spasms, back pain, migraine headaches, fibromyalgia, and other forms of chronic pain."[7] Also, the release of stress hormones into our bloodstream very likely plays a role. The experience of threat can be real or imagined, happening right now or connected to memories. It's all the same to our brain and body because any perception of threat releases hormones like adrenalin and cortisol. Adrenaline will increase heart rate and blood pressure. The release of cortisol will increase sugar in the bloodstream and switch off systems not immediately needed for survival, such as the digestive and reproductive systems. If the release of adrenaline and cortisol happens occasionally and for brief periods, your physiology is unlikely to be disturbed. However, recall that one of the common features of C-PTSD is a generalised experience of threat, which of course connects to emotions such as fear or anger. If you are walking around for much of the day swimming in a soup of your own stress hormone, it makes sense that this will eventually get expressed through any number of medical complaints.

It's important to make a couple of points here. First, if you have a history of trauma and some physical problems, it doesn't necessarily mean the past trauma *is causing* the physical problem. Your physical problems might have a very real physical causation, i.e. your back pain is caused by an actual injury. However, in some instances, the past trauma *is* being expressed through pain or other bodily problems. Or, perhaps there is some underlying physical difficulty, but a traumatic past worsens the experience of a physical problem. Second, if your past trauma expresses itself through your body, it doesn't mean the physical problem is 'all in your head'. With somatisation, your experience of pain or other physical difficulties is very real; it's just not being *caused* by physical illness, disease or impairment. The underlying cause of the physical problem is psychological.

Exercise 5: Somatisation may or may not be relevant to you. What do you think?

Emotional dysregulation

Children who experience trauma are introduced to experiences of threat and fear, *and* they often lack supportive adults who can soothe those painful emotional experiences. Consequently, people who experience childhood harm can be quite emotionally reactive to stressors, e.g., bad news, criticism, or a perception of threat. Some might react to a stressful event by feeling 'flooded' by strong or overwhelming emotions, or they might deal with the situation by 'shutting down' emotionally or feeling numb. In other words, emotional reactions can be so strong that some lack confidence that they can 'regulate' or control them.

Emotionally dysregulated states are often really problematic because some people can become afraid of their own emotional lives. Painful states of emotional dysregulation are *not* the fault of people who experienced childhood harm – these states are a common consequence of being exposed to genuine threats in childhood and lacking stable and caring people who can consistently soothe those states. We focus specifically on emotion regulation in chapter 14.

Exercise 6: Can you identify with the idea of emotional dysregulation? In other words, are there times when you feel overwhelmed by powerful emotions or emotionally 'cut-off' or numb?

Dissociation

Dissociation is something we all do to a degree. It refers to a strategy where we cope by 'shutting off' or 'tuning out' from feelings or a situation. You can spot it in other people when their gaze loses focus. They're not connected anymore – they've gone somewhere else. Dissociation is a way of coping so we don't get overwhelmed by a situation. However, because people who experienced childhood harm were exposed to more threats and fear, they are more likely to develop a pattern of dissociating in order to shut off from dangers or emotional pain.[8] This was an understandable means of coping when you were being hurt.

Dissociation is the experience of being detached from the world, other people, your feelings or physiological sensations. It's 'being numb' or 'spaced out'. Dissociation is the *opposite* of being present, of feeling the wind on your face, hearing the sounds around you, and being able to listen and connect to others. Dissociation occurs along a continuum from mild (i.e. daydreaming while driving) to more severe, i.e. having little awareness of external events or feelings and having no memory of recent events. If you sense that what is happening isn't real, this is called *derealisation.* If you have the sense that what is happening isn't really happening to you, this is called *depersonalisation.* Derealisation and depersonalisation are just particular expressions of dissociation. Dissociation can be a problem because what started in childhood as a way of coping can end up separating us from our feelings, others or life.

Exercise 7: Can you identify with this description of dissociation? In what manner?

The human family

Many people who experience childhood harm can feel like they 'don't belong'. *I'm odd; I don't fit in; there is something really wrong with me; I'm just so different; why can't I cope like other people?* Reynold, a 35-year-old who experienced abuse and periods of abandonment, put it like this:

> **"I can have this weird fantasy that a space ship arrives and they get out and explain that I am an alien. I'm like, excellent – let's go. It's sort of funny but I feel sad about it too."**

In chapters 2 and 3 we explored universal human needs and common psychological symptoms, and before we end it's important to emphasise the connection between these topics. People who experienced childhood trauma *are* often different from those who did not. The difference usually is experienced through the impact that trauma and the lack of an enduring and safe relationship in childhood had. In other words, people who encounter childhood trauma are much more likely to experience painful psychological symptoms.

However, people who experience childhood trauma are absolutely a part of the human family because they have the same universal human needs as everybody else. If we only think about psychological symptoms, we miss the bigger picture. Of course people who were abused will experience problems with anxiety *because* their universal need for basic safety went unmet. If you were uncared for or abandoned, of course you will struggle with anxiety, depression or dissociation *because* your universal needs for belonging or a secure sense of self were not attended to.

There are many connections between painful psychological symptoms and unmet needs which can be drawn, and you will have further opportunities to do this as we go along. So, there are two take-away points here. One, despite your unique and painful experiences, you are very much a part of the human family in respect to universal human needs. Reynold's quip about feeling like an alien was humorous, but neither Reynold nor anyone who experienced childhood harm is an alien. Two, if you want to make progress concerning painful psychological symptoms, you will need to look at how needs when unmet in childhood and how they remain unmet today. Getting universal human needs met reasonably well is an unavoidable feature of recovery.

References

1. Herman, J. (1992). *Trauma and Recovery: The Aftermath of Violence – From Domestic Abuse to Political Terror*. NY: Basic Books.
2. To explore *The Adverse Childhood Experiences Study*, go to: https://acestoohigh.com/got-your-ace-score/
   If you wish, you can fill out the Adverse Childhood Experiences (ACS) questionnaire which formed the basis of this study. This will offer you feedback concerning the extent of your own abuse or neglect history.
3. Van Der Kolk, B. (2014). *The Body Keeps the Score: Mind, Brain and the Body in the Transformation of Trauma*. Milton Keynes: Penguin.
4. Rowe, D. (2003). *Depression: The way out of your prison*. Oxford: Routledge.
5. May, R. (1969). *Love and will*. New York: Norton.
6. Gupta, M. A. (2013). Review of somatic symptoms in post-traumatic stress disorder. *International Review of Psychiatry*, Feb, 25(1): 86-99.
7. Van Der Kolk, B. (2014). *The Body Keeps the Score: Mind, Brain and the Body in the Transformation of Trauma*. Milton Keynes: Penguin.
8. Sar, V., Akyuz, G., & Dogan, O. (2006). Prevalence of dissociative disorders among women in the general population. *Psychiatry Research*, 149, 169-176.

Chapter 4

Childhood Harm and the Body

"Sometimes it's like my nervous system is playing for a different team."
Terry

When a psychotherapist collects their client,
all too often the client's body gets left in the waiting room.[1]

People who experienced childhood harm are usually frustrated and even exhausted by the psychological problems they encounter. They are often desperate to change, either for themselves or the people they care about. But getting away from familiar painful experiences can feel difficult, and the fact that change is so hard can be confusing as well.

Bob was neglected by his mother and physically abused by a stepfather. As an adult, he had struggled with a mix of social anxiety and depression for many years.

> **"My wife and friends say, *Bob, you've got to think differently. Bob, you've got to stop reacting like that. Bob, snap out of it.* I don't want to be the way I am... but... it's just not that simple."**

Marion experienced childhood abandonment and neglect, and had a long history of coping through eating-disordered behaviours.

> **"I hate the way I keep making a mess of things, but it's like there's something in me that just keeps going in the same direction."**

The fact that people like Bob and Marion so often feel stuck with their psychological problems is not because they don't want change, but because the effects of childhood harm have deep roots. Roots are hidden beneath the ground, and they can be very stubborn. One of the most important and helpful ways of understanding these deep roots of childhood trauma is to appreciate how a developing body and brain is effected by repeated distressing experiences. More specifically, we need to know how the *autonomic nervous system* develops in relation to the care or lack of care a child experiences.

No one has been more helpful in clarifying the relationship between childhood harm and the development of the nervous system than Dr Stephen Porges, who developed a model called *polyvagal theory*.[2] We will be relying on this model to help explain why emotional and body-based problems can be so challenging for those who were harmed in childhood, but it's worth making a few brief comments upfront. While many of our clients have found polyvagal theory to be *really* useful for their recovery, some have struggled to connect with the medical terminology it uses. Some clients have expressed confusion or frustration in therapy sessions. This has been the single most challenging chapter to construct, and several rewrites have been necessary as we received ongoing feedback from our clients. While we provide the important medical information, we substitute simplified language in order that Porges' essential insights can be accessible and memorable.

The three neurological pathways described by polyvagal theory

Polyvagal theory describes the three neurological 'pathways' which make up our nervous system and helps us understand why healing body-based distress is such an important feature of recovery. We will explore this model in a moment, but you may already have an intuitive understanding of what these three pathways are all about because you were introduced to *the window of tolerance* previously. In a sense, the window of tolerance and polyvagal theory are different ways of describing similar experiences. However, Polyvagal theory adds a lot of value because it provides a medical basis to our understanding and offers important ideas for how we can respond to distressing states.

The autonomic nervous system controls all of our vital functions, like breathing, digestion, and heart rate – often in ways we aren't consciously aware of. However, the autonomic nervous system has another important job – responding to threats and keeping us safe. On the surface, people who experience childhood harm seek help for many different reasons. However, if there is one thing they all seem to struggle with, it's that they don't feel safe. To understand why people who experienced childhood harm have a problem feeling safe, we need to understand how the autonomic nervous system develops and operates.

Polyvagal theory teaches us that our nervous system contains three separate but linked 'pathways', each evolving to help us respond to threats and meet our core need for safety. These pathways run throughout our body from our brain to our toes, and it's important to note that the word body indeed includes the brain.

Sympathetic Nervous System (SNS): When activated, the SNS pathway represents a MOBILIZED state. Heart rate, blood pressure, breathing, and hormones such as adrenaline all increase. We tend to 'flip into' this pathway if we are threatened or perceive we are threatened but imagine we can defend ourselves. Emotions of fear or anger are common. To simplify language, we will refer to the sympathetic nervous system as the *Fight or Flight Pathway.*

Dorsal Vagal System: When activated, the Dorsal Vagal pathway represents an IMMOBILIZED state. We experience low heart rate, muscle tone and energy. We tend to move into this pathway in instances where a threat seems so overwhelming that active defence seems impossible. Hormones and neurochemicals are released to protect us through 'shutting down' and we experience emotional numbing. This happens to conserve energy or to prevent an escalation of threat, and we may feel disconnected, dissociated, hopeless, or depressed. To simplify language, we will refer to the dorsal vagal nervous system as the *Shut-Down Pathway.*

Ventral Vagal System: When activated, the Ventral Vagal pathway represents a RELAXED state. We experience moderate heart rate, respiration and muscle tone. It's fundamentally a state of safety and hormones or neurochemicals are released which encourage social connection and creativity. We are present and connected. Co-regulation becomes possible (i.e. the giving and receiving of soothing and support within relationships). To simplify language, we will call the Ventral Vagal system the *Present and Connected Pathway.**

In a moment, you will have a chance to reflect on how you experience these three pathways within daily life. But first, it's important to point out that there are three reasons why understanding these neurological pathways can be so important for recovery.

1. Polyvagal theory may use *ideas* to describe experience, but these descriptions are based in medical science and research.[3] It's a developing field, but it represents the leading edge in providing us with a solid medical explanation concerning the impacts of childhood trauma on the body, as well as recovery.

* The Sympathetic System and Dorsal Vagal pathways can work differently if we are in safe circumstances. If safe, we can experience the mobilisation of the sympathetic system as playfulness or excitement, as for example when we are engaged in competitive sport. When feeling safe, the Dorsal Vagal System can be experienced as a state of tranquillity.[4] However, we focus on ways these pathways operate as part of our threat response as it is most pertinent to childhood harm and recovery.

2. Polyvagal theory helps us understand how essential it is to work with body-based and emotional issues with respect to creating experiences of safety and connection. Safety and connection can be created within relationships and the world, but as polyvagal theory tells us, they also need to be found within our own bodies. Recovery means being able to feel safe and comfortable 'within our own skin'.

3. Many adults who experienced childhood harm blame themselves for the fact that they have struggled with coping and psychological problems for many years. Polyvagal theory provides a genuine explanation for *why* trauma produces such damn difficult challenges, and this can encourage individuals to be more self-compassionate (and less self-punishing!).

Below we provide examples of clients who experienced activation of the *fight or flight*, *shut-down*, and *present and connected pathways*, and then you will have an opportunity to reflect on your experiences. Mary Kay took a 3-hour train journey with two friends to London which unfortunately activated her *fight or flight pathway*.

> **"My friends we're lovely, but there were so many people on the train, and I kept looking around the carriage. We played cards but my heart was pounding, my chest hurt and I was shaking for most of the trip. I just wanted to get off the train and I went to the bathroom 4 times just to get away."**

Charlie experienced a lot of emotional abuse as a child. He was dealing with a number of stresses and when he saw an envelope from the gas company it seemed like one too many problems, and he felt overwhelmed. His experience is a good description of responding to threats through the *shut-down pathway*.

> **"I'm watching a movie with my daughter but I'm not hearing any of it. Later, when she went to bed, I was sitting on the couch just staring into space. I don't even know what I was thinking about or how long I sat there for. When I get like this I'm just numb and I lose track of time."**

June had no memories of early childhood and had been abandoned to the care system. However, her experience of meeting her son's new partner allowed her to access the *present and connected pathway*.

"I'd been worried about meeting my son's new girlfriend, but she had such a warm and friendly smile on her face. She said she was really happy to finally meet me and asked me about my indoor plants. I just felt so relaxed with her that I forgot about being anxious."

How can we know when we are largely in one pathway or another? As we will explore, pathway responses get triggered quickly and automatically. We often just find ourselves in a pathway response. However, there are typical physical, emotional, and behavioural clues which can help us 'work backwards' and figure out which pathway is active. Chart 1 can help you with the exercise which follows.

Chart 1

NERVOUS SYSTEM PATHWAY	PHYSICAL INDICATORS	EMOTIONAL INDICATORS	SOCIAL AND BEHAVIOURAL CLUES
Fight or flight pathway (Sympathetic nervous system pathway)	Increased heart and breathing rate, trembling, muscle constriction, flushing, hyper-alertness	Fear, anxiety, anger, rage	Raised voice or shouting, direct staring, tightened facial expressions, racing thoughts, threatening physical gestures, avoidance or fleeing, confrontation
Shut-down pathway (Dorsal Vagal Pathway)	Lower energy, slumped body, physically inactive, flaccid facial tone	Numb, disconnected, depressed	Socially cut-off, can't think, don't take in situation or conversation, don't defend oneself, gaze into middle distance
Present and connected pathway (Ventral Vagal pathway)	Alert, calm to moderate energy levels, soft or responsive facial tone.	Feel safe, calm and connected emotional tone	Socially engaged or content in solitude, playful, creative, laughter, can listen and notice

Exercise 1: Reflection of your experience of 3 pathways

There are no 'right' or 'wrong' answers to the three questions below – only answers you will understand. 1. Comparatively speaking, do you have a sense of how much time you spend with the *fight or flight*, *shut down*, and *present and connected* pathways activated, i.e. how prominent a role each state plays in your life? 2. Do the fight or flight and shut-down pathways keep you safe and work as they should or are they a problem in your life? 3. Is it difficult for you to access the *present and connected* pathway when you need to?

How the nervous system operates is 'shaped' by trauma

During childhood, how the nervous system develops relies on the quality of care received. Infants and babies are incapable of 'regulating' or soothing their distress when the fight or flight pathway is triggered, and children have limited capacity in this respect. Imagine a baby who is hungry or wet, a young child frightened by a dog or distraught by an ice cream which has fallen onto the pavement, or an older child who is angry at a rejection. They will experience physical bursts of distress, fear or anger, and the baby or child may have little capacity to soothe these states of physical and emotional dysregulation. The baby or child requires the presence of a caregiver to co-regulate or soothe these states. Reassuring and soft words or physical contact assist the child's nervous system to shift from the distress of a *fight or flight state* (sympathetic pathway) to being *present and connected* again (ventral vagal pathway). Through many such experiences, the baby or child learns to *trust* that distress can be soothed within caring relationships. And, they are learning that there are ways they can soothe their own distress over time.

However, children who experience abuse or neglect will experience many more situations where the fight or flight pathway is triggered *and* there is often no one there to soothe this reaction and help them shift into the present and connected pathway. Over many such experiences, the brain and body gets 'shaped' or 'toned' to favour the fight or flight pathway (sympathetic pathway). This can become a pattern of reacting, so it's not surprising that those who experienced childhood harm spend more time in fight or fight responses and have a difficult time finding present and connected experiences when they need it.

But what about the shut-down response (dorsal vagal pathway)? If threats are deemed as overwhelming and insurmountable, shut-down responses may be triggered and a child may freeze up, go numb, or cut off from experiences. This is a form of dissociation, where you are being desensitised to what is occurring, and it is a way our body is trying to provide protection. If a child experiences emotional or physical abuse which is overwhelming often enough, their nervous system will be 'shaped' to favour a pattern of emotional numbing, 'shutting down' or dissociation. As with the fight or flight response, the shut-down response can become a pattern of coping.

In summary: multiple instances of childhood harm can 'shape' how the nervous system develops and operates. Fight or flight (Sympathetic) or Shut-down (dorsal vagal) pathways may become more sensitive, easily triggered and harder to shift out of. The safety of the present and connected pathway (ventral vagal) can seem less familiar and harder to access. These patterns often endure into the adult years.

How polyvagal theory encourages insight and self-compassion

We have an entire chapter later in the programme that focuses on self-compassion, but here is a brief definition: *Self-compassion* means being able to speak to yourself with kindness and support when it makes sense (special note: if you intuitively don't like the idea of self-compassion, you are in good company – lots of people who experienced childhood harm feel uncomfortable or annoyed just reading or hearing the word).

Many people with trauma histories have a genius for self-blame in situations where they find it hard to appreciate that past trauma 'set them up' for problems. Appreciating how past trauma leads to emotional distress getting expressed through your body can help you access self-compassion in a genuine way.

Consider Nigel, a kind-hearted middle-aged man who had been physically abused by a step-father and neglected by his mother. As a consequence, Nigel spends a lot of time stuck in a *fight or flight* pathway response, and this occurs to varying degrees when he is in group therapy. During certain sessions we could see he was visibly shaking and stammering as he spoke. During one check-in he told the group:

> **"I'm so sorry. This shaking I experience must be so distracting for everyone and it's hard for me to get words out. It's this way at home too and sometimes my wife has to take the kids to clubs because I just can't do it. When it gets bad, I'm just so useless."**

Nigel's shaking was in fact not very distracting, but he felt so badly about it that he needed a lot of encouragement to prevent him from ending his work with the group. Like many people with trauma histories, Nigel was not only suffering by being stuck at times in a *fight or flight pathway* response, but he was also generating a lot of self-blame and worry with respect to group members, his family, etc… It's bad enough that those who experienced child trauma over-react to events through a *fight or flight* pathway response, but beating up on yourself amounts to 'pouring salt in a wound'. Others can get stuck in a state of *shut-down*. They may withdraw from life and relationships, or be unable to face stressful situations. Being unable to recognise how trauma set them up, they may punish themselves for difficulties with coping.

Polyvagal theory provides a couple of further explanations which encourage you to think about your reactions in a more insightful, realistic, and self-compassionate way. Let's explore them.

1. You don't choose your body-based reactions when triggered

No one who experienced childhood trauma wakes up and decides they are going to have a powerful anxiety reaction when out shopping or that they are going to go into emotional shut-down when faced by a demanding customer at work. Fight or flight and shut-down pathways get triggered automatically. Stephen Porges coined the term *neuroception* to explain how we shift into fight or flight (sympathetic), shut-down (dorsal vagal), or present and connected (ventral vagal) states.[5] At a subconscious level, we constantly scan the environment, searching for signs of threat or safety. Imagine how your smart phone continuously searches for a phone signal or a ship searches the sea floor using sonar. If someone shouts, if someone is suddenly behind us, or if we sense a warm smile on someone's face, our nervous system scans this information and makes nearly instantaneous decisions about threat or safety. Before we can determine through conscious awareness whether something is a threat, our nervous system has already shifted our physiology in preparation for defensive mobilisation, defensive collapse, or social connection. In other words, before we can assess danger or safety through reflection (thinking), our heart may be pumping and our breathing may have quickened (fight or flight), we may experience numbing and cutting off (shut-down) or we may feel relaxed and interested (present and connected).

2. "Story follows state"

Neuroception means *detection* which happens at the level of our neurology. Neoroception is much faster than conscious reflection (thinking). What this means is that the information our bodies provide us through neuroception will influence how we *think* about our situation, relationships and ourselves. Deb Dana uses the phrase 'story follows state' to describe this process. Dana explains, "Your autonomic [physical and emotional] state comes to life and *then* the information is fed up to your brain and it's your brain's job to make sense of what's happening in the body, so it makes up a story."[6] This represents a further idea which can encourage insight and self-compassion. Below are three examples of how 'story follows state' can operate. See what you can identify with.

Mary is at an adult art class and the teacher is asking students in turn to talk about the paintings they have been working at. Other students are speaking and she is waiting to be called on. Mary's heart is pounding, she is perspiring, and her breathing is quick and shallow (a fight or flight state). Thoughts come to mind such as *people are going to criticise my art; my art is rubbish; I will make a fool of myself when I try to speak.* This is the *story* which follows from Mary's physical/emotional state.

Mark's wife asked for a divorce recently, he is having serious financial problems, and he is responsible for solving problems at work for which he has no answers. He's having lunch with some work colleagues who are talking. He isn't really taking in what is said, his gaze is unfocused, his body slumped, he's disconnected and can't think (a shut-down state). A colleague asks Mark a question and he mumbles a response and realises he misunderstood the question. Thoughts come to mind such as *I'm useless, I'm making a mess of everything, I can't cope*. This is the *story* which follows from Mark's physical/emotional state.

The finding that physical reactions can strongly influence the stories we create is not something which should depress or demotivate. Quite the opposite, really. Through learning about these processes we can begin to consciously identify both our nervous system state and the stories it encourages us to tell ourselves. This can be a basis for change which can provide a greater sense of control and support your recovery. More about this in a moment.

What can this mean for adults who experienced childhood harm?

Some reassurance may be necessary at this point. For individuals who experienced childhood harm, it's not the case that your nervous system is 'damaged' or 'broken'. If we scan your nervous system we will see that everything is as it should be. However, it's likely that it just *operates* differently than for many people who experienced safety and received emotion regulation in childhood. Three common dilemmas can develop for those who experience childhood harm – dilemmas which (fortunately) you can work on in positive ways.

First, a person with a trauma history may 'flip into' the fight or flight response in situations where they are largely safe. In other words, their body-based reaction and the 'story' they tell themselves about an event is an *over-reaction.* Julie experienced childhood neglect and abuse and lacked a secure 'attachment' to provide the safety she needed. You can almost hear 'the voice' of the fight or flight system in her description of an encounter with her partner Jim.

> **"Jim said that he'd bumped into his ex-girlfriend at Tescos and they had caught up. My heart started pounding and it felt hard to breathe. I got really angry at Jim, and I know that wasn't right. Jim loves me and it doesn't make sense to feel scared and angry like this... but it's like I can't stop it."**

The preconscious process of neuroception signalled a serious threat, and Julie's heart began pounding and her breathing quickened almost instantaneously. Her physiology also instigated 'a story' which was unrealistic.

Second, some people will find that the shut-down pathway gets triggered in situations where they need to be assertive or protect themselves. We mentioned Charlie earlier. Charlie was on the receiving end of physical and emotional abuse from both parents and was bullied at school. Unfortunately, his wife had quite a temper.

> **"When Linda gets angry it's like I disappear. I can't think or say anything or even move. I just stand there, like an idiot."**

For Charlie, the process of neuroception often signals that a threat is so overwhelming that escape or active defence will not suffice, so a shut-down (dorsal vagal) pathway gets activated. His emotions are numbed and his capacity to think or respond is blunted. Dissociation (cutting off from experience) occurs along a spectrum, and Charlie often dissociates to a degree. Sometimes there is a genuine threat that the individual should respond to through active defence. If a company overcharges you, if someone insults you, if you see someone stealing your wallet or mistreating someone you care about, the activation of the fight or flight (sympathetic) system and feelings like fear or anger make sense. However, for some people the numbing of the shut-down (dorsal vagal) pathway prevents them from responding adequately.

Adults who experienced childhood harm can sometimes blame themselves for not stopping abuse when it was happening as a child. However, the disengagement and emotional numbing that occurs when the shut-down pathway is triggered can explain why a child did not resist or run. At a preconscious level, the mobilising of the fight or flight (sympathetic) pathway was seen as too dangerous, and the shutdown pathway was deemed as a better bet for safety. Because the body and brain shut-down for protection at a preconscious level, the inability to fight or run was not a 'decision' the child made.

We need to honour and respect the child's attempts to find protection – they were doing the best they could at the time. Defensive mobilization through the fight or flight pathway or 'shutting down' may have protected an individual during childhood. Being able to resist, run, hide, or numb the impact of harm may have shielded the child from further harm. However, as an adult the fight or flight or shut-down pathways can now be easily activated through neuroception. *On a physical and emotional level, the individual can experience the present moment as if it were the past.*

Third, whereas the fight or flight and shut-down pathways may become overly sensitive, the good feelings, safety and social connection associated with the present and connected (ventral vagal) pathway may be harder to access. Such people often lacked childhood experiences where a parent soothed their distress, they lacked opportunities to learn how to soothe their own distress (self-regulation), and they lacked opportunities to appreciate how people can soothe each other's distress (co-regulation). The headline here is that the individual may come into adulthood with little trust that emotional difficulties can be soothed through relationships with others or confidence that they can soothe their own distress in healthy ways. Without being able to trust in themselves or others to soothe distress, attempts at self-soothing are likely to happen in more extreme and isolated ways.

Exercise 2: Problems responding to events

Below is an opportunity to journal how past trauma may have set you up to have difficulties responding to events. The questions below can act as a guide.

1. Are there experiences where you 'flip into' the fight or flight pathway when you are likely quite safe (as was the case with Julie).

2. Like Charlie, are there instances when you experience a shut-down response (can't think, emotional numbing) when you need to be assertive, get to safety, or protect yourself?

3. Are there times when you know you are safe but you nevertheless find it difficult to access the calm feelings of the present and connected pathway?

Applying polyvagal theory in real time

It may be interesting that we have a medically-based theory of our nervous system which describes the way people can be affected by childhood trauma – but how is this meant to be helpful? The remainder of this chapter will support you in getting a start on using polyvagal theory to observe and respond to body-based distress and related 'stories' about our experience. We hope this is a good start, but a note of realism is probably in order. As mentioned previously, childhood trauma has deep roots, and this is especially true with respect to how our nervous system was 'shaped' to operate. Neuroception is a preconscious experience, so our bodies react to events before we have conscious control. And, the 'stories' we begin to tell ourselves to explain experience often happen quickly and automatically. You can respond to these experiences in ways which supports your recovery, but it is neither a simple or easy process. We hope that what follows is helpful in supporting this work, but there is no 'quick fix' to healing trauma which has found its way into body-based reactions to events.

Despite this note of realism, there are therapeutic ways you can respond to body-based distress when it occurs: 1. You can develop your ability to observe and label the nervous system pathway you are experiencing. 2. You can develop your capacity to notice the 'story' which bubbles up in your mind about your circumstances. 3. You may be able to respond to a body-based reaction and story in ways which will help you in the moment. Let's break these steps down.

1. Observe and label the nervous system pathway you are currently in

When you are triggered and get 'whacked' by a trauma-based fight or flight or shut-down response, it's easy to slip into an automatic response. As one theorist described it – there is a tendency to be most aware of our behaviour, somewhat less aware of our thoughts, and least aware of what's happening in our bodies.[7] However, you can develop a habit of observing the physical sensations and related emotions in your body, and then labelling the pathway. It's not hard to do, but difficult to remember to do. It can be as simple as, *'ah, this is a fight or flight response'*. At other times, it may be helpful to notice that you are experiencing the *present and connected pathway*. It's good to be able to label and appreciate that as well. Towards the end of the chapter we will provide you with a structured exercise to help you gain confidence in this task.

2. Notice the 'story' you are telling yourself about your situation. Is the story realistic or does it need some healthy editing?

Recall Deb Dana's notion of 'story follows state'. If a background of trauma is eliciting a fight or flight or shut-down state at the moment, this may encourage a story which is trauma-based rather than reality-based. Ask yourself – is the 'story' (way you are making sense of things) reality-based or being driven by past trauma?

3. *Can you work to shift your body-based reaction or a trauma-based 'story' in ways which feels supportive and healthy?*

If there is a serious and genuine threat of physical or psychological harm, then of course you need to resist, run, hide, etc... However, if a fight or flight or shut-down response is trauma-based, then managing your body-based response and challenging unhelpful stories is important. Every situation is different so there is no simple advice which can be given. However, if you have gone into fight or flight, deep breathing and grounding (described previously in the Guidebook) can help. Noticing and releasing muscle tension is also useful.

If threats are minimal and you have gone into shut-down, the key is to increase breathing (get more oxygen), think, and move. A shut-down state is like when your computer goes into 'sleep mode' in order to save energy. But if you require your computer, it needs activating.

Unrealistic trauma-based stories which are driven by body-based reactions require healthy editing (or rewriting). How you go about doing this will require creative thinking on your part because every person and each situation is unique.

SPECIAL NOTE: The above suggestions for responding to body-based reactions and 'stories' may seem insufficient. However, providing real-life examples may be the most powerful means of illustration. We hope Mary Ann and Charlie's experiences described below will support your confidence in this respect.

The words of Mary Ann and Charlie are not verbatim but represent a fairly accurate account of what occurred. Mary Ann experienced physical and emotional abuse from her mother and a step-father. She had been introduced to the polyvagal model and had worked with a therapist for a few sessions on how she might respond to difficult trauma-based reactions. The below is her description of an experience which occurred spontaneously.

> **"I'm sitting in a café with my two best friends and they are talking away. My heart is pounding and I feel sick in my stomach. I spill some of my coffee on the table. I keep looking at the other customers and all I can think is *everyone is staring at me and thinking I'm a mental case.* I can't cope and I have to get out of here."**

Mary Ann's reaction to sitting in a café and spilling her coffee is a good illustration of the *automatic* nature of body-based responses and trauma-based 'stories'. Given the seriousness of her trauma history, it's unrealistic that Mary Ann could prevent this reaction from occurring. However, she became conscious of what was occurring and exerted control with respect to *how she responded.*

> **"I remembered my therapy at one point and paid attention to my body. My heart was pounding, my breathing was fast, and there was this pain in my chest. I'm in fight or flight, definitely. I needed to slow things down so I took a deep breath and held it and then let it go. I did that a few times and I was calming down a bit. There was loads of muscle tension in my shoulders and so I let it go. I thought about the story I'm telling myself, this idea that people think I'm nuts and are staring at me. It's over the top, no doubt. People are just eating their lunches and talking. I can cope with this. I told my friends what was happening and Patty [friend] held my hand."**

If Mary Ann made this look easy, keep in mind that she had been working on this three step process with a therapist and had been practicing at identifying the pathway state she was in by using chart 2 (found later in chapter) at home and in sessions. However, you can see the three steps in her description. She identified the pathway response she was in ("I'm in fight or flight, definitely"). She noticed the 'story' being driven by this fight or flight state ("people think I'm nuts and are staring at me… I can't cope…"). She found ways to respond to body-based distress and create a heathier story – this included deep and slow breathing to reduce oxygen in her bloodstream, telling herself that "people are just eating their lunches… I can cope with this," and letting her friends know what was going on. By bringing awareness to what was happening in her body Mary Ann had been able to shift out of a trauma-based fight or flight response and into the present and connected pathway. The danger was in the past, not in that café at that moment, and the safety of the present and connected pathway is where she needed to be.

We mentioned Charlie a couple of times in this chapter. The way he managed a situation with an Amazon delivery woman is a good example of how to shift out of a shut-down state. This delivery person had been dropping off their packages at their neighbour's house for a while, and Charlie's wife had asked him to address the problem.

> **"I was in the garden when I heard her delivery van stop a couple of doors down. I put the rake down and went out on the street and saw she was about to put a package into this bin our neighbours have. I said, *excuse me, is that for number 9?* She said *yes*, and I pointed to our house and said *we are number 9 – I think you have been delivering our packages to our neighbour's place.* There is this pissed-off expression on her face. She said *you need to have your house number marked – we can't know where to deliver without number markings.* My mind went blank and I felt numb. I stared past her and it's like I couldn't move or do anything. She stood there holding the package, looking angry. I thought *this must be my fault. I'm so useless.*"**

For people without a trauma history this situation might not seem like a big deal, but for many people like Charlie, simple confrontations can be challenging. His body and mind had gone into shut-down ("My mind went blank and I felt numb"). An unhelpful story had followed ("This must be my fault. I'm so useless"). Like Mary Ann, Charlie had been working to understand body-based reactions and the 'stories' they throw at him.

He had been using chart 2 (see below) to practice identifying which pathway he was in at home and in situations outside the home, like when shopping. How he responded in the moment to the above situation is a heartening example of how to work with a shut-down reaction. In his words:

> **"I realised my body was stuck in shut-down and I was hardly breathing. *This isn't my fault and it needs sorting*, I thought. I have got to think and stay with this. I took a large breath and blew it out. She's was still staring at me. *Can I show you*, I said, and she followed me to our gate. I pointed to the number 9 which is on the gate post. *The house number is here*, I said. She said, *I didn't see it and your neighbour doesn't have a house number. That's true*, I said. She handed me the package and smiled and said *I'm sorry – I didn't see your house number."***

Charlie identified he had gone into shut-down. As a child, his body had gone into shut-down countless times as a way of protecting him from emotional abuse, and it was an automatic response to conflict these days. Taking a large breath helped activate and mobilise Charlie's body. He challenged the trauma-based story ("This isn't my fault and it needs sorting"). He asserted himself and felt damn good about the outcome, shifting into a pleasant *present and connected* state following the encounter.

Exercise 3A: Identifying what pathway state you are in

Step one in recovering from body-based and emotional difficulties is being able to observe and label what is going on under your skin. The chart below can help you practice identifying the nervous system pathway you are in at any one time. Sit quietly whenever it suites you and have **chart 2** close by. Close your eyes if it helps and pay attention to what is happening in your body, such as heart rate, breathing, muscle tension, energy levels, etc.... When you get a sense of the signals coming from your body, place a finger along the spectrum in chart 2 which identifies which pathway you are in. This is practice for when life triggers a body-based reaction. What did you discover doing this exercise?

Chart 2

FIGHT OR FLIGHT	PRESENT AND CONNECTED	SHUT-DOWN
(Sympathetic) ------------------------	(Ventral Vagal) ----------------------------	(Dorsal Vagal)
Heart beating harder, breath quick and shallow, high or 'prickly' energy, can't settle, constricted muscles	Calm but alert, able to attend, comfortable sensations, moderate energy levels	Low energy levels, mind unable to focus, numbness, flaccid muscles, slumped, disconnected, in a fog

Exercise 3B: Responding in real time when triggered

If you find yourself triggered by a real-time situation, the challenge is to respond with the three-step process described above, illustrated by Mary Ann and Charlie. The chart below can help you keep these steps in mind and can be used to journal your experiences after the event, or if possible, when an event is occurring. Journaling in this way may feel odd at first. When you are in a fight or flight or shut-down response it may not seem natural to start journaling what is going on. But it can be really helpful with respect to getting some distance from the reaction and allowing an opportunity for reflection.

If you sense you are flipping into a fight or flight or shut-down response, see if you can start journaling as soon as possible. If you are standing at the check-out at the supermarket, we understand you may need to wait a bit. The challenge is to work with the experience in really time and journal as soon as you are able. It can be very exciting and encouraging to have a clearer view of these experiences and to begin experimenting with ways of responding. And, you can also journal experiences where you are experiencing the present and connected pathway. If you are doing well to be present and connected when you are safe, it can be encouraging to track this too.

Chart 3

What pathway am I in now (fight or flight, shut-down, present and connected?)	Is there an unhelpful trauma-based story I'm telling myself? What is it?	Is there a way I can work with my body-based reaction and edit the story which will support me?

Final encouraging thoughts

Polyvagal theory is a big topic and it needs acknowledging that we have packed a lot of ideas into a brief space. Some who work with this chapter appreciate the model but lack confidence that they have the necessary skills to respond to problematic states of fight or flight or shut-down. Here are a couple of encouraging thoughts: There are a number of skills you will find later in the Guidebook which will provide further support in responding to challenging states of distress as well as difficult 'stories'. Also, if you found Polyvagal theory exciting and want to go deeper into it, there are a couple of books which can provide more detail. Stephen Porges' *The Pocket Guide to the Polyvagal Theory* provides further explanation of the theory and Dana's book *Anchored* is a personal development styled book which can be useful.

References

1. This was an idea the author came across many years ago when reading a book on therapy, but despite the author's best efforts, the quote cannot be found.
2. Porges, S. W. (2011). *The polyvagal theory: Neurophysiological foundations of emotions, communication, and self-regulation.* Norton series on interpersonal neurobiology. New York, NY: W. W. Norton.
3. Porges, S. W. (2018). *Polyvagal Theory: A primer*, in Clinical Applications of the Polyvagal Theory, S. W. Porges & D. Dana (Eds.). pgs 50-60.London: Norton.
4. Sunseri, J. (2023). Personal communication to the author.
5. Porges, S. W. (2004, May). *Neuroception: A subconscious system for detecting threats and safety.* Washington, D.C.: Zero to Three.
6. Dana, D. Youtube interview with Justin Sunseri. Deb Dana: Story follows state, climbing the ladder and diagnosing #polyvagaltheory.
7. A. Lowen. (1994). *Bioenergetics: The revolutionary therapy that uses the language of the body to heal the problems of the mind.* London: Arkana.

Chapter 5

Retraumatisation and Relationship Patterns

"I wish I could be attracted to nice guys. I was in a relationship with a nice guy last year, but I found him so annoying. He was always touching me and wanting to talk. I think I even turned him into a bastard. Why do I do this?"
Shelly

People who experienced historical trauma had childhood relationships and experiences which were frightening, confusing or inadequate – experiences where core needs for safety, love, self-esteem or self-expression were not met properly. These childhood experiences were painful. If painful experiences were simply something which happened in childhood, then historical trauma would not be the problem that it is. If these individuals grew into their young adult years with a positive self-concept and created healthy relationships, the wounds of the past would stand a better chance of healing. Sadly, this is *not* what usually happens.

The term retraumatisation captures the tragic reality that childhood pain seems to find a way of continuing into adulthood. This chapter is consistent with an idea we have mentioned more than once – we want the traumas of your past to have as little control over you and your life as possible. This chapter will help you explore how retraumatisation and relationship patterns are relevant for you, and whether you can exert some control concerning these issues.

Retraumatisation

Retraumatisation refers to the finding that people who experienced childhood harm are at substantially more risk of experiencing traumatic events as adults than those who did not have such childhood experiences. The evidence for retraumatisation is supported by considerable research[1,2,3]. Retraumatisation is normally discussed in terms of repeated harm occurring within adult relationships. However, retraumatisation can also occur through one's thoughts and behaviours, which is important to consider. Perhaps the simplest way to understand retraumatisation is to point out that it involves emotional states which just seem to re-occur. During childhood, an individual may have felt frightened, distressed, humiliated, lonely or bad about themselves. In adulthood, the context may be different, but this individual discovers that they continue to experience similar emotional, cognitive and behavioural patterns. While we will use the word retraumatisation throughout this chapter, the term *traumatic re-enactment* has a very similar meaning. Below we explore *how* retraumatisation seems to happen.

Retraumatisation through relationships (and an idea from 1914)

The ideas of psychoanalysis have permeated popular culture to such an extent that it's difficult not to come across them in movies, TV, radio or everyday conversation. While some psychoanalytic ideas have fallen out of favour with the passing of time, there is certainly one idea that has had remarkable 'staying power'. It's an idea first mentioned by Sigmund Freud in 1914, and for some people, it can help explain quite a bit. This idea is referred to as the *repetition compulsion*, and it serves as one way of explaining how retraumatisation occurs.

The repetition compulsion refers to the idea that we have a need to create circumstances in our adult life which are similar to those we experienced in childhood. We don't do this by conscious design, but it tends to occur anyway. As adults, we tend to end up in relationships that *mirror* the relationships we had when we were children. Furthermore, this may not occur only once in adulthood – it might be recognised as a pattern. If others hurt me as a child, I might end up in adult relationships with people who frighten or hurt me. If people ignored me or didn't care about me, I might find I end up in adult relationships with people who are selfish or incapable of caring for others. If I was always expected to put my needs last and care for others as a child, I might end up doing the same thing in my adult relationships. If I was abandoned, perhaps I get left by people, or I end relationships suddenly. If I felt lonely in my childhood, perhaps I have ways of re-creating this as well.

Claudine experienced significant childhood neglect and periods of abandonment, and had a history of choosing relationships with men who mistreated or left her. She was making a lot of insight in therapy and had established a good relationship with a man who treated her well and was committed to her. Then, one night she got drunk at a pub and had sex with a man she met. She was confused and distraught over her behaviour.

> **"I just don't know why I did it. I wasn't even attracted to this guy really. I know I was drunk but that doesn't really explain it. I've made such a mess of things."**

Claudine was able to make sense of her behaviour through the lens of retraumatisation. Whether in childhood or as an adult, all she had known was insecure relationships where you might get hurt and where abandonment was likely. She knew that her partnership was what she needed, but at some level she found it uncomfortable and hard to trust. Being drunk may have played a role in her one-night stand, but she was creating insecurity and risk within her relationship, an experience she knew only too well. Claudine's behaviour is a good example of how retraumatisation is often driven by unconscious forces. She hadn't consciously decided to undermine the security of her new partnership, but her behaviour had done just that. Fortunately, she was able to be honest with her partner, and despite a difficult period, the damage was eventually repaired and trust renewed.

Fear and excitement can go hand-in-hand in healthy ways, as when you go on a roller coaster or take some calculated risk in sport. But for some who experienced childhood abuse or neglect, fear and excitement get tied together in unhealthy ways. These individuals might feel excitement or enthusiasm when taking risks which can land them right back where they were as a child – scared, alone, humiliated, hurt, etc… They might also feel bored or frustrated when they have milder experiences which offer security and contentment.

Just the places or situations a person ends up in can invite trauma to happen all over again. Being inebriated in precarious settings can expose a person to harm by others. Some people end up in prison, where retraumatisation by others is likely. Others may end up in prostitution, creating circumstances 'mirroring' earlier sexual and physical abuse. Whatever the context, retraumatisation rarely happens once or by conscious design.

Retraumatisation through your thoughts

Physical, sexual or emotional abuse sends a message to a child that they are bad, shameful or defective. As discussed in chapter 2, children can absorb these messages. The people who originally hurt you may not be around today to continue to send these messages, but they don't need to be. Many people who experienced childhood harm can take on the role of 'beating themselves' with their own thoughts and mental images. It is possible to keep trauma active via your thought processes.

Donald was emotionally abused by both parents throughout childhood. His capacity for self-denigration in response to even small mistakes was quite extraordinary. Donald drove a bus, and while hanging out with three female colleagues in a staff room, he made a joke which contained a mild reference to female stereotypes. The women didn't laugh, and Donald spent the next three days punishing himself for the imagined offence. "I'm rubbish, they hate me, I'm so stupid, they probably don't want to work with me anymore," and so on. More than just verbal thoughts, he kept visually imagining the scene, the joke and his female colleagues. He hardly slept. When he explained the self-denigrating nature of his thoughts in therapy, his clinician said: *So all these horrible things you have been saying to yourself – who does that sound like from your childhood?* He smiled in recognition. "Yeah," he said, "that's how my mom and dad used to talk to me." Donald no longer spent time with his parents, but he could take on the role of his parents and create the same horrible feelings through how *he* talked to himself. Though unaware that it was happening, Donald was retraumatising himself through his own thoughts and images.

For many people who experienced childhood harm, there is often a 'trauma drama' happening inside their heads. By using the word 'drama', we are in no way suggesting that what is occurring is trivial, and we are certainly not suggesting that such individuals are 'being dramatic'. But these recurrent thoughts and images are a drama in that they contain characters, plots and powerful emotions like anger, fear, guilt and shame. Even though the drama is being played out in the form of thoughts or images, it certainly *feels real* and can have a profound effect on a person's life, e.g. stopping them from being able to concentrate or sleep. If a child is being hit, shouted at or sexually abused, trauma is happening through *actual* life events which are deeply disturbing. As adults, such individuals are more likely to experience *mental* events which are also disturbing, and this is one way in which trauma keeps occurring. That's what retraumatisation means: trauma is happening again.

Individuals who experience childhood harm can also encounter distressing and intrusive thoughts or images. This is a feature of post-traumatic difficulties which we look at in more detail in a future chapter. It's worth saying that memories of what happened that are intrusive and distressing are another way that retraumatisation is happening through our thoughts.

Retraumatisation through behaviour

Through their behaviours, people who experienced childhood harm can keep traumatic experiences going within adulthood. There are many ways this can occur, including:

- Using deliberate self-harm, e.g. cutting, burning, punching walls, etc…
- Harming yourself through poor self-care, e.g. not looking after your body.
- Harm inflicted through drugs or alcohol.
- Harm occurring through a poor relationship to food or eating.
- Behaviours which tend to lead to injury.
- Reckless financial decisions.
- Criminal behaviour or prostitution.
- Getting into fights or being in situations where they are likely.

Exercise 1: How does retraumatisation happen for you, either past or present?
If it sounds like we are blaming people who experienced childhood harm for acting in ways that keep trauma alive, we certainly are not. For one thing, retraumatisation is usually an unconscious process. People don't consciously plan or choose for retraumatisation to happen. No one thinks:

"I was in relationships with people who hurt, neglected or abandoned me as a child – I think I'll get into relationships with people who treat me in similar ways."

"I was abused as a child in ways which induced bad feelings about myself – I think I'll continue to punish myself with my own thoughts."

"People hurt me when I was a child – I think I'll act in ways which ensure that I continue to feel pain."

While retraumatisation may have been an unconscious process, below is an opportunity to tic what you can identify with.

___ I can see a pattern of retraumatisation through what happens in my relationships (either in the past or present)
___ I can experience retraumatisation through my own thoughts
___ I can experience retraumatisation as a result of my behaviours

Below, you can describe in further detail how these forms of retraumatisation operate for you. Later in the chapter, you will have opportunities to consider how to repair this pattern.

Traumatic bonding

We've explored three ways through which retraumatisation can happen. But we haven't really looked at *why* it happens. Why do we keep ending up feeling the way we used to feel when we were a child? It doesn't seem rational, does it? If you were scared, unsafe, felt bad about yourself or were ignored, why would this keep happening now that you are an adult? Traumatic bonding is one way of making sense of this.

The term traumatic bonding (or trauma bonding) was first used by Patrick Carnes in his book *The Betrayal Bond*.[4] Humans have a powerful desire to bond with others to meet needs for safety, social belonging and self-esteem. As an infant and child, it is essential to bond with those who are meant to care for us. Being unable to bond with these carers could mean the difference between life and death. But what if the person who should be caring for and protecting us is neglecting or hurting us? A child is likely to still feel a powerful need to bond with this person despite the fear of harm or rejection. Furthermore, it can be the case that an abusive adult will alternate affection or attention with abuse and rejection, which is confusing for a child. A young child may continue to seek the attention and affection they need in the context of rejection and abuse. As a child enters their teen years, some may experience anger or hatred mixed with a continued need for acceptance and love.

So what exactly is a traumatic bond? It means that a child or adult experiences a contradictory desire to be close to and accepted by someone who (at least part of the time) is hurting or rejecting them. There is a bond, but the quality of the relationship is traumatic. Trauma + bond = a traumatic bond. Traumatic bonding is one of the reasons many people we work with feel guilty or disloyal for even speaking about what happened to them as a child.

Van Der Kolk captures the quality of traumatic bonding vividly in describing his clinical work with children. "I have never met a child below the age of ten who was tortured at home (who had broken bones or burned skin to show for it), who, if given the option, would not have chosen to stay with his or her family rather than being placed in a foster home. Of course, clinging to one's abuser is not exclusive to childhood."[5]

Traumatic bonding in childhood helps to explain why many are vulnerable to retraumatisation in adult relationships. As a child, the need for love and acceptance got tied up with pain and rejection, which of course is the basis for a traumatic bond. This pattern of love and pain being bound together is then more likely to repeat itself in adulthood relationships, i.e. the compulsion to repeat. So having traumatic bonds in childhood simply makes having traumatic bonds more likely within adult relationships.

We often hear 'the voice of a traumatic bond' when speaking with people who experienced childhood harm. It can sound like Marsha, who was physically and emotionally abused by her father and then continued to be abused by a string of male partners in adulthood. Discussing her current relationship, she tells us:

> **"I know it's not right that he shouts at me and takes money off me. I'm not an idiot. But it's not always like that. I know I should leave him but... I love him."**

I know I should leave him... but I love him. Marsha feels a strong bond with someone who is hurting her, which is just what she experienced in childhood. Traumatic bonding in childhood relationships can 'prepare the ground' for traumatic bonding in adult relationships. Adults will often accept a relationship characterised by a traumatic bond today because it's what they saw as 'normal' in childhood. Recall that we said retraumatisation means that the painful patterns that happened in childhood find a way of repeating. Traumatic bonding in childhood can encourage traumatic bonding as an adult, so it's another way of explaining retraumatisation.

Exercise 2: Traumatic bonding

Did traumatic bonding occur for you in childhood, i.e. did you want acceptance and care from someone who was rejecting or hurting you? Have you noticed a traumatic bond in adulthood, i.e. someone you had strong feelings for who was hurting, ignoring or rejecting you?

Chemistry and compatibility

Jeffrey Young and Janet Klosko made a fascinating observation about childhood trauma, 'chemistry' and compatibility.[6] It's an observation that seems closely related to traumatic bonding. They suggest that people who were abused or neglected in childhood can feel 'chemistry' when they meet the sort of person who might hurt or neglect them as an adult. For example, if we are physically abused in childhood, we might feel 'chemistry' if we meet someone who seems 'a bit dangerous'. If neglected, we might feel 'chemistry' towards someone who seems self-contained and aloof. In other words, we can feel attraction for someone who (on an unconscious level) triggers memories of past trauma. To our knowledge, there is no research which demonstrates this is true, but it is certainly a phenomenon we have observed many times.

Young and Klosko's point is that 'chemistry' is not the same as compatibility. Particularly for those who experienced childhood trauma, we can be attracted to the wrong people. Of course we need to feel 'some chemistry'. But chemistry needs to co-exist with compatibility, and this means we need to be with someone who will not evoke the old awful emotions we experienced as a child. Compatibility means, among other things, being with someone who will not retraumatise us.

Further ways of understanding why retraumatisation occurs

There are other ways of making sense of retraumatisation. They all overlap with and help to explain trauma bonding and are worth exploring.

"It's what I'm 'comfortable' with"

Strangely, people who experienced childhood harm can be more 'comfortable' with what is painful than with what might be otherwise. When we experience something hundreds or thousands of times, it can just seem like *the way things are*, and to experience it another way 'feels wrong'.

Quick Exercise 3: Folding your arms

Fold your arms as you normally do. Keep them folded for a few moments to get a sense of what this feels like.

Unfold your arms. Now, we'd like you to fold your arms again, but fold them the other way around, i.e. if your right hand is normally over your left arm, do it so your left hand is over your right arm. Keep your arms folded for at least 30 seconds to see how it feels.

What was that like? Most people discover two things. One, folding your arms the other way around was something you had to *think* about and expend effort to do. Second, it didn't feel natural or comfortable. The fact that you have folded your arms in a particular way on thousands of occasions means that doing it differently is hard, unnatural and feels uncomfortable. This experience is neurological. Your brain and body have coordinated folding your arms so many times that there are well-trodden neurological pathways which make this habit simple and easy. To do otherwise is asking a lot of your brain and body.

There is even evidence that a frightened mammal will leave pleasant circumstances and return home, even if the circumstances at home are very unpleasant. In one study,[7] animals such as mice were raised in circumstances which were loud and where food was scarce. They are then allowed to go to pleasant circumstances with plenty of food. If you introduce a loud noise, they will run for home (a place which is loud and has little food). The study suggests that in times of stress, mammals return to what is familiar, even if it doesn't make sense – even if it means returning to a bad situation.

What if a child is told thousands of times, in one way or another, that they are useless? What if a child is physically or sexually abused on numerous occasions? And what if there is also an *absence* of experiences characterised by safety, nurturance, affection, and positive messages? As an adult, these individuals may be more 'comfortable' with mistreatment and less comfortable with trust, intimacy, affection, etc.

Mary Ann was physically and emotionally abused by her parents. She entered therapy because she was having difficulty being affectionate with her newborn daughter, which was disturbing for her.

> **"I don't really like being touched. If my husband or other people try to hug me, my skin sort of crawls. I can enjoy sex, but just the sex part. I don't like it when it becomes intimate or emotional."**

A consequence of childhood abuse meant that Mary Ann felt more 'comfortable' when people didn't touch or were intimate with her. But at a deeper level, Mary Ann still has the same need for affection and intimacy as everyone else. *She is uncomfortable with what she needs*. For Mary Ann, part of overcoming the consequences of childhood abuse is about learning to be comfortable with physical affection and intimacy. Learning to trust it. For Mary Ann, learning to accept affection is like becoming comfortable folding her arms the other way around.

Brandon had been physically and emotionally abused by his mother and bullied at school. When we knew him, he was socially isolated.

> **"I only go out once a week to go shopping and otherwise I don't see anybody. I mean, I don't have friends or family I hang out with. But**

I read a lot of books, and I follow the news every day. I'm happy with my own company."

Brandon is clinically depressed and suffers from insomnia and nightmares. To be frank, Brandon is not really happy with much of anything. We are not convinced by the idea that Brandon is 'happy with his own company'. When Brandon says, 'I'm happy with my own company', what we are really hearing is 'I'm very *uncomfortable* being around other people'. Brandon is uncomfortable with something which is a natural human need.

"It's what I expect"

Circus troupes discovered many years ago that you could train baby elephants to stay put simply by using ordinary rope or light chain to fix them to a stake. The baby elephants will try to break the rope or chains, but after some frustration or anger, they accept that they are just not strong enough. As full-grown elephants, they certainly could break away from a normal rope or light chain, but it doesn't occur to them to try as they have come to 'accept the situation'. This is apparently good news for travelling circus troupes because they don't need to carry around heavy rope or chains.

Human beings are incredible regarding their capacity for abstract thought and the richness with which they can communicate with one another. But in certain ways, human beings share much with other mammals, including how we often accept something today because it's what happened in the past. People who experience childhood harm are just like everyone else in this respect, but what makes them different are their past experiences. People who were loved and safe within their childhood relationships *expect* love and safety, and if they are frightened or hurt as an adult, they will experience this as shocking and unacceptable. If this happens, many such individuals will get out of that relationship fast and put an end to the trauma because it's *not what they expect to happen*. But if a person is physically or emotionally abused as a child and it starts to happen in an adult relationship, they may think, "okay, this is what happens in relationships. It's awful, but that's relationships." So they may stay, and the hurt continues. In this way, they are more vulnerable to retraumatisation.

"It's what I deserve"

Molly's case is extreme, but it serves as a powerful example of how childhood trauma can damage self-concept and lead to further trauma in adulthood. Molly was emotionally abused and neglected by her mother, a woman who was a heroin addict and prostitute. She never knew her biological father and was exposed to dangerous situations due to a string of 'johns' her mother had contact with. She was unsafe and unloved. As a young woman, she developed a masochistic sexuality and only seemed to be attracted to men who would hurt her physically and demean her emotionally. When we began working with her, she was a member of a group of people who practised sadomasochistic sexuality, and she was 'popular' within this group. These masochistic experiences gave her a role and allowed her to have some relationships, but her contact with the group inevitably fuelled her self-loathing.

> **"I try not to let these guys know I'm available and I can keep that up for maybe a week. But I can feel so distressed and lonely and then I will just send out a text to a few of them. One of them will be around within an hour. Afterwards, I just feel calmer for a day or so, but it's a trap because I also feel awful about what I let them do to me."**

When you ask Molly what it would be like to have a relationship with a man who didn't hurt or demean her, she will tell you she's just not attracted to that sort of man. Occasionally, she would even try to convince her therapists that sadomasochism is a lifestyle choice and that it's not necessarily unhealthy. But when you explore this deeper, Molly can acknowledge that there is more to it: she appreciates that her sense of self was so damaged in childhood that she doesn't feel she *deserves* to be treated with affection or love. Her difficulty believing that she deserves to be cared for properly traps her in a cycle of retraumatisation.

Exercise 4: Other explanations for retraumatisation

Have you tolerated hurtful or neglecting relationships as an adult for any of the following reasons?

___ It's what you are 'comfortable' with, i.e. safety, intimacy, and love can feel 'uncomfortable'.

___ It's just what you expect to happen in relationships (it seems 'normal').

___ It's what you believe you deserve?

If you wish, describe what you may have ticked in further detail below.

Retraumatising vs reparative relationships

Retraumatising relationships are adult relationships which keep trauma going. If you were frightened, hurt, ignored, or humiliated in childhood, this is traumatising. If you are having a relationship as an adult, and the relationship regularly elicits some or all of these old feelings, this is a retraumatising relationship.

Reparative relationships are often a very important part of an individual's recovery. These are relationships which serve to repair at least some of the original harm. People who experience childhood harm are fortunate when they can have a reparative relationship which is sustained over time, and it is not unusual for us to work with adults who have not (as yet) had a reparative relationship. Reparative relationships come in many forms – partnerships, friendships, family members, and even pets.

Creating or allowing reparative relationships to occur in adulthood seems like an obvious thing to do. However, for many people we work with, this may not be obvious at all. Some have only known relationships characterised by neglect or threat, so why would they imagine reparative relationships can happen? And, when there is an opportunity for a reparative relationship to develop, many don't trust what is on offer or 'feel uncomfortable'. As a result, some people may avoid or push away people who could potentially offer them a reparative relationship. We will come back to the need for reparative relationships in more detail in chapter 18.

Getting control of retraumatisation

This chapter has looked at three ways trauma can be kept going. Trauma can continue to be experienced through:

- A repeated pattern of painful relationships in which needs for safety, love, acceptance and esteem get frustrated.
- Thoughts and images which drive feelings like fear, shame, stuck anger, or inappropriate guilt.
- Behaviours which leave us with bad feelings or physical sensations.

Emotional or physical pain was bad enough during childhood. Having to carry on with psychological pain in adulthood adds 'insult to injury'. We believe many people can limit the impact of retraumatisation in ways which make a real difference. But it's also important to be realistic. The roots of childhood trauma run deep. Impulses to think and act in ways that invite retraumatisation represent habits that do not wish to go away on their own. There are no simple or magical solutions, and we are not fond of approaches that suggest there are. However, below are some ideas about how you can end or at least minimise retraumatisation.

Protecting yourself from unhealthy relationships

A simple way to understand if a relationship is healthy is to reflect on how you typically *feel* during and after you spend spent time with someone. Do you feel safe and do you feel good about yourself, and do you have more positive feelings about life? Or do you feel afraid, exhausted or angry? If there is 'chemistry' in a relationship, but the experience is typically painful, this is worrying. Whatever the event, if you recognise that you are in a relationship that 'mirrors' painful childhood relationships, there are a few ways forward. Either (1) the relationship can somehow get repaired or improved, or (2) you need to *get out* of the relationship. If the relationship can't be repaired or improved, but you feel you can't end it (as is sometimes the case with family members), then it may be a matter of (3) protecting yourself by creating boundaries or limiting contact.

If you were neglected and felt alone in childhood, it's possible that what is repeating are feelings of isolation. This is a more subtle form of 'the compulsion to repeat' or retraumatisation, but it can be just as relevant. The challenge in this instance isn't repairing or ending unhealthy relationships, but finding the confidence to *develop* healthy relationships.

If the above information seems simplistic or you need more support with this area, there is an entire chapter concerning relationships later on, and we will return to these ideas in more detail.

Managing retraumatisation occurring through your thoughts

Obsessing on events in ways that drive painful feelings and disturbing physical states can be a form of retraumatisation. We offered the example of Donald, who told a joke to female colleagues that misfired and then experienced a stream of thoughts and images which frightened him.

The way to deal with retraumatisation through your thoughts and images is both simple and difficult. If you find that you have powerful thoughts and images which are out of proportion to current triggers and represent past abuse, you just need to recognise what is happening, let it go and soothe yourself. Perhaps you can find words such as: "the thoughts I'm having about this are driving anger or fear in ways which are out of proportion and are just hurting me. I got traumatised in the past – this situation is different – I need to keep this in proportion." In practice, it's often very difficult to do this because anger or fear can be powerful, and the threat or slight you experienced can seem momentous.

Putting an end to retraumatisation which occurs through your thoughts can be a powerful means of addressing past abuse, but it can be a difficult task for some people because these thoughts can be very insistent and hard to challenge. If distressing yourself through your thoughts is really difficult for you, chapters 15-17 may be especially helpful.

Managing retraumatisation through self-care

We mentioned that some people who experienced childhood harm retraumatise themselves through their behaviours, and that this is often an unconscious process. They were hurt, demeaned, ignored, scared or told they were a failure in childhood. Today, these individuals may act in ways or put themselves in situations which make it likely they will continue to experience these feelings all over again, though in some new context. Self-harm, dangerous behaviours, criminal activity, substance abuse, not caring for your body properly, poor nutrition, starting fights, sabotaging relationships, self-isolation, addictive behaviours, and so on.

If you recognise these patterns, self-care is a way to help yourself. What constitutes self-care can be different for everyone who retraumatises themselves through their behaviour. Marjorie is a young woman who was emotionally abused by a stepmother and sexually abused by a babysitter.

> **"When Robert [partner] doesn't call me, I can feel so angry and scared, and horrible thoughts go around in my head. That's when I usually cut myself. But I know that if I call Janet [a friend], she will come over or we can go and get a drink, and I can get through it."**

Calling her friend was a means of self-care Marjorie found helpful. How trauma keeps going and what represents good self-care for you will be unique. Nurturing self-care is anything you can do which leaves you feeling better about yourself or life. Self-care will get more attention in chapter 19.

Exercise 5: Journaling opportunity (Getting control of retraumatisation)

People who experienced childhood harm can get control over retraumatisation in at least three ways:

- Protecting yourself from unhealthy relationships.
- Noticing thoughts and images which are retraumatising you. Letting them go and self-soothing.
- Recognising when you are retraumatising yourself through behaviour and coping through better self-care.

But these are generic ideas. How they apply to you is unique. Below is an opportunity to explore specific ways in which *you* want to get in control of retraumatisation.

References

1. Duckworth, M. P., & Follette, V. M. (2011). *Retraumatisation: Assessment, treatment, and prevention*. New York: Routledge.
2. Widom, C. S., Czaja, S. J., & Dutton, M. A. (2008). Childhood victimisation and lifetime revictimisation. *Child Abuse and Neglect*, 32 (8), 785-796.
3. Classen, C. C., Palesh, O. G., & Aggarwal, R. (2005). Sexual revictimisation: A review of the empirical literature. *Trauma, Violence and Abuse*, 6, 103-129.
4. Carnes, P.J. (1998). *The betrayal bond: Breaking free of exploitive relationships*. Deerfield Beach: Health Communications.
5. van Der Kolk (2015). *The Body Keeps the Score: Mind, Brain and Body in the transformation of trauma*. London: Penguin.
6. Young, J. E. & Klosko, J. S. (1993). *Reinventing Your Life*. New York: Plume.
7. Mitchell, S., Koleszar, S. & Scopatz, R. A. (1984). Arousal and t-maze behaviour in mice: A convergent paradigm for neophobia constructs and optimal arousal theory. *Learning and Motivation*, 15, 287-301.

Chapter 6

Seeking a Secure 'Attachment'

"Because children grow up, we think a child's purpose is to grow up.
But a child's purpose is to be a child."[1]
Tom Stoppard

"I hate it when someone gives me a compliment."
Sally

Attachment theory may sound terribly academic, but this theory explores some of the most vital features of human development and has direct implications for those who experienced childhood harm. In fact, much of what it describes is so fundamental that it not only applies to human beings, but to mammals that care for their offspring. This material has been quite 'eye-opening' for many people we have worked with.

A word of encouragement for those who are parents

For people using this programme who are parents themselves, it isn't easy to read this chapter without reflecting on their role as a parent. For many people who experienced childhood harm, parenting is very important, often because they feel a need to provide for their children what was missing in their development. However, it's not unusual for these individuals to be self-critical concerning their role as a parent. They often know what it feels like to have a parent who didn't keep them safe or caused harm, so they can be very sensitive to making parental mistakes. It's important to point out that all a child needs is to be fundamentally safe and loved. Beyond that, parents can make many mistakes and still provide 'good enough parenting'. Some recognise that the complex trauma they experienced made being a parent more challenging. For example, some people we work with can feel conflicted about providing normal boundaries or discipline to their children. Others may experience complex feelings concerning physical intimacy with their children, especially if they experienced abuse or never received safe physical intimacy themselves. For these individuals, reading this chapter may trigger difficult thoughts or feelings about how they have coped with their role as a parent.

If you feel you have struggled with your role as a parent in any way, we encourage you to look at this *psychologically* and with self-compassion rather than through any lens of self-blame. Also, remind yourself that you are engaging in a challenging model of help to support your personal development, which you deserve credit for.

Attachment theory

It is essential that a child has a relationship with a carer that is characterised by enduring safety and care. This is the main idea behind attachment theory, and as obvious as this sounds, there are some very significant findings which come from this area of study.

Let's have a brief definition of attachment, and then we will get into the helpful detail of what this theory is all about. The attachment between two human beings refers to the quality of the emotional bond. In a secure attachment, there are experiences of safety, warmth and trust. To say *an attachment* is just an academic way of saying *a relationship*. So if we refer to a secure attachment, we just mean a secure relationship. Attachment is often considered with respect to the bond between a carer and an infant or child. However, as we will see, attachment is an essential human experience throughout life. And the quality of attachment you experienced in infancy and childhood tends to impact the experience of attachments in adulthood.

Attachment theory is not a 'perfect science', and while the ideas can seem clear-cut on paper, for some it can seem messier when you apply them to your experiences. Despite the scrappiness of this theory, it really does try to get at important aspects of child development and adult well-being. At any rate, the way in which *you* identify to the ideas you will find here is what really matters. As you read, try and connect your childhood and adult experiences to the ideas you encounter. See what memories you can manage to work with.

Attachment theory was developed in the 1950s by British psychiatrist and psychoanalyst John Bowlby.[2,3] Before Bowlby, there was a prevalent view that human development was driven by feeding experiences or a child's inner fantasy life. Today these ideas seem out of date, and most people naturally assume that the developing bond between a caregiver and a child is far more important for healthy development. No one deserves more credit for this shift in thinking than Bowlby, and his theory has had a profound influence on hospital visitation to children, the shift away from orphanages to foster care, the need to support young mothers suffering from mental health problems and how therapy is provided.[4]

Attachment theory indicates that the infant and child have an instinctual need to bond with or 'attach' to a caregiver. This instinct to attach to a caregiver is based on the biological need for survival. The infant and child will naturally express *attachment behaviour*, which is any behaviour designed to form a bond with a caregiver. Infants and young children monitor adults and experiment with strategies to stay close to or attached to a carer. The form that attachment behaviour takes can depend on the age of development. A newborn will cry and stretch out their arms, a 6-month-old will cling onto a carer or smile in delight, a 1-year-old may hold onto a carer's leg or express a wish to be picked up, a 2-year-old may want to hold a hand or cry. As a child begins to move about independently, they may bring the carer something to show them. Attachment behaviour is about staying in close physical proximity to the carer. This inborn need for a secure attachment is so basic that it's thought to be shared with other mammals. A chimpanzee and a human baby will cling to their mother in a remarkably similar way. A puppy will follow its owner all over the house to stay in close proximity. Ducklings ride on mom's back or swim behind her in an orderly queue when they get too big. What a mammal infant will *not* do is allow a caregiver to get too far from them.

The mammalian brain evolved in layers. The first and innermost layer to develop is sometimes called the 'reptilian brain' because it performs the most basic functions for survival – functions we still share with replies. Later formations of mammalian brain development underlie our essential need for contact and care from those within our species. Bessel Van Der Kolk makes an amusing point which illustrates this finding.[5] He points out that any trip to your local pet shop will vividly depict the difference between the reptilian and the mammalian brain. Reptiles will happily exist alone in their glass enclosure, focusing on hunger and body temperature. A group of hamsters will typically play with one another and explore until they get tired, and then they will all form into a big furry pile and rest or sleep. The mammalian brain is wired for connection.

A *secure attachment* to a caring adult provides the child with what is referred to as a *safe base*. If the child feels secure within the attachment, then they will have the confidence to venture away from the safe base, knowing they can return if they are frightened or confused. This means a child can explore the world, experiment, play spontaneously, and take healthy risks. If something gets scary, they can run (or crawl) back to the secure base, confident that the carer will soothe their distress or explain something. Having a safe base within a secure attachment will support the development of independence, self-confidence and exploration. Those experiencing childhood harm often didn't have a safe base through a secure attachment. They may have formed some attachment to a carer, but it is referred to as an *insecure attachment*. As adults, they can find it much more difficult to take healthy risks, expose themselves to new experiences, and tolerate disappointments. Or, because they expect harm or disaster, some may just act recklessly or place themselves in vulnerable situations. Why not take senseless risks if you'll just get hurt in any event? Without the consistent experience of a safe base in childhood, your experience can narrow through avoidance or the danger may continue.

There are thought to be three different styles of insecure attachment, which we will look at in a moment. However, to keep things simple, let's first summarise some of the main differences between a *secure attachment* and an *insecure attachment* which forms in childhood. As you read through chart 1, you may wish to highlight or circle what seems relevant for you. The word 'child' covers birth to 18.

Chart 1

SECURE ATTACHMENT BETWEEN CHILD AND CARER	**INSECURE ATTACHMENT BETWEEN CHILD AND CARER**
Enduring presence of safety for child	Experiences for child of insecurity, danger, or threat. Walking 'on egg shells'
A close, warm and intimate bond	Bond may be minimal or missing. Or, there may be a bond but it's volatile or unreliable.
Carer is able to understand and respond to the child's feelings and needs	Carer either ignores or at times can't understand or respond to child's feelings and needs.
Child provided with a safe base which allows them to explore and play	Safe base is not provided and child may not explore their world with confidence or safety.
Carer able to soothe child's distressed emotions. Child is learning to soothe (regulate) own emotions.	Carer does not consistently understand or soothe child's emotions. Child has difficulty learning to soothe (regulate) own emotions.
Carer encourages positive self-concept in child.	Negative self-concept often produced. Where positive self-concept develops, it's often based on excessive self-reliance.

Exercise 1: Secure and insecure attachment during childhood – your thoughts?

As you consider the chart above, keep in mind the central point of attachment theory: it is essential that a child has *a relationship* with a carer that is characterised by enduring safety and care (enduring means throughout infancy and childhood). The chart may seem a bit complex for you because you may have had more than one carer – two parents, a step-parent, a foster parent, some other family member, etc.… . Please reflect on chart 1 below relative to your childhood experiences.

Enter Mary Ainsworth and attachment styles

While we can consider attachment in terms of secure and insecure (as in chart 1), a colleague of John Bowlby's named Mary Ainsworth illuminated 3 different insecure attachment styles. Ainsworth discovered these insecure attachment styles through an ingenious experiment run during the 1970s called *the strange situation*.[6] Where Bowlby was the theoretician, Ainsworth was the exacting scientist who wanted to get to the detail of how secure and insecure attachment styles actually work.

The strange situation experiment involved a room with various toys and a one-way mirror the experimenters could look through. A mother and her 12 to 18-month-old child are shown into the room by an experimenter who leaves after about 1 minute. For 3-minute periods the child has different experiences: the mother is left alone with the child; a stranger then joins them; the mother leaves the child with the stranger; the mother returns and the stranger leaves; the mother leaves and the infant is left alone; the stranger returns; the mother returns and the stranger leaves.

This experiment will have caused some anxiety for the child, and we are sorry if this is upsetting for some readers. From Ainsworth's perspective, causing some anxiety in the child was necessary to understand the quality of the attachment between child and mother. The experimenters were interested in observing the child's reaction to the above events in various ways. Was the child able to use the mother as a 'safe base' to explore the room and toys? Was the child distressed when the mother left? Did the child search for their missing mother? Did the child seek comfort when the mother returned? Was the child comforted by the mother or did they resist the mother's efforts to comfort?

Through her experimentation, Ainsworth identified four *attachment styles* in children: secure, anxious (or ambivalent), avoidant, and disorganised. You will have an opportunity to explore these styles in a moment, but we need to make a couple of general points. Recall that a child has an instinctual need to form an attachment to a carer, and they will try different strategies to achieve some form of attachment. You may not remember how you went about this as an infant and young child, but you will have made attempts. The style of attachment you will have been able to form is thought to largely result from the carer's response to you. In order to form a *secure attachment*, you needed to have at least one person who could consistently understand and respond to your needs and who you felt safe with. If this did not occur, you may well have developed an *insecure attachment style*. If these attachment styles were only present during childhood, this information would be less relevant. However, the attachment style you developed in childhood to primary carers tends to endure and show up within adult relationships.[7,8] In other words, the style of attachment you were able to develop with a carer as an infant and child will 'colour' the quality of attachments you tend to form within your adult relationships. So, when we are discussing the different attachment styles, you can consider both your attachment to carers (i.e. parents or others) and adult relationships.

As you read about the attachment styles below, see what you can connect with. Accessing memories and some creative reflection may be useful. Bowlby originally felt that an infant and child would only bond with one 'attachment figure', typically the mother, and Ainsworth experimented with mother and child bonds. However, later research suggests that fathers can be important attachment figures, as can other individuals acting in a nurturing role.[9] You may have had more than one carer that was relevant as a child, and the attachments may have been quite different. For some, an attachment to one caregiver may have helped to reduce the harm experienced with other carers. The section below looks at how attachment can develop in childhood, and later we will draw out how this can manifest in adulthood relationships.

The attachment styles

Secure attachment style

For a secure attachment to develop, the child will have largely felt safe with a caregiver. The caregiver will have understood their own emotions and been largely emotionally stable, and they will have been able to tune in accurately to what their child is feeling and needing. They will have been responsive to the child's feelings and needs. The child experiences the carer as 'a safe base' from which they can explore, knowing they can return and be soothed by their carer if something goes wrong. The child is learning through experience that people can be trusted to understand and meet needs. The child is encouraged to develop a positive sense of self and will largely see others in a positive light. No parent gets it right all the time and every parent can have bad days. The quality of time spent with the child may be more important than the amount of time.

In the strange situation experiment, children who were securely attached to their mothers felt distressed when their mothers left the room, avoided the stranger when the mother was not present, but were friendly with the stranger when the mother was, and were positive and happy when the mother returned. If upset, the child could seek and be comforted by the mother.

Anxious (ambivalent) attachment style

The infant or child who develops an anxious attachment style will often *not* know what to expect from a carer. The carer may have been quite unstable, sometimes involved or connected with the child but other times insensitive or unavailable. Affection or attention may alternate with abuse or neglect. The child wants an attachment but also fears an attachment. The *key* here is inconsistency and instability on the part of the carer. The child may feel needy and dependent on the caregiver but also fearful or angry towards them. This attachment style is sometimes referred to as *ambivalent*. The word ambivalent means to have contradictory or conflicted feelings. This captures how the child's neediness for an attachment is mixed with fear of rejection and abandonment. The child is insecure and develops a largely negative view of self, imagining that others will reject or abandon them because they are inadequate. The child can have a positive view of others, perhaps even seeing them as a saviour or remedy.

In the strange situation experiment, children thought to have an ambivalent attachment show *intense* distress when the mother leaves the room, they are fearful of the stranger, approach the mother when she returns but may push her away. The child explores the room less and cries more.

Avoidant attachment style

The infant and child may have experienced more consistent neglect, rejection, or abuse concerning a caregiver. The caregiver may have been unavailable, abusive or preoccupied with their needs or problems. The child will have wanted a safe attachment, but at some point they decide that ignoring their own needs and feelings and not trusting in others might be the best strategy. The developing child will learn that they must be independent of attachment figures and that relying on others will be a disappointing or harmful experience. The *key* here is consistency, but it's a fairly consistent lack of safety or nurturance. Ironically, the child may develop positive aspects of self, but it will be based on notions of independence, self-reliance or certain personal skills.

In the strange situation experiment, children with an avoidant attachment style show little distress when the mother leaves the room, are okay being alone with the stranger, play normally with the stranger present, and show little interest in the mother when she returns. If the child accepts any comforting when distressed, they are equally likely to accept it from the mother as the stranger.

Disorganised attachment style

Mary Ainsworth initially identified the first three styles indicated above. However, as numerous trials of the strange situation experiment continued, she identified a 4th – the disorganised attachment style. The abuse and neglect these children experienced were thought to have been severe and consistent to the point that they were left dazed or confused, with little strategy for attempting an attachment. The adult's behaviour was likely very erratic but consistently negative – alternatively abusive, distant, intrusive or controlling. The child can experience dissociation, anger, distress, or passivity. Their experience of themselves is very negative, and they are fearful of others, who they also see as negative or harmful. This is why it's sometimes called the 'fearful attachment style'. At least with the anxious and avoidant styles the child is developing some strategies for dealing with their experiences. With the disorganised style, the child is simply overwhelmed and confused. They can't seem to discover any strategy for attachment or control within relationships.

We mentioned that the attachment style which forms in childhood tends to endure into adulthood and shows up within adult relationships. How does this happen? Bowlby said that through childhood experiences, a child develops an *internal working model* to help them achieve a sense of security and control within relationships. The internal working model is like a story people keep telling themselves about relationships. You can sometimes hear 'the voice of' the internal working model in the way people describe themselves and their relationships.

Alice experienced consistent neglect and emotional abuse, and was placed into care at 13. She had one friend who she spoke with about twice a month, though that relationship wasn't that close. Ironically, Alice worked as a human resources officer, but she had developed what we saw as an avoidant attachment style. You can get a sense of her internal working model as concerns others through her words.

> **"I don't like people. I have so little tolerance for all the bullshit and stupidity. You can't rely on anyone."**

Danial was raised by a single mother who was emotionally unstable, sometimes loving and attentive, but other times absent or rejecting. He had a series of childhood illnesses and would intermittently spend weeks in a hospital, separated from all his family. He was a military veteran who now worked as an ambulance driver. Danial loved his wife intensely but often imagined she was having an affair, and when she went out of town for work he became desperate and would call and text several times a day. He struggled with low self-esteem and could feel a sense of emptiness and desperation, often when alone. His childhood experiences would predict an anxious attachment style, which we saw. His words also express an internal working model about himself and others.

> **"I'm such an idiot and I hate acting the way I do with Karen [wife] and I know I'm messing everything up. I really love her but I just keep thinking she is going to leave me in the end."**

Jerry was a young man who experienced frequent and extreme physical and emotional abuse from his father, who was his main caregiver. With a complete absence of any safety in childhood, he presented with a disorganised attachment style. He appears frightened, confused, and sometimes dissociated within our sessions, and he can't remember much of his childhood. His only social connections are through gaming sites, and he has been unemployed for five years. His spaniel is literally the only thing he seems to trust. He has little strategy for attaching, reflecting how overwhelmed he was as a child. His words also give clues to his internal working model concerning self-concept and how he sees others.

> **"I don't want to be alone but I can't cope with people. I want to have friends but I get paranoid that people hate me and then I leave a gaming site. I've left three sites now."**

As you read through chart 2, see what you can connect with. You may identify clearly with a particular style, or it may not feel that simple.

Chart 2

Attachment style	*View of self and other*	*Intimacy or closeness*	*Self-reliance and dependence*	*Internal working model*
SECURE ATTACHMENT STYLE	Positive and stable view of self and of other	Consistently seeks intimacy/closeness and is comfortable with it.	Interdependence. Self-confident and self-reliant but can ask for/accept help.	"I can largely trust in myself and other to get needs met." Safe, content, comfortable.
ANXIOUS (AMBIVALENT) STYLE	Negative and unstable view of self. Can hold positive but unstable view of other. Highly sensitive to other's state and may feel love, neediness, anger, or fear.	Pursues intimacy/ closeness but is fearful of rejection or abandonment. Jealousy, possessiveness. Must keep other close or there is danger.	Insecure about relying on self and feels dependant on other. Doesn't like being separate from other and uncomfortable on own.	"The other is important and capable but there's something wrong with me." "I must find ways of keeping the other close to me because I might get rejected or abandoned." Excited, anxious and needy.

AVOIDANT ATTACHMENT STYLE	Some positive views of self, especially about independence or skills. But this positive view can be unstable when there is stress. Tends towards negative, critical views of other.	Tends to avoid intimacy. Keeps other at a distance. May experience need for intimacy, but uncomfortable and untrusting if it happens. Puts up walls.	Strives for self-reliance and doesn't trust relying on other. Tries to solve problems and get needs met on their own. Relying on others is "weak" or exposing.	"You can't trust other as they will hurt you or let you down, so you have to rely on yourself." Anxious, angry and feel sad.
DISORGANISED ATTACHMENT STYLE	Negative view of self and other.	Confused. Alternatively wanting and fearing intimacy. May attempt and then reject attachments.	Feelings of defectiveness so unable to rely on self. Highly mistrustful of being harmed, so difficult to trust in other.	"I'm defective and can't rely on myself, but others will harm me." "I'm confused about wanting or avoiding other." Afraid, Dissociated.

Below is a brief summary of the main points concerning attachment theory.

1. The infant/child has an *instinctual need* to form an attachment with a carer to ensure survival.

2. A secure or insecure attachment will form as a response to the carer's sensitivity and care for the child. A secure attachment is considered, well, a *secure attachment style*. Anxious, avoidant and disorganised styles are considered *insecure attachment styles*.

3. A secure attachment provides *a safe base* from which a child can explore, experiment and play, knowing they can receive comfort and reassurance if they become distressed. Insecure attachments do not provide a safe base, which can limit exploration and the development of confidence.

4. The development of attachment style in childhood tends to endure into adulthood and adult relationships. This occurs due to the *internal working model* the individual forms during childhood.

Exercise 2: Reflection on attachment styles

Chart 2 and the descriptions above are ways of helping you reflect on attachment styles and how they might connect to your childhood and later adult relationship history. The space below can be used for further reflection. Can you identify with an attachment style or styles in a way which provides any insight?

How might attachment theory help you?

If attachment theory were merely a set of ideas, it wouldn't have much use. However, this theory can directly support personal development in a couple of ways. First, a deep appreciation of how adverse childhood experiences led to an insecure attachment style and related relationship difficulties can allow you to be *more compassionate with yourself.* A child will have developed an attachment style as a way of trying to stay safe and feel some control within relationships. At the time, *it made sense* for a child to orientate themselves to carers in an avoidant, anxious (ambivalent) or disorganised fashion. If you can appreciate that the attachment style which developed in childhood can 'rear its head' in unhelpful ways within adult relationships, it's important to be compassionate with yourself. The three insecure attachment styles have unique expressions and challenges, but they all share something in common: a difficulty trusting that you are safe in relationships. This is an understandable consequence of childhood abuse, neglect or abandonment. If your lack of trust expresses itself through an insecure attachment style, you are not 'failing'. You may sense that you need to find ways of developing more secure attachments. But, it's important *to understand* and work on relationship difficulties – *not punish yourself for them.* An insecure attachment style develops over many years at the most vulnerable time in a person's development, so it's important to be patient with yourself. An insecure attachment style won't shift without a struggle.

Second, if you can identify with an insecure attachment style, this might *point you in the general direction of recovery.* We mentioned Danial earlier, an individual largely struggling with an *anxious attachment style*. He was the military veteran who experienced abuse and neglect from a single mother. He loved his wife intensely and could be caring and attentive. However, his low self-esteem, jealousy and fears of abandonment led him to be controlling and invasive, and his behaviour was creating a crisis in the marriage. Danial's appreciation of an anxious attachment style helped him see that he would need to work on self-esteem, develop skills for dealing with his insecurities in ways which would not undermine his marriage, and cope better with his feelings when he was separated from his wife. He also needed to appreciate that one person can't meet all his relationship needs and that developing friendships outside his marriage was safe and healthy.

We mentioned Alice earlier, the HR officer who had experienced emotional abuse and neglect before being placed into care. She had developed an *avoidant attachment style* in childhood which she continued to rely on as an adult. Alice kept people at a distance, was overly self-reliant, felt uncomfortable with intimacy, and was quite critical of others. Alice's avoidant attachment style seemed to protect her and prop up her sense of self, but she often felt depressed, lonely and angry. Alice was coming to recognise that if she was going to create secure attachments, she would need to trust others more, let people know who she was, allow others to help her, and let others get closer to her. She would have to be more vulnerable in relationships with the right people. She needed to realise that she just couldn't sort all her problems or soothe her emotions on her own. This was a scary insight for Alice because she had decided long ago that trusting and being vulnerable with others meant she was going to get hurt or abandoned. Recovery was going to require time, taking risks in developing relationships and experimentation.

And then there was Jerry, the young man with a *disorganised attachment style* who experienced severe and ongoing abuse as a child. He related to himself, others and life in a largely confused, disconnected, and overwhelmed fashion. Crushingly low self-esteem and intense fear of social situations meant he could only connect to others through gaming sites. The avoidant and anxious attachment styles can certainly be problematic, but at least they represent some strategy for staying safe and having control within relationships. Mary Ainsworth theorised that people with a disorganised attachment style may have experienced more extreme trauma and a complete lack of care, so attempts to form attachments are just disorganised or muddled. Individuals such as Jerry may require professional help for some time because they have little inner resources they can rely on to direct personal development. For Jerry, a lot of work will focus on rebuilding a damaged sense of self and slowly developing trust in others and the world.

Danial, Alice and Jerry represent unique examples of how insecure attachment styles can express themselves. Your attachment style will get expressed somewhat differently. To further help you reflect on how your attachment style may help you understand personal development needs, we offer generic descriptions in chart 3.

Chart 3

ATTACHMENT STYLE	COMMON PERSONAL DEVELOPMENT NEEDS (OR, STEPS TOWARD MORE SECURE ATTACHMENTS)
Anxious Attachment Style	Self-esteem or self-concept often requires repairing or building up. Trusting that you are lovable and acceptable and that you won't necessarily be rejected or abandoned. Closeness or intimacy is important, but being able to trust when others are separate or need space. Having a safe base in a relationship, but also being able to separate for periods, explore new experiences, or spend time alone. Developing skills to regulate your emotions. Developing more self-reliance and reducing unhealthy dependence on others. Challenging internal working models suggesting that *you are not acceptable/lovable or will get rejected.*
Avoidant Attachment Style	Self-esteem or self-confidence may be in better shape, but it relies on your own efforts, so it could be fragile if you struggle to cope on your own. Finding ways to lower barriers that keep people at a distance. Allowing others to help you regulate fear, sadness or anger. Allowing yourself to be more open with the right people so they can see who you really are. Learning to feel more comfortable with closeness or intimacy when it happens with the right people. Asking others for help with practical and emotional needs. Realising that you can't entirely be your own safe base, and that you need someone to help you with this. Challenging internal working models such as *you can't trust others as they will hurt you or let you down, so you have to rely on yourself.*
Disorganised Attachment style	Serious harm was probably done to self-concept, so a lot of support and time is probably necessary to form a more confident sense of self. The fearfulness of people and places where people are is probably significant, so learning to feel safe when you actually *are* safe is a big project. Confusion, disconnection, or dissociation needs a lot of work because it leaves you cut off from life and intimate relationships. You may need help just knowing what a safe relationship is and how people form one. Being able to challenge working models such as *I'm defective and can't rely on myself, or others will harm me.*

Exercise 3: Can attachment theory help in any way?

Below is space for self-reflection on how attachment theory may be useful. However, we need to briefly mention something. If you can connect with attachment theory and attachment styles, this may offer insight which can feel helpful. Perhaps these ideas will support you in being more self-compassionate concerning self-concept or relationship problems you have experienced. Perhaps being able to connect with a particular attachment style helps point you in a direction of personal development. However, it's important to appreciate that insecurities in attachment have deep roots. Insight of the sort offered by attachment theory can be really important, but repairing the harm of childhood and creating secure attachments in adulthood requires time, trial and error, and patience.

Much of the remainder of the programme can help build on this chapter, but recovery is normally neither easy nor simple.

In the space below, you have an opportunity to reflect on how attachment theory may help. Chart 3 may offer some guidance. If you have been able to identify with an attachment style, does this help point you in a particular direction concerning personal development?

Final note

Attachment theory and the four attachment styles are not 'a perfect science'. For example, some people who experienced childhood harm can quite clearly identify with one of the attachment styles, and the insight this offers can make things simpler. Others can recognise the value of considering secure and insecure attachment but find it harder to identify clearly with a specific attachment style. If this is true for you, be aware that some research suggests certain people may not fit neatly into one attachment style.[10] And, some people we work with feel that in addition to experiences of trauma, their inborn biological temperament plays an important role in their attachment difficulties. There is some research to support that this experience can also be true.[11]

However, despite the criticisms and ongoing debates, attachment theory has been going strong for over 70 years and is the predominant theory for explaining how childhood harm impacts child development and the patterns of relationship difficulty which can later emerge.

References

1. Stoppard, T. (2007). The coast of utopia: Voyage, shipwreck, salvage. New York: The Grove Press.
2. Bowlby, J (1969. *Attachment. Attachment and Loss (vol. 1) (2nd ed.).* New York: Basic Books.
3. Holmes, J. (2014). *John Bowlby and Attachment Theory*. London: Routledge.
4. Berlin, L., Zeanah, C. H. & Lieberman, A. F. (2008). *Prevention and Intervention Programs for Supporting Early Attachment Security*. In Cassidy, J. & Shaver, P. R. (eds.). Handbook of Attachment: Theory, Research and Clinical Applications. New York: Guilford Press.
5. Van Der kolk, B. (2015). *The body keeps the score: Mind, brain and body in the transformation of trauma*. London: Penguin Books.
6. Ainsworth, M. D. S. (2015). *Patterns of Attachment: A Psychological Study of the Strange Situation*. London: Routledge.
7. Bretherton, I. & Munholland, K. A. (1999). *Internal Working Models in Attachment Relationships: A Construct Revisited*. In Cassidy, J. & Shaver, P. R. (eds.). Handbook of Attachment: Theory, Research and Clinical Applications. New York: Guilford Press.
8. Hazan, C., Shaver, P. (March 1987). *Romantic love conceptualised as an attachment process*. Journal of Personality and Social Psychology. 52 (3): 511–24.
9. Marshall, P. J. & Fox, N. A. (2005). Relationship between behavioral reactivity at 4 months and attachment classification at 14 months in a selected sample. *Infant Behavior and Development*, 28 (4): 492–502.
10. Fraley, R. C. & Spieker, S. J. (May 2003). *Are infant attachment patterns continuously or categorically distributed? A taxometric analysis of strange situation behavior*. Developmental Psychology. 39 (3): 387–404.
11. Harris, J.R. (1998). *The Nurture Assumption: Why Children Turn Out the Way They Do*. New York: Free Press.

Chapter 7

The Challenge of Memory

"If there's any way you guys can get me a different brain, I'd appreciate it."
Kurt

The idea of reading about traumatic memory may evoke some anxiety for you. After all, it's disturbing memories that many people want to avoid. So, here is a message of reassurance: we are going to be exploring this area in a gentle and gradual way. Also, this chapter will hopefully 'normalise' difficulties you may have with traumatic memories. We will explore the difference between 'normal memory' and traumatic memory, and understand why traumatic memories can feel like a challenging issue. We will look at the difference between *protecting yourself from memories* and *'processing' memories*, and explain why it's important to be able to do both. We hope this chapter will aid your understanding and provide you with more confidence in managing the effects of traumatic memories.

Appreciating the complexity of traumatic memories

A traumatic event is a frightening situation in which a person experiences physical or emotional harm, or the threat of harm. Attacks on one's physical safety or 'sense of self' can be traumatic. Trauma involves serious stress which overwhelms an individual's capacity to cope or to integrate emotions and sense-making. In this respect, childhood physical, emotional and sexual abuse, neglect or abandonment is normally traumatising. The emphasis here is on the word *normally*. When children experience significant threats, it is normal for such experiences to have traumatic effects, including traumatic memories. Traumatic memories can be thought of as a normal consequence of highly abnormal events. Dealing with traumatic memories can be one of the most difficult and yet important aspects of recovery.

Most people who experience childhood harm appreciate that there are memories of what happened that are problematic. In a sense, the problem of childhood trauma *is* the problem of traumatic memories. What's different about someone who grew up with safety and love from someone who grew up with experiences of threat? Well, obviously the experiences are different. But, the experiences happened in the past. What is different today is that traumatic memories live on in the individual who experienced harm. The legacy of childhood trauma is kept alive for adults through memories encoded in the brain, felt in the body, and represented in the habitual ways the individual thinks about self, others and life.

However, the way in which individuals are affected by traumatic memories is complex and can vary from one person to the next. Many do struggle directly with *re-experiencing* of traumatic memories. If you recall, in a previous chapter we explored Complex Post-Traumatic Stress Disorder (C-PTSD), a common diagnosis for those who experienced childhood harm. There were six features of this diagnosis, one of which is referred to as *re-experiencing.* Re-experiencing occurs when intrusive and unwanted memories of a traumatic event come into a person's mind. The memories often come with difficult emotions, distressing physical sensations and disturbing thoughts. An individual may respond by avoiding events, people or places which might trigger re-experiencing. If re-experiencing comes with *very* powerful physical sensations and emotions and the person loses contact with the present moment, isn't sure what is real, or even feels that something awful is happening again, this is called a *flashback.* A flashback can be scary. Only some individuals who encounter childhood trauma experience flashbacks, and if this has not happened to you by now, it probably won't. *Nightmares* can be thought of as re-experiencing when asleep, often in symbolic form. Whether re-experiencing occurs through intrusive images, flashbacks or nightmares, the individual is dealing with significant emotional and body-based distress connected to memories.

While re-experiencing as described above is quite common, it's just not this simple. There are others who can recall events and talk about what occurred, but they seem disconnected from the emotion or physical sensations that ought to be a feature of the memories. In therapy sessions, they might tell you about awful childhood or adult experiences through 'deadpan' expressions, almost as if what occurred happened to someone else. This does *not* mean that they were unaffected by events or that traumatic memories are not an issue. It can mean that the emotional and sensory content is disconnected from the memory of what occurred. Some of these individuals can struggle with depression or distress they feel in their bodies.

And, the complexity of traumatic memory does not end there. Certain individuals can really struggle to recall traumatic memories, and they can feel quite confused about the past. They may have a sense of abuse or neglect occurring, or they were told about such events by others, but there are significant gaps in memory. In more extreme cases, certain trauma memories are completely repressed in ways that the individual does not consciously direct. However, memories that are repressed or lost can resurface later in life. The issue of 'recovered memories' was controversial at one point, but we can now be quite sure that this is a genuine phenomenon.[1] For some, it really is possible to remember an event later in life that had been unconsciously repressed, and when this occurs, people need to be believed. Recovered memories can occur with any form of trauma, but appear to be especially likely in instances of childhood sexual abuse.[2] Again, difficulties in recalling what happened or total repression does not mean that trauma memory isn't significant. What can't be recalled can be experienced within the body and emotions, or 'acted out' through difficulties in relationships or coping.

Here is another complexity to consider. How difficult traumatic memories are can vary for a particular individual over time. For periods in their lives, often when things are going better or they are in a good relationship, traumatic memories may ease up or even disappear. But, if a person faces new stressors, experiences a relationship loss, or encounters something from their past, traumatic memories can 'wake up' for a period of time. This was the case for Mary Ann, who had been physically abused by her stepfather.

> **"My relationship to John [partner] was great and I was really focused on training as a massage therapist. I was doing so well. And then I saw him [her step-father]. I thought he was living up north or maybe even dead, and suddenly there he was – walking in the high street. All these memories started coming back to me."**

Fortunately, this was a temporary setback for Mary Ann, and with support from her partner and friends, she regained control over re-experiencing. However, her experience illustrates how memories can recede and then wake up.

The fact that traumatic memories can be experienced so differently from one individual to the next can also relate to how people have tried to cope with the problem. There are many different ways individuals can attempt to suppress or push memories away. Examples can include drug and alcohol misuse, manic behaviour, perfectionism, eating-disordered behaviour, OCD, or deliberate self-harm. It's not unusual for individuals to present initially to mental health services with the above issues which then need to be traced back to childhood harm and associated traumatic memories.

We are going to be exploring traumatic memory in ways which will hopefully support you in developing insight and your recovery. However, here is an important thought. Clinicians and researchers have made some useful discoveries about the problem of traumatic memories and what can help, which we will explore. However, given the complexity of this issue, we will not be explaining *how traumatic memory works for you* or *what you should necessarily do about it*. It will be necessary for you to see what you can identify with and explore the best way to use certain ideas or strategies.

Traumatic memory and 'normal memory'

Let's consider the way memory normally works in the case of non-traumatic events. Suppose you go to a birthday party – it's a nice event with largely pleasant emotions and low stress. The event is likely to be properly 'processed' and stored away in memory. What does this mean? It means that 1. You were connected to the event when it was happening. 2. You were not overwhelmed by physical sensations and powerful feelings like fear, terror, disgust, or rage. You had access to both your emotional brain (limbic system) and your thinking brain (prefrontal lobe). 3. Because your emotional brain and thinking brain were 'online' and working together, the birthday party events were encoded into memory in a straightforward way. These memories can be recalled and form the basis of a coherent 'story' you can think about or explain to others without problems.

Traumatic memory tends to operate differently than 'normal' memory in a couple of ways. First, there is a difference in the level of emotional and physiological arousal when we experience traumatic events. Adrenalin is released when we experience a threat, resulting in memories being strongly encoded. The fact that we strongly encode threatening events in memory is our mind's way of trying to ensure safety in the future. As well-intentioned as traumatic memory is meant to be, there is often a real problem with how it works later in life. Traumatic memories may keep reoccurring when we are quite safe. For some individuals, they show up in nightmares, often in symbolic form. The memory of the pleasant birthday is something we might think about occasionally and we do not feel compelled to re-experience it. Rather than acting as a helpful guide and protecting us from further problems, memories of trauma have become a problem!

Second, how traumatic memories get stored can work differently than non-traumatic memories. Memory involves storage systems (thalamus and hippocampus), our emotional brain (limbic system), and thinking brain (prefrontal lobe). With normal memory, these systems are 'integrated' and work together to process and store away experiences in a coherent way (as with the pleasant birthday party). If an event is threatening, our emotional brain may take over while our thinking brain gets shut down. We experience shock and powerful physical sensations and get flooded by emotions such as fear, terror, disgust or anger/rage. The sympathetic nervous system we discussed in in a earlier chapter is activated. Images and powerful physical responses and emotions can be stored away, but without access to our thinking brain during the event, we may not have a coherent story. The storage of the memory can be fragmented and laden with disturbing emotional and sensory aspects. By shutting off our thinking brain we are defending ourselves by repressing or dissociating from some of what is happening.[3,4] Repression or dissociation are ways of 'cutting yourself off' from the event so that you don't experience the full awfulness of it. If you recall the traumatic memory today you may experience emotions and physical sensations, but might find it hard to access a coherent and helpful story about what happened. It's common for people who experienced childhood harm to tell us that their traumatic memories come to them in 'flashes' or fragmented 'bits' rather than in a chronological way. Because of this, some can feel upset about having difficulties recalling events in a coherent way, and they may worry that others won't believe them if they can't describe it confidently. These individuals need to be believed and to feel reassured that they are recalling what happened as well as they can.

This is how traumatic memory often works, but it can go in another direction as well. If an individual was truly overwhelmed by a terrifying event, it's possible that their thinking brain *and* emotional brain got switched off. They can be deep in a Dorsal Vagal response where everything is shutting down for protection. The experience will certainly have impacted them but they may have limited or no access to the events, emotions or physical sensations. This can sometimes explain the confused and 'deadpan' descriptions we sometimes hear from clients. It can also explain the fact that a memory can be lost and then recovered later in life.

So, when an individual experiences trauma, the emotional and thinking parts of the brain found it hard to work together so that a memory could get stored away in an integrated and coherent fashion. In other words, the event wasn't 'processed' thoroughly at the time. The result is that later in life the individual does not simply *recall the event* – they may *re-experience it.* The images often come with the same old feelings of fear, terror, anger, shame, etc… In a sense, the individual is going through it again. The individual is not able to look back on the event with a sense of distance; the memory can feel frozen in time. The sense an adult may make of the event – the 'story' they tell themselves – may also be frozen in time; they may still, in certain ways, explain what happened through the eyes of the child.

Many people who experience childhood harm feel badly that they are continuing to struggle with traumatic memories well into adulthood. For this reason, it's important to make the point that such individuals are not 'weak' or failing. They are struggling with traumatic memories because this is what childhood trauma produces. *The problem of traumatic memory is better thought of as a 'condition' rather than a choice.* No one who experienced childhood harm gets up in the morning and decides they are going to have distressing and intrusive memories that illicit emotional and body-based distress, undermines their sense of self, and pushes them towards unhelpful coping. When it comes to considering traumatic memories, self-compassion and self-acceptance make a lot of sense.

Should you protect yourself or 'process' traumatic memories?

This is a common question. Let's look at what we mean by 'protecting yourself' from memories and 'processing memories'. By protecting yourself from traumatic memories, we simply mean exerting control so you are not getting harmed (or re-traumatised) by them. This can include, for example, deciding *not* to deal with memories at a particular time. 'Processing' traumatic memories is a term that clinicians and researchers use. It just means allowing yourself to recall events, safety experience sensations and emotions attached to memories, and to think about, talk about, or write about what happened. Processing traumatic memories means allowing yourself to experience them, but in a way which is relatively safe and hopefully allows for better 'integration' of emotions and thoughts (that story we tell about what happened).

Before we look at protecting yourself from memories vs processing memories, let's explore a bit further why traumatic memories can be such a problem. For many, re-experiencing childhood events through memory can feel like a trap. For some, these memories can be intrusive, and the individual may feel compelled to re-experience them. The memory feels harmful and difficult to get away from. As one client we knew put it, 'it's like having to listen to this extremely annoying person saying the same horrid things over and over again. It's like – shut up already!'

On the other hand, some will find ways of strongly suppressing traumatic memories. They may blot out memories through substance misuse, manic behaviour, self-harm, filling their mind with 'noise', or other behaviours. If you constantly push away or suppress trauma, trauma often expresses itself indirectly through generalised anxiety, nightmares, or through the body, e.g. headaches, frozen muscles, fibromyalgia, IBS, etc.[5] The trap looks like this: re-experiencing traumatic memories can feel disturbing, but running from traumatic memories can be exhausting.

We mentioned Donald earlier, a man who was emotionally abused by his parents. He provided us with an analogy which beautifully illustrates the dilemma of traumatic memory.

> **"I don't want to remember what happened and I know I have all sorts of ways of forcing it out of my head. But it can be exhausting. It's like I'm standing in this swimming pool and I'm pushing a large ball under the water. I can't see the ball, but I can feel it pushing itself back up, and after a while your arms get tired."**

So suppressing or running from the memories doesn't get rid of them. On the other hand, it's no good allowing yourself to get *flooded* by distressing memories that leave you feeling out of control, make living your daily life very hard, give you panic attacks, etc… Many people intuitively know that suppressing memories doesn't get rid of them, yet they can be very anxious about facing them.

Let's return to our original question: Are you supposed to protect yourself from these memories, or are you supposed to face and process these memories? *We believe you should be able to do both.* Sometimes it's important for you to control and protect yourself from memories. However, it's also important to process memories when possible – to safely recall what happened, allow for manageable emotions and sensations, think about it, talk about it, and make sense of it in ways that help you feel stronger. Below, we explore methods of protecting yourself, *and* we look at informal and formal ways of processing memories.

Protecting yourself from traumatic memories

Recovering from a traumatic childhood will require being able to face what happened in childhood. However, there are times when it's better to protect yourself from memories. Why might it be important to protect yourself, and when might you want to do this? There are three ways of answering this question.

1. You might be having intrusive memories at a time when you need to function or help someone else. It's just the wrong time to experience and think about childhood memories.

2. There may be times when you feel that a particular memory is too disturbing, and you are worried about being overwhelmed. This can sometimes be the case if an intrusive memory comes with very distressing emotions and physical reactions. It is always the case with flashbacks. A flashback is something to manage and protect yourself from. Jerry was physically and emotionally abused by his father. He told us, "I can think about a lot of what happened when I was growing up, but there are a few memories which, if I remember them, I feel like I'm being mugged." At this stage in his recovery, those were memories he needed to protect himself from.

3. There is evidence that the more you think about something (or recall a memory), the stronger that memory becomes.[6] This is helpful if we are studying for a test or want to improve our tennis serve. However, recalling a traumatic memory over and over again can also strengthen the memory trace. Making progress with childhood trauma does require being able to access memories safely in order to develop insight and create change, but recalling a traumatic memory numerous times is not required. If you are repetitively recalling a distressing memory in ways which do not support insight or recovery, this isn't helping you move forward.

So, if you realise that you need to protect yourself from a disturbing memory or a flashback, what can you do? Below are some strategies to consider. Perhaps some will appeal to you more than others. Practicing them when you need to can provide feedback about what works best.

Distance yourself from a trigger

Sometimes, an intrusive memory can 'come out of the blue', and it's difficult to know what triggered it. Other times it's quite obvious what is triggering the memory. If you feel it's best to protect yourself from the memory, you can get distance from the trigger. If the trigger is something you hear on TV or radio, you may want to turn it off or switch the channel. If you see someone in the street that triggers you, you may want to avoid them. If it is something in a magazine you are reading, you may want to put it down. Many will do this naturally as it just makes sense.

Use an anchoring object

Intrusive images or flashbacks pull you out of the present moment and into the interior world of memory. Some people will use an anchoring object, sometimes called a grounding object. It's ideal if the object is something small enough to fit into a pocket or purse. If the object has personal and pleasant associations, that helps. It might be a small stone, a gift from someone important to you, a ring, a small stuffed animal, etc… If it's a good time to protect yourself from intrusive memories or a flashback, then holding, feeling and looking at the object can get you out of your head and into the world again.

Using movement

When a person is sucked into an intrusive memory or flashback it can feel like everything *stops*. The world disappears and a person might find themselves immobilised and staring into space as the memory gets hold of them. Getting yourself moving can help. Walking, singing, stretching, or yoga, etc… can work. Intrusive memories or flashbacks disconnect you from your body and the world; movement can shift you out of the internal space of memory and get you reconnected.

Grounding exercises

We introduced the technique of 'grounding' during the introductory pages, but it can be such a useful strategy it's worth highlighting again. Grounding can be handy for intrusive memories, but it's especially useful for flashbacks. Any time you struggle with flashbacks or strong intrusive memories, you can circle back to the grounding exercises we described in the previous section entitled *Preparing for a safe and productive experience*. As mentioned, some people find it helpful to write out the text of a grounding exercise and keep it with them at all times.

Reassure yourself strongly

Intrusive thoughts and flashbacks can leave individuals feeling that something awful is happening *right now* and that they won't be able to cope. They need reassurance that they will get through it. Michelle was prone to strong intrusive memories and even flashbacks when she was strongly triggered. To prepare herself for these moments, she wrote a reassuring statement on a 3 X 5-inch card that she kept in her purse and would read if she had a powerful intrusive memory: *What's happening is not real. This is just a strong memory I'm having. This is really upsetting but I'm safe and nothing bad is happening to me. It happened a long time ago and it's not happening now. I'm completely safe right now. This will get easier and in a few minutes I will feel okay again.* She didn't need to use the card that often, but just having the card with her offered some reassurance.

Breathe and relax your muscles

An intrusive traumatic memory will kick breathing and muscular tension into high gear. If you really focus hard on slowing breathing and relaxing your muscles, it serves not only to distract you from the memory but also to calm down the physical/emotional response. As with grounding, the technique of controlled breathing was discussed in the section entitled *Preparing for a safe and productive experience*. You can review and practice controlled breathing as a way of protecting yourself from memories. If you can manage it, combining controlled breathing with other strategies found here can help too.

Connect with someone you trust

Some people feel most vulnerable to intrusive memories or flashbacks when they are alone. These individuals may feel safer if they get in contact with someone they trust. You don't have to talk about the intrusive memories when you contact someone, unless this works for you. For some, just getting in touch with someone you trust will distract you or minimise the effect of the intrusive images.

Pay attention to the world 'out there':

Intrusive thoughts and images are happening in your mind. The world you are experiencing is happening around you, out there. An intrusive thought or image says, *forget what's going on out there in the world – pay attention to what is happening inside your head and body*. If now is not the right time to attend to the memory, force your attention *outward*. Stay connected to reality. The extent you can keep your attention on what you are doing will drain away the power of the intrusive memory. Janet told us about an intrusive memory that occurred while she was washing up.

> **"I was listening to the radio and this song came on. It was a song which was popular when I was young and it immediately triggered bad memories from when I was a kid. I was going out to my book club soon and I didn't want to be a mess. I turned the radio over to the news. I focused all my attention on the feel of the warm soapy water and the dishes and what they were saying on the news."**

Exercise 1: Techniques for protecting yourself from memories or flashbacks

We briefly described eight strategies for protecting yourself from intrusive memories or flashbacks. Some will have more appeal to you than others. Scan back over the headings for each strategy. Which strategies do you intuitively imagine will work best for you? Knowing what works best can require some practice. When you need to protect yourself, we suggest practicing those strategies you are most drawn to. The space below can be used when appropriate to record what seems to work.

What is meant by 'processing' traumatic memory?

'Processing' a traumatic memory may sound technical or complicated, but it's quite straightforward. *Processing trauma memories involves 1. recalling a memory, 2. experiencing manageable emotions and physical sensations attached to the memory, and 3. thinking about, talking about, or writing about the memory.* Through remembering and allowing for feelings and reflection, you may be able to create a more realistic and supportive 'story' about what happened, how you were affected, and who you are. As mentioned, 'processing traumatic memories' is a phrase clinicians use, but if you prefer, it can be thought of as *working with* or *responding to* traumatic memories. While processing traumatic memories may not be difficult to understand, it is often difficult to do. We are going to look at what happens when you are processing distressing memories in more detail and explore why it can be so challenging. Also, there are 'informal' ways you can process memories and formal processing strategies that happen when you are working with a qualified therapist. We will explore both.

As mentioned, when a person experiences a shocking event, the emotional brain can take over, the thinking brain can shut down, and the memory can get stored away without a coherent story about what took place. So, processing traumatic memory involves remembering, having access to some feelings, and being able to construct a story which is helpful and healing. Constructing this story can involve thinking about it, talking about it, writing about it, or even drawing or painting about it. In other words, you are trying to integrate feeling and thinking – you are putting it back together, but in a way which is tolerable and supports a coherent and healing story.

While this process is important and can support healing, it is *normally* challenging. Let's explore some of the common issues. First, just having access to memories stored in the hippocampus can be difficult. Traumatic events may have happened many years ago. And, you may have dissociated ('cut-off') from some of what was happening at the time to protect yourself. Second, the emotional brain will very likely have coloured traumatic memories with disturbing emotional tones which can be felt throughout the body. When you recall a traumatic memory, the painful associated emotions and physical sensations can also be present. The main reason those who were harmed avoid memory is because they don't want to re-experience these difficult emotions and body-based sensations. Third, being able to think, talk, or write about an upsetting memory in healing ways (through the use of the frontal lobe) can be challenging. Even if a person can begin reflecting on a traumatic memory, previous stories featuring self-blame, guilt, shame, etc… may just override more supportive and recovery-focused ways of sense-making. Robin was a woman who experienced neglect and emotional harm within the family home before being abandoned to an aunt at eight. You can sense in her words that she is struggling to develop a realistic and healing story with respect to memories.

> **"The fact is, no one wanted me. I was always just a problem. Maybe I shouldn't feel like a reject or ashamed about what happened. But, that's just not what my brain tells me."**

So, on the one hand it's important to acknowledge that processing memories can be challenging. On the other hand, if you are able to process memories with reasonable safety, there are good reasons to do it. Let's look at this.

Why process memories?

If you are going to deal with painful memories, it can be helpful to know what the point is. Why allow yourself to recall an event which was disturbing and has led to a number of psychological problems in later life? Wouldn't it be better to try and never think about what happened again? The problem is that continually forcing the memories away can be exhausting (recall Martin's description of holding a big ball underwater).

An important reason to process traumatic memories is to reduce the negative impacts they are having on your sense of self and life experiences – to feel a greater sense of control. The collegial team of Christine Courtois and Julian Ford are highly respected academic authorities on complex trauma. While discussing the neurobiology of childhood trauma, Courtois made this point: "The true antithesis to intrusive re-experiencing is not freedom from trauma memories or trauma-related distress, but the capacity to choose whether, when, and how to recall and make sense of… those memories."[7] What Courtois means is this: by processing memories, your aim isn't to have complete freedom from intrusive trauma memories and related distress, but to gain control over these experiences by choosing 'whether, when, and how to recall and make sense of… those memories'.

By allowing yourself to process painful memories, you are facing those memories, and when you face something you are afraid of, you can take the fear out of it. In a sense, facing distressing memories is no different than facing anything people are frightened of—spiders, heights, crowded places, water, the dark, public speaking, etc. However, the key is that you not only face what you are afraid of but also feel relatively safe and successful by facing it.

We've discussed intrusive memories and flashbacks, but what about nightmares? At least some nightmares can be considered re-experiencing of traumatic events in symbolic form while you are sleeping. Night terrors are a form of nightmare where an individual may scream, shout, thrash about, fight something, or jump out of bed. Nightmares are one way in which a mind is trying to process traumatic events. If nightmares are a frequent problem and you worry about going to bed or feel tired all day, this may be an argument for processing trauma during your waking hours. We have nightmares about what we suppress or repress during our waking hours. If we can find ways of processing what we are struggling with during our waking hours, we may be less exposed to nightmares while sleeping.

Here is another reason why processing trauma matters. For many years you have been telling yourself a story about who you are, what value you have to others, whether people can be trusted, whether life has a point to it, or whether you are safe in the world. This story very likely continues to be driven by the traumatic memories you still hold. It's as if the traumatic events and the memories they produced are co-writers of this important story you are telling yourself. A feature of processing memories is being able to shape this story about yourself, relationships and life in healing and self-supportive ways.

The goal of 'processing trauma' is *integration*. As mentioned, while trauma was happening, your emotional brain may have overwhelmed your thinking brain. When you recall the event today it may therefore come with the old disturbing emotional and body-based distress, but there is no realistic and healing story which can support you. This is why it's called *re-experiencing*. You are re-experiencing the event in a way which can be frozen in time. Processing heals this split between the emotional and thinking brain so they can work together. This may help you feel like you are in 'one piece' – the experience is more 'integrated'. Processing memories takes practice and patience, but with practice can come a growing confidence that you can look at your past with safety, success, and a sense of integration.

Processing memories informally

There are formal methods of trauma memory processing that occur when you are working with a qualified therapist. Later in the chapter, we will describe two of these models. For some people or for certain memories, doing trauma memory processing with a therapist may be a good idea. However, many people can work at processing memories informally on their own or with someone they trust.

If informally processing traumatic memories seems daunting, here's something which needs saying: surprise – you're already doing it! In your own way, you've probably been doing it for years. Let's remind ourselves what processing difficult memories involves:

1. Recalling an upsetting memory. This will often happen automatically. You're walking the dog, taking a shower, watching a film – and boom – the memory is there. Or, it's possible for you to decide to recall a memory to process.
2. Having access to the emotions and physical sensations which come with the memory (but in a relatively safe and manageable way).
3. Reflecting on and making sense of the memory in a way which feels helpful. This can involve thinking about it, talking about it, or writing. The point is to create a story which feels realistic and healing in respect to the memory.

You may not have used language like 'processing traumatic memory', and you may not have divided it into three steps, but it's likely that you can identify with this process. You have probably had many occasions where you found yourself recalling something painful from the past, experiencing associated emotions and physical sensations, and trying to make sense out of it. That's informally processing a traumatic memory. In this respect, processing memories is not new. This chapter may just be supporting you with the challenge from a particular perspective.

Also, reading this Guidebook and doing related exercises will no doubt 'stir up' difficult memories, associated feelings and physical sensations. And, you will find yourself making sense out of these memories. So just engaging with the programme encourages you to process memories from a number of different perspectives.

When might you informally process a painful memory? If the memory just spontaneously appears and it's a safe and good time to deal with it, you can work with it in the moment. Or, you can sit down when it's quiet and decide you are going to recall a difficult memory and work with it. You can work with a memory on your own or talk through the process with someone you trust. It may feel weird at first to think of working with memories in this way, but it can feel more natural as you practice. If this all sounds too theoretical, Mary's experience of informally processing a memory may make it feel more real. She described it like this:

> **"I was sitting in my car in a supermarket parking lot and this guy walks by who looked like my stepdad. This memory comes into my head of when I was about 12 and I'd got a bad report card and my step-dad is just screaming at me, his face all red. I feel scared again and kind of frozen, just sitting in the car remembering it. I can recall how stupid and useless I felt. My breathing is going fast and I slow it down, breathing deeper. I know I need to see this differently. I'm feeling more angry now at my step-dad and I think, *he shouldn't have screamed at me like that. I wasn't stupid, I was having problems learning because I had dyslexia and nobody even knew it. Somebody should have taken the time to talk to me and to help me. I wasn't bad – I just needed help.*"**

This was an intrusive trauma memory that got triggered and happened spontaneously. Mary did some processing right in the moment, and you can see all three components of processing at work. She *recall*s the memory and *accesses feelings and physical sensations* that happen quite automatically. There were also some quite automatic negative thoughts attached to the memory, such as thinking of herself as useless and stupid. But there is this moment where Mary starts to take control of how she wants to *think about the memory*, her stepdad, and herself. She begins to see events in a way that is realistic, self-supportive and healing. She is shaping a story to support her recovery. Concerning this intrusive memory, all Mary needed to do was to think about it in a particular way. In addition, some people may find talking through how they see it with some they trust helpful, or writing about it. Whether thinking, talking or writing, you are using your frontal lobe to support processing. The emotional and thinking aspects of your brain are online together - that's integration.

Processing means that you are giving new meaning to what happened which supports you and your recovery and changes how you relate to the memories. Just reliving a memory repeatedly strengthens it and keeps you stuck in the past, unable to free up emotion and energy for the present. This was a distinction which a client really helped us understand. Darnell had been physically and sexually abused by an uncle. Making matters worse, as a black child growing up in a predominantly white neighbourhood in the 1980's, he'd experienced significant racial abuse. Now in his 50s, at one point he had worked on shooting commercials. He put it like this:

> **"I'd never heard of processing a memory, but it made intuitive sense. It's sort of like working on a set for a commercial shoot. There's a lot going on that is just a part of what needs to happen, but I can also direct the scene in ways that make sense. I have a lot of intrusive memories that just pop up, and at a certain point I just direct part of it, mostly how I want to think about what happened or how I should feel about it."**

So, like Mary, you can process a memory which occurs spontaneously. However, it's also possible to proactively decide to do some processing with a particular memory. You can sit in a quiet place and recall the memory, get in touch with feelings and physical sensations, and then shape your story about how to make sense of it in a realistic and self-supportive way. You can talk to someone about your experience or do some writing if you wish. If the memory feels like it has a bit less control over you, you are on the right path.

Whether you do some processing for memories which occur spontaneously or choose to recall a particular memory, there are a couple of guidelines which can help.

1. Work at processing memories when it's practical and you feel safe enough. If it's the wrong time or the memory seems too powerful, then it may be better to access any of the skills for protecting yourself from memories.

2. Keep in mind the distinction between *processing a memory* and *re-experiencing a memory*. You will be recalling the memory with some associated feelings and physical sensations. But, as Darnell suggests, processing means that you can act as a director. The

story you tell through thinking, talking or writing should support your recovery, not keep you and the memory frozen in the past.

Exercise 2: Informal traumatic memory processing

There are two ways you can do this exercise. First, you can go about your life and wait for an intrusive memory of past trauma to catch up with you. Depending on who you are this may take 3 minutes or 3 days, but such experiences are common enough that you probably won't have to wait long. If it's the right time and you feel safe enough to manage it, see if you can work at processing in the moment. Or, rather than waiting for an intrusive memory to arise spontaneously, you can sit quietly and choose a memory to recall, ensuring it is one you feel you can manage safely. Whether you work with a memory which arises spontaneously or choose to work with a memory, you will be:

A. Recalling the event. B. Allowing for tolerable feelings and physical sensations, and C. working with the thoughts which arise. See if you can work at thinking about the memory in a way which is realistic, self-supportive, and healing. Like Mary's experience depicted above, shape a story of the memory which helps you feel stronger and better about yourself and life. Talk or write about it as well if that helps you.

Following processing of a memory, you can use the space below to describe your experience and anything helpful you may have learned.

Formal therapeutic models for trauma memory processing

This chapter suggests that it's important to be able to protect yourself from re-experiencing *and* develop confidence in informally 'processing' memories. With practice and perseverance, a combination of protection and informal processing may feel adequate for some. However, others may find that re-experiencing is really stuck and painful. If this is the case, you may want to consider seeing a clinician who has specialist training and experience in providing formal therapeutic interventions for traumatic memories. You may want to seek professional clinical help if:

1. You are struggling with intrusive traumatic memories frequently.
2. Memories come with intense emotional and physical responses that you just don't feel confident you can deal with on your own or with support from people you trust.
3. You feel strongly compelled to see past events in ways which produce shame, guilt, or self-blame. It's just difficult to shift this 'story' on your own.

There are a couple of formal models of therapy that have been shown to help certain individuals make progress with re-experiencing difficulties. These are models that have a good evidence base. Keep in mind that re-experiencing is one of the core problems associated with PTSD. So, if you specifically want professional help with re-experiencing, you are asking for help with PTSD.

Trauma-focused Cognitive Behavioural Therapy (TF-CBT)

Trauma-focused CBT has been established for decades, is evidence-based, and is one of two recommended therapeutic interventions for PTSD in the UK by the National Institute of Care and Excellence (NICE). Therapy is typically 8-25 sessions. There are a variety of techniques which you and your therapist may use. With TF-CBT, you will likely be exposing yourself to traumatic memories in a safe and gradual way with a view to processing and overcoming their painful impacts. A therapist offering TF-CBT should thoroughly explain from the outset what therapy will involve, the therapist and client's roles, any risks, and the potential benefits.

Eye Movement Desensitisation Reprocessing (EMDR)

EMDR has also been established for many years, is evidenced-based, and is recommended for PTSD by NICE. As with TF-CBT, an EMDR therapist should thoroughly explain what therapy involves, the therapist and client's role, any risks, and the potential benefits. Clients will be asked to recall traumatic memories while making rapid, precise movement of their eyes that the therapist facilitates. We don't precisely know why EMDR is helpful. However, it's thought that through the use of rapid eye movements and guided instruction, trauma is reprocessed in a manner that allows for a greater sense of control over disturbing emotions and sensations.

References

1. van Der Kolk, B. A. & Fisher, R. (1995). Dissociation and the fragmentary nature of traumatic memories: overview and exploratory study. *Journal of Traumatic Stress*, 8 (4), 505-525.
2. Loftus, E. F., Polonsky & Fullilove, M. T. (1994). Memories of childhood sexual abuse: remembering and repressing. *Psychology of Women Quarterly*, 18 (1), 67-84.
3. van der Kolk, B. A. (1994). The body keeps the score: Memory and the evolving psychobiology of post-traumatic stress. *Harvard Review of Psychiatry*, 1, 253-265.
4. Terr, L. (1991). Childhood traumas: An outline and overview. *American Journal of Psychiatry*, 148, 10-20.
5. Roelofs, K. & Spinhoven, P. (2007). Trauma and medically unexplained symptoms: Towards an integration of cognitive and neuro-biological accounts. *Clinical Psychology Review*, 27 (7): 798-820.
6. Buchsbaum, B. R., Lemire-Rodger, S., Bondad, A. & Chepesiuk, A. Recency (2015). Repetition and the Multidimensional Basis of Recognition Memory. *Journal of Neuroscience,* 35 (8), 3544-3554.
7. Ford, J. D. (2009). Neurobiological and developmental research: Clinical implications. In C. A. Courtois & J. D. Ford (Eds.), *Treating complex traumatic stress disorders: Scientific foundations and therapeutic models*. (pp. 31-58). NY: Guilford.

Chapter 8

The Complexities of Coping

"Hurting myself or hurting others… means they won. Life shouldn't hurt."
Bobby

This chapter encourages you to explore the important area of coping, but we want to mention something at the outset. Many people who experience childhood harm have a genius for self-blame. They not only experience the pain associated with what happened to them, but they can also punish themselves for how they have coped.

It's likely that reading this chapter and doing the exercises will stir up some difficult feelings because it asks you to explore patterns of coping. Here is what we think is important – as you read this chapter, we want to encourage you *not* to beat up on yourself for how you have coped in the past. Looking at coping from the standpoint of self-blame may boost self-loathing, but does little to enhance recovery. Of course it's important to take responsibility for your recovery, but it's better to explore coping *psychologically*. In other words, if you have acted in ways which have made things worse or caused difficulties, there will be reasons for this. Punishing yourself is simply unhelpful and misses the point. And what is the point? The point of this chapter *isn't* to give you all the skills necessary to cope. Much of what happens through the remainder of the guidebook will focus on that area in one way or another. This chapter encourages you to develop insight into how you have coped, and why you may have developed certain ways of coping.

If you are doing the work in this chapter and find yourself lapsing into self-punishing thoughts, or if you start dredging up memories of times you made mistakes, we want you to notice that this is happening. See if there is a way you can look at this with insight and self-compassion.

What is meant by coping?

If human beings are in enough pain, they are likely to do whatever is necessary to escape pain. How we go about getting away from pain is coping. However, the need to cope with pain can be a more complex and insistent issue for those who experienced childhood harm. For one thing, these individuals are likely to experience more significant psychological pain (symptoms) such as anxiety, depression, anger, intrusive memories, sleep disturbance, and so on. And, this emotional pain often goes deeper than this. As we have explored, these individuals did not get important needs met in childhood – needs for safety, affection, belonging and self-esteem. Related to unmet needs, these individuals sometimes describe the feeling of a void or an emptiness. A sense that something is missing. Those who experienced childhood harm were 'set up' to develop problems with coping, which is something which really needs to be appreciated.

Clinicians sometimes use the terms *maladaptive coping* and *adaptive coping*. While these terms may sound overly technical, they can be helpful in the way they connect coping with human needs. If an individual copes in a way which seems to help in the short term, often by reducing or numbing pain, but means that 'deeper' needs don't get met, we'd say that's maladaptive coping. For example, getting drunk, isolating yourself, or self-harming might reduce short-term pain quickly, but may also prevent someone from meeting needs for safety, belonging or self-esteem. If individuals cope in a way that leads to soothing some pain *and* supports getting important needs met, that's adaptive coping.

The distinction between adaptive and maladaptive coping might sound simple and easy, but in practice it's often not. For one thing, distinguishing adaptive from maladaptive coping is not always straightforward. Also, adaptive coping is often not as powerful and immediate as maladaptive coping, and many people who experienced childhood harm have come to depend on their particular manner of maladaptive coping. Developing insight into coping and the confidence that you can get important needs met often requires patience and trial-and-error.

Why might unhelpful ways of coping develop?

We are going to look at four specific reasons why those who experienced childhood harm are more likely to develop maladaptive means of coping, but first we need to make an important point. Most behaviours that today can be considered unhelpful means of coping started out as a way to get safety, regulate painful emotions, or get very human needs met. We will use the term coping in this chapter, but we could also use the term *traumatic adaptations*, which has a very similar meaning. If you experienced abuse, neglect or abandonment, you had to adapt to (or cope with) these frightening and lonely experiences. You will have done whatever was seen as necessary at the time. Some turn to obsessive-compulsive behaviours, others develop eating disordered behaviours, others learn to avoid people or places, some fight, lie or steal, some develop phobias, others begin picking at their skin or pulling hair out, and so on.

No child or adolescent has a moment where they think, *I'll develop some really unhealthy coping behaviours to become a problem to myself and annoy others.* You developed unhelpful coping because you were trying to get safety, manage emotional pain, or get understandable needs met. You were just trying to *adapt* to traumatic experiences. So, unhelpful coping can also be seen as a traumatic adaptation. Suggesting that you look at unhelpful coping psychologically and with self-compassion rather than through the lens of self-blame is not about 'being nice' – it's literally a more valid way of seeking understanding.

So, let's look at four specific reasons why those who experience childhood harm may develop unhealthy ways of coping. First, as children, many *were not soothed or cared for well when they were in emotional or physical pain.* Imagine a 4-year-old girl. She is running, trips over, and skins her knee on rough tarmac. Blood comes oozing out of the wound, and she begins to sob in pain and shock. Her father runs over, picks her up, and brings her into the house, reassuring her that he will sort it out. He then carefully stops the bleeding and cleans and bandages the wound, all the time soothing his daughter with his words. She becomes calm, and the pain and shock go away. Soothing the emotional and physical pain that children experience is what many parents do, and it's essential for children to experience this support many times as they are developing.

However, something else is happening to this 4-year-old girl. She is learning that pain can get soothed, and that this often happens through caring relationships. She is learning that she can trust others to help soothe her pain. And, if her physical or emotional pain gets soothed by caring adults consistently, she learns from these experiences and is therefore more able to soothe and care for herself. *Being cared for and soothed allows her to develop an internal model of self-care and self-soothing.* Those who experienced childhood abuse and neglect were often at a big disadvantage. Their emotional and physical pain was often not soothed and may have been caused by the very people who should have been helping them with pain. As adults, they may have little understanding of how to soothe their own pain in healthy ways. The result is that, as adults, they may cope with emotional pain in rather isolated, extreme and ultimately less healthy ways.

Second, *many had parents or carers who themselves did not cope well with pain.* Especially for children, we learn about how to manage or cope by watching others. This is a powerful form of learning called modelling.[2] A child learns how to cope by watching important adults in their lives and how they cope. If those adults are coping and trying to get their needs met through substance abuse, aggression, withdrawal, etc… this is the template a child has for knowing how to cope with their own lives.

Third, *extreme pain may seem to require more extreme coping.* People who experience childhood harm tend to experience more extreme psychological pain in response to life events. If an adult who was well cared for as a child gets some really disappointing news or experiences a rejection, they may feel upset, drink a couple of extra beers that evening or vent to a friend. If someone who experienced childhood abuse or neglect has a similar experience, they may feel utterly distraught or abandoned, and they may experience a need to cope in more extreme ways, e.g. heavy intoxication, isolation, self-harming, etc...

Fourth, *some people who experience childhood harm don't trust others to help them with their emotional pain and so lack an important means of coping.* This is an understandable reaction. Someone who didn't get helped with pain and confusion as a child can have a harder time trusting others as an adult. So rather than seeking support from others when they are in pain, they may feel they need to cope in an isolated way. If you have a history of being harmed by people, the idea of getting pain soothed through intimate relationships can evoke anxiety. The problem is that there are times when *everyone* needs someone else to help them through something painful.

If you can identify with any of the above explanations, this may not only enhance insight, but it might help you feel more compassionate with yourself in relation to coping problems you have had previously.

Exercise 1: Why might you be vulnerable to coping in less helpful ways?

Those who experienced childhood trauma often had experiences which 'set them up' to cope in less helpful or maladaptive ways. We described four possible explanations which are summarised in the statements below. Tick any statement that you think is relevant in explaining why you may have developed less helpful ways of coping.

___ I didn't get soothed or cared for well as a child when I was in emotional or physical pain, so it was difficult to develop an internal model of how to care for myself or soothe pain.

___ The adults around me as a child coped in unhealthy ways, so I may not have been shown helpful ways of coping.

___ Because the emotional pain I sometimes feel can be quite extreme, I seem to need powerful or extreme ways of coping to get rid of it.

___ Because I've been hurt or let down in the past, I don't trust others to help me. So, it's made more sense for me to cope in isolated or secretive ways.

This exercise can 'stir up' unique thoughts or feelings for many. Do you want to add any thoughts you have or describe how this has left you feeling?

Blocking and numbing strategies

Every infant, child and adolescent will have many experiences of being scared, angry, sad, lonely, confused or in physical pain. They should feel safe enough to cry or ask for help. An adult should be attuned to their emotions and needs and should respond to soothe distress or bring understanding. If this does not happen, the child or adolescent will have to find ways of soothing or numbing distress on their own. The problem is that they are not developmentally equipped to do this.

Below are coping strategies people who experience childhood harm often rely on to block, avoid, or numb painful feelings. Such strategies may have developed at any point – childhood, adolescence, or young adulthood. They often become a pattern of coping. See what you can identify with, either in the past or present. As mentioned, you may feel badly about how you cope, or you might worry that if you acknowledge how you cope, someone may try to stop you. And, there is almost certainly a part of you that doesn't want to stop because you rely on how you cope to get rid of painful feelings. So, here is some reassurance – the reading and exercises below are *for you.* This chapter will not try to convince you to be different. We all need our defences and our coping strategies. This chapter is simply an opportunity to reflect on coping and whether you may wish to make some changes.

Drugs and alcohol

Traumatic experiences usually lead to painful psychological experiences such as PTSD, chronic anxiety or depression. It should not surprise us that many who have experienced historical trauma will rely on coping through substance misuse or addiction. Between 30-50% of people who experience significant historical trauma will develop substance abuse problems.[1] All coping strategies represent an attempt to control emotional states, and of course drugs and alcohol will do the job, although often with negative consequences to health, relationships and self-esteem. Drugs such as alcohol, heroin, barbiturates or ketamine have the effect of depressing or calming states of distress. Drugs such as cocaine, methamphetamine or amphetamine can act as stimulants, allowing access to deadened emotions and physical sensations. Some drugs, like cannabis, don't fit neatly into one category. So-called 'legal highs' represent a broad range of substances, are not well understood by many clinicians (or users, for that matter), and are a growing concern within mental health and medical systems.

Those who experienced childhood harm are more likely to feel overwhelmed by emotions or emotionally numb, so, understandably, they may be vulnerable to drug and alcohol abuse. Some seem to keep drug or alcohol use under some measure of control. For others, either past or present, it can have very destructive effects on self-concept, relationships, education/work or health.

Food

A surprising number of women and men who experienced childhood harm can develop an unhealthy relationship with food, developing eating difficulties or even a full-blown eating disorder. As explored in the chapter on childhood harm and the body, those who experienced historical trauma are often disconnected from the physical sensations or signals coming from their bodies, or they may simply get signals of distress much of the time. Some don't experience hunger because they are just not in touch with the physical signals of hunger. Some may overeat as a way of trying to manage chronic states of emotional distress.

Food can become a way of feeling a sense of control in a world which is otherwise perceived as dangerous. These individuals usually lack the sense of control that should get experienced through a secure self-concept, secure attachments, and confidence that they can regulate their emotions. So, they develop a relationship with food which goes way beyond the role food is supposed to play in one's life. Food is no longer just about the pleasure of eating and nutrition – it's about feeling in control. Food restriction, food binging, use of junk food, laxative misuse, over-use of diet sodas, diet pills, or over-exercising can play a role. All of this can be tied to an intense sensitivity about whether we are acceptable to others or a need to stay in control emotionally. For some, food can act like any drug.

Obsessive-compulsive behaviours

Uncertainty is a core feature of human experience. We may plan our time and order our lives, but there will always be features of experience that are simply outside of our control. For people who experienced a secure attachment and protection from harm in childhood, tolerating the uncertain nature of experience is likely to be easier. They may think, *if something unplanned or difficult crops up, we'll just have to deal with it and things will probably be okay in the end.* However, for some people who experienced childhood trauma, the uncertain nature of existence is very hard to tolerate. For them, the nature of control takes on a rather 'black and white' quality – if they are not feeling *in control*, then they are *out of control.* If they do not have lots of reassurance, then something bad or terrible is likely to happen to them or those they love. This is an understandable reaction to experiences of childhood abuse or neglect. Threat and harm were very real when they were young, and they did not feel the sense of security and control which comes from being cared for and protected. They learned that the world is a dangerous place and that they must cope by doing everything they can to get control and prevent harm.

Obsessive-compulsive difficulties can be a way of trying to be in control and prevent harm. The 'obsessive' part of this problem just means worrying like mad or imagining everything that might possibly go wrong. By imagining everything bad that might happen, you are trying to control potential danger and therefore achieve reassurance. The 'compulsive' part of this problem means doing something (often repetitively or ritualistically) to gain control over imagined threats. For example, repetitively checking on things like locks or appliances, repetitive hand-washing or excessive cleaning, continually checking that loved ones are safe or arranging things in 'exactly the right way'. As with obsessing, compulsive behaviours are a way of trying to get control and reassurance.

The problem is that all the obsessing and compulsive behaviours are never enough to really get reassurance, and the individual can become exhausted by their attempts. And, they are missing out on life and relationships in the process. It's a difficult journey, but learning that the danger was in the past and that the world really is safer now is necessary. For those with obsessive-compulsive difficulties, learning to tolerate normal levels of uncertainty is part of recovery.

Manic behaviour, perfectionism, or workaholism

For many, thoughts or feelings associated with the past are always in the background, waiting to pop up and disturb them, either in their conscious thoughts or in their dreams. Some will cope by throwing themselves into projects, activities, or work with an intensity designed to distract them from their past. They may strive for perfection in the process. It's as if they imagine *if I can run fast enough, the memories can't catch me*. This can work as a coping strategy to an extent, but it can also be exhausting, and some will 'crash-out' after a while. Pete was a victim of severe physical and sexual childhood abuse, and he's a good example of this type of coping. As he put it:

> **"I'm a self-employed bricky [brick-layer]. There's loads of jobs available so I'd work for about twelve hours a day and six or seven days a week. People on the work sites were amazed at how fast I'd go and they thought I needed the money, but I didn't. I just needed to keep going."**

And then, after one particularly full week of brick-laying, Pete damaged a ligament in his shoulder and had to stop work. Having lost his main means of coping, he was more exposed than ever to painful memories and feelings, and he broke down. Had he not torn that ligament, Pete may not have found his way to therapy.

Self-harm

For some who get flooded by powerful feelings (often anger or emptiness), self-harming can seem like the only way to get some relief. For those who don't rely on self-harm, it can seem odd that cutting, burning, hitting yourself, or pulling hair out can provide comfort and soothing. However, for some people who experienced childhood harm, that's how it works. Juliet, an individual who experienced childhood sexual abuse, put it like this:

> **"I try not to cut myself because I know I'll feel rubbish about doing it later on. But when I get to a certain point of feeling terrible, it seems like the only way out. When I do self-harm, it's like my emotional pain turns into physical pain, and then I feel calm for a while. I really want to stop, though."**

After the relief from a self-harming episode, the individual can feel guilt and regret. We rarely meet someone who relies on self-harm and genuinely wants to self-harm. Many describe self-harming as having an addictive quality they want to be free from.

Other addictive or compulsive behaviours

Blocking or numbing strategies are anything we might do which (at least temporarily) calms painful feelings or memories. We've mentioned some of the most common strategies, but the variety of methods is pretty wide. Compulsive spending or shopping, gambling, hoarding, compulsive sexuality (i.e. promiscuity, affairs, or addictive use of pornography), addictive video-gaming and internet use, dangerous thrill-seeking, etc.... It's not necessarily *what* you do that matters; it's *why* and how *driven* you feel to do it. It's whether the behaviour is helping you meet important needs or becoming another problem on top of the past trauma.

Exercise 2: Blocking and numbing strategies

Common blocking and numbing strategies mentioned include drugs and alcohol, food, obsessive-compulsive behaviours, manic behaviour (including perfectionism and workaholism), self-harm, and other addictive/compulsive behaviours. However, the ways in which pain can get blocked or numbed are probably endless. You are unique in how you block pain. What blocking strategies are especially relevant to you, either in the past or currently?

Relationship style as a way of coping

Blocking and numbing strategies are often ways of coping on your own. However, it's also *essential* that coping is understood relationally, i.e. the pattern of how you cope and get needs met through your relationships. Below is a model adapted from the very helpful work of Jeffrey E. Young and Janet S. Klosko.[3] However, before describing these styles, there are a few important caveats we want to make clear.

First, the four relationship coping styles we explore below represent *a model* for understanding human experience, and models never truly capture an individual human being. As such, people who experienced childhood harm often do not fit neatly into one style of coping. You may recognise yourself coping in a particular style within one context or relationship, but may slip into a different style in another context or relationship. Or, perhaps one style was more prominent at one time but not another during your life.

Second, it's important to point out that many people who experienced childhood trauma can at times cope within relationships in healthy, enlivening and productive ways. They do not always cope through the four styles indicated below.

Third, if you do fall into coping in one or more of these styles, there are usually understandable historical reasons why this is the case, as will be pointed out. If you recognise yourself coping through the styles below, please try to see this with self-compassion.

Having mentioned these caveats, many people who experienced childhood harm can identify with certain relationship coping styles. As you read, see what looks familiar to you.

The avoidant/isolating style

How it works: The avoidant/isolating style of coping is characterised by withdrawing from people or society. This individual may be socially phobic, and so avoids situations or places where there are many people, e.g. shopping centres, public transport. They find excuses in order not to attend social events and may spend much time on their own. They are mistrustful and quick to imagine people will harm, use or manipulate them. Avoiding people or places seems like the best bet for *staying safe* and in *control*.

Rarely, however, is any individual completely avoidant/isolating. They may allow some limited relationships with others, just as long as it doesn't get too close or intimate. Ryan is a young man we worked with who had very limited relationships in the 'real world', but online gaming allowed him a degree of connection to others (though only through anonymous pseudo-names). He ran into a crisis when a longer-term fellow gamer (who by coincidence lived locally) wanted to meet up with him for coffee. The idea seemed threatening, so he considered cancelling his account with his favourite gaming site (something his therapist managed to talk him out of).

While some who struggle with an avoidant/isolating style live alone, some may live with family members or others. However, despite living with others, they may isolate themselves in particular ways, perhaps creating private worlds within the context of family or flatmates.

Some with an avoidant/isolating style can show self-sufficiency. However, in a relationship, others tend to become excessively *dependent* on another person or the state for many years. Developing a dependency on one other person or the state allows them to avoid the rest of the world of relationships. These individuals usually have a genuine desire to be independent and self-reliant, but the abuse or neglect they experienced damaged their self-confidence.

Some with an avoidant/isolating style of coping may develop very important relationships with pets. Pets (often though not always dogs) can provide the individual with affection and a sense of purpose, but manage to do so in a way which is not threatening.

Why it developed: These individuals were often harmed by others in childhood and had good reasons not to trust. As a child, they may have coped by trying not to be seen, 'fading into the woodwork' or keeping their heads down. They may have learned that by avoiding or hiding from those who harmed them, they could reduce or have some control over the trauma. This pattern of being mistrustful, assuming others will harm you, and avoiding people and social situations developed as a means of trying to meet a need for safety.

The dilemma: Individuals with an avoidant/isolating style of relationship coping have the same core needs as everybody. Social isolation/avoidance may seem to offer a semblance of safety, but needs for *belonging or intimacy* go unmet. If unhealthy levels of dependency also are a feature, this undermines the individual's need for self-esteem. Depression and underachieving in life are common.

The challenge: The challenge is to see that the fear response to social situations is often disproportionate to any actual threats. The challenge is also to learn to develop trust for situations and relationships where it is well placed. For those who are safe, the challenge is often about recognising that current experiences are **not** the same as what happened to you when you were a child. And the challenge is to choose to be with people who will not repeat a pattern of hurting you.

The rigid/controlling coping style

Some people who experienced childhood harm are less socially avoidant. Perhaps they have a partner and children, and they might have relationships outside of the home. But, like the avoidant/isolating style, they experienced threat or neglect in childhood. As such, they don't trust others, and they may imagine life is a dangerous place. Those with a rigid/controlling style believe that if they are not *in control* – they are *out of control!* If others show independence, assert themselves, or have other important relationships, this can feel threatening. If they receive criticism, they experience it as humiliating rather than just feedback. To cope, they feel a strong need to be in control of their environment and their relationships. Their attempts to be in control can sometimes feel suffocating to others.

If people they are closest to assert themselves, have other friendships, or express independence, they can feel threatened. If they are put under stress, they can even react with outbursts of anger or aggression. They are more likely to cope by what clinicians Lubin and Johnson refer to as *dumping*.[4] This person was dumped on by people who abused or neglected them in childhood. There is anger and frustration which has built up over the years, feelings which are difficult to find an outlet for. The people who hurt them normally cannot or will not acknowledge what they did or make amends. At times the frustration is too much. They can regret it later on, but when under stress, they can dump on others too.

If this style of relationship coping sounds unattractive, there are two things to keep in mind. First, as long as they feel in control, they may be lively and fun and have a range of attractive attributes that shine through. Second, despite how difficult their behaviour can sometimes be for others, their manner of coping needs to be seen with empathy. They don't really want to cope as they do. Underneath the rigid and controlling style of coping is someone who is scared that history will repeat itself and they will get hurt, humiliated, or abandoned all over again.

Why it developed: As a child, they were abused or neglected, and they may have felt humiliated. But, at a certain point they began to fight back. They learned that by fighting back and doing whatever they could to be in control, they could get some needs met. They don't ever want to be humiliated again. This means of coping became a pattern which they took into adulthood relationships.

The dilemma: These individuals want to feel emotionally safe and have a sense of belonging, just like everybody. However, their controlling behaviour can push important people away from them, and they might even get left in some instances. They can also feel guilty about their behaviour within relationships.

The challenge: The challenge for these individuals is to let go of some control and appreciate that those close to them need to have a degree of independence. They often need to accept the normal 'give-and-take' within relationships. They often need to see that opposing views or criticism is not humiliating but a normal part of what happens in relationships.

The subjugating/passive coping style

The subjugating/passive coping style is in many ways the opposite of the rigid/controlling style. This sort of individual tends to want to have relationships, but they subjugate their needs to others. In other words, they put everyone's needs before their own. They tend not to assert themselves or say what they want, and if they do, they often feel *guilty*. They have a tendency to feel overly responsible for the well-being of others. They may choose relationships with more dominant people. They tend to get abused or neglected within their adult relationships, which may reflect what happened to them when they were young. They may fear that others will leave or reject them, so subjugating their needs to others is a way to prevent this. They fear and try to prevent conflict. Beneath their subjugating behaviour, they may feel *angry*, but they rarely express it, scared that people will hurt or leave them. They may soothe their anger in private ways, e.g. food, substance misuse, obsessive-compulsive behaviours, etc…

Why it developed: The abuse or neglect this individual experienced in childhood may have been so overwhelming that they concluded that the only way to be safe or get any needs met was *not to have any needs or assert themselves*. Subjugating their needs to powerful others was seen as the only option. Or, these individuals may have had parents who were ill, drug addicted, or unfit, and they learned that they had to put aside their needs to care for family members.

The dilemma: These individuals have the same core needs as everyone for self-esteem, self-respect and self-expression. However, if they begin to access and express their needs, they imagine they might get hurt or be left, and this is scary. But the manner in which they subjugate their needs to others leaves them feeling sad, resentful, and prevents them from getting the respect and recognition they really crave. Like the avoidant/isolating style, they may be underachieving.

The challenge: The challenge for these individuals is to feel they deserve to have and express their needs in relationships. To find their voice. Some may need to learn to avoid relationships with domineering people and to choose to be with people who will encourage the self-expression which is so important to their development.

The unstable style

Thus far, we have seen three relationship coping styles. The first tends to avoid others, the second to control others, and the third to subjugate themselves to others. We also recognise a fourth style, which is not explicitly described as part of Young and Klosko's original model. This style can seem like a mix of other styles, but is also distinct. The other three styles may be unhelpful in certain ways, but there is more stability in the pattern of coping. Those with an unstable style can feel 'all over the place', often veering from clinging to others to becoming angry and challenging.

Individuals with an unstable style of relationship coping definitely want to have relationships. In fact, they often really don't like being on their own. On their own, they can feel quite empty, distressed or sad. But relationships can feel scary for them as well. They can feel needy and clingy, and they tend to fear abandonment. They work hard to keep people close to them, and they might idealise others or see them as a saviour. However, if there are even subtle signs that a partner or friend is becoming distant or might abandon them, they can get 'flooded' by powerful emotions which seem overwhelming. They might blow up with anger at their partners, friends or family members. Or, they might feel they need to do something dramatic to keep people close to them. If distress or anger really gets out of control, they might self-harm or do something reckless. They really struggle with self-worth or self-image, and some even will say they hate themselves.

Why it developed: Childhood trauma is common for this style of coping, but it's difficult to know why this level of instability develops. It can be challenging to have a relationship with someone who copes in unstable ways. But, we need to see those who cope in unstable ways with understanding and empathy. It's possible they may have had a more sensitive biological temperament or the harm they experienced occurred at a younger age, before a sense of self had a chance to begin forming. More research is likely needed to answer this question.

The dilemma: More than anything, those with an unstable style of coping want to feel emotionally safe and loved. But their fear of abandonment can mean that they cope in ways that frighten others or create distance in their relationships.

The challenge: Those with an unstable style of coping often have a very poor self-image and are quick to imagine they will be left or that others hate them. Developing self-compassion and self-esteem is important. Also important is finding ways of coping with powerful emotional states so they don't get out of control and end up damaging relationships.

Exercise 3: Reflecting on relationship coping style

You may find that you can identify quite closely with one of the above relationship coping styles. Or, perhaps you can identify with more than one style, or you cope differently depending on the relationship or situation. You know your experience best. Please describe your thoughts about the above relationship coping styles and how they might apply to you. *The relationship-based coping styles we're described are:*

The avoidant/isolating style
The rigid/controlling style
The subjugating/passive style
The unstable style

Why does a relationship coping style develop?

Why would one individual develop a particular relationship coping style and another develop a different style? There are a couple of possible explanations. First, how individuals cope in relationships today may have been something they *learned to do* as a child. The way individuals cope in their relationships today may not appear to make a lot of sense in certain circumstances. However, as a child, this way of coping may have made *a lot* of sense. Bertrand was physically and emotionally abused by his father and bullied in school for many years.

> **"When my dad was at home, I would hide. I'd hide in the airing closet or in the garden shed. At school I tried not to be seen and at break times I would hide in a bathroom stall."**

For Bertrand, avoiding people as a child made very good sense. To some extent, it probably reduced harm. However, Bertrand developed an *avoidant/isolating style* of coping, which today gets in the way of making friends, dating, and work. A style of coping which made sense in the past is now preventing him from getting needs for intimacy and self-esteem met.

Molly's mother was a heroin addict, and she had no relationship with her biological father.

> **"Mom was gone a lot and if she was at home she was strung out or shouting at us. I had two little brothers. I cleaned the house and cooked and looked after my brothers. I couldn't afford to have any needs of my own."**

It made sense to Molly to *subjugate* her needs to her mother and brothers in childhood. The family had to survive somehow. But subjugating her needs to others became deeply ingrained into who she was, and today she can feel guilty when she asks for help. A subjugating style of coping in relationships was the result.

A second explanation for why an individual develops a particular relationship coping style can relate to the *biological temperament* they were born with. While the quality of our childhood relationships is important, part of our personality is a product of our biological temperament. Most all parents with two or more children can see that there are aspects of who their children are that came 'pre-packaged'. That's temperament. If a child was born with more of a sensitive or anxious temperament, they might be inclined to develop an avoidant/isolating or subjugating/passive style of relationship coping. If they were born with more of a fiery or assertive temperament, they might be inclined to develop a rigid/controlling style as a response to abuse/neglect. The sort of temperament someone with an unstable style was born with seems less clear. If you think as far back into your past as possible, perhaps you can see that certain aspects of your personality have always just been a part of you.

Exercise 4: What's your view?
Did you learn to cope through a particular relationship style as a way to stay safe in childhood? How did this occur? And, do you think you were born with a particular temperament which inclined you to cope in a certain way?

An unfortunate consequence of relationship coping styles

There is something rather gloomy that often occurs as a result of the way people who experienced childhood harm cope. *A relationship coping style may bring about exactly what they fear the most.* Through no fault of their own, individuals may end up 'shooting themselves in the foot'. The avoidant/isolating individual really wants intimacy, but their avoidant behaviour can leave them feeling alienated and lonely. The controlling/rigid individual wants to feel safe, but their behaviour can create distance within their relationships, which is scary for them. The subjugating/passive individual wants to be treated with respect and care, but their coping style can invite mistreatment or neglect. The unstable individual wants to avoid abandonment, but they may act in ways which eventually drive people away. The sort of feelings or relationship dynamics you had in childhood has a way of showing up in later life. We will explore later how you can get yourself out of this trap, especially during chapters on traumatic core beliefs and healthy relationships.

Coping with trauma: What's worked for you?

We recall working with a man named Barry. When we asked what coping strategies worked well for him, he replied with this: "Hey, if I knew that, I wouldn't be in therapy!" It was quite funny the way Barry said it.

The purpose of this chapter has been to explore coping generally and how it has worked for you, not to recommend specific coping skills. This programme will offer many opportunities later to consider what healthy coping means for you (especially in part three, *A Focus on Recovery*). However, our experience is that many people who encountered childhood harm have discovered healthy ways of coping long before they showed up for therapy. They may still feel troubled by what happened, but they have found some ways of getting relief which can seem helpful and healthy. So, despite the plausibility of Barry's remark, you have an opportunity below to explore what seems to work for you.

In order to consider what may represent healthy coping, it may be helpful to mention again the ideas of adaptive and maladaptive coping. If you respond in a way which offers short-term relief, apparent safety or control, but fails to get more important needs met (e.g. safety, connection to others, self-esteem and meaning), that's maladaptive coping. Adaptive or healthy coping should offer some short-term relief (though not always as powerfully) but should help you get these important needs met as well.

Exercise 5: Adaptive/healthy coping

Are there adaptive (healthy) coping strategies which currently work for you or that you imagine could work for you?

References

1. Kessler, R. C. (2000). Post-traumatic stress Disorder: The burden to the individual and to society. *Journal of Clinical Psychiatry*, 61 (5), 4-14.
2. Bandura, A. (1963). *Social learning and personality development*. New York: Holt, Reinhart, and Winston.
3. Young, Jeffrey E. & Klosko, Janet E. (1993). *Reinventing Your Life*. Plume: NY.
4. Lubin, H. & Johnson, D. R. (2008). *Trauma-centered group psychotherapy for women: A clinician's manual*. The Hayworth Press: London.

PART II

EXPLORING THE PAST

Over three chapters, Part II will ask you to recall and work with childhood memories. This is sometimes referred to as the 'processing' part of therapy or personal development work. It can be really helpful in terms of developing insight and understanding your needs today. But, for many people, this is the hardest part of the programme, and it will likely stir up difficult feelings. Please keep yourself safe and access support if you need to. Also, if you start to lose stability, you may wish to circle back to the section *preparing for a safe and productive experience* before picking up the work again.

Chapter 9

The Child's Point of View

"He always told me and my sister that we were bad. And he would hit us.
I guess I thought we got hit because we were bad."
Laurence

It's worth pointing out that there are two *very different* perspectives from which you can view the abuse or neglect you experienced. As an adult, you can look back on what occurred and have views about your childhood. In other words, from your *current perspective,* you can explore why it happened, who was at fault, what sort of child you were, why you did or did not get protected, and whether it was 'normal' or 'abnormal'. But this is not the same thing as how you viewed all of this from the perspective you held as a child *when it was occurring.*

For much of this chapter, we will ask you to rely on your memory. We will be asking you to get back inside yourself as a child at whatever points in time are most relevant to the abuse/neglect you experienced. There are two thoughts we want to share. First, this can be an emotionally challenging chapter, so please go at a pace you can manage. Remember to keep the right distance from distressing memories. Accessing and working with memories is normally an important part of this work, but if you feel worried you are losing stability or may fall into destructive coping, get some distance for a while or talk with someone

Second, if you're having problems accessing memories or feel unsure that what you are remembering is not factually correct, don't worry. Memories of historical trauma are often incomplete, or different events can blend together in confusing ways. The events may have occurred many years ago, and traumatic memories tend to get encoded in ways which can be difficult to recall in a linear or complete manner. It's not necessary for you to access your past with absolute certainty in order to derive therapeutic benefit from this work.

Some guidelines about choosing memories

During this chapter and the two that follow you will at times be recalling memories from childhood. What you choose to recall does *not* have to be the worst or most terrifying thing that occurred. It should be something you are fairly sure you can cope with. If you think you can cope with remembering some detail of actual abuse, then do that. But if that seems too difficult, you can access a memory of what was happening *after* the abuse occurred. For example, one individual did not want to remember either the sexual or physical abuse perpetrated by her step-father, so she accessed a memory from the point where she was in her bedroom *after* the abuse had happened. Also, some people find that *looking at a photograph* of themselves as a child can help them access memories in a more vivid way or in a way which evokes emotions attached to memories. This is optional.

Occasionally, someone we work with will say something like… *but there were so many incidents of abuse, neglect or abandonment – is it necessary to remember and try to work with all of them? There's a lot I don't remember well and some events blend together.* It is not necessary to recall every memory of harm, which may come as a relief. What you are trying to do is safety access a limited number of memories in in order to develop insight and find a way of thinking and talking about what happened in a way which supports your progress. By accessing a limited number of memories which were typical of the type of difficult experiences you encountered, you can do what is necessary.

The question of blame or responsibility

The issue of responsibility can be more complicated for the child. Something dreadful is happening, but who is at fault? Typically, the issue of fault or blame is not only complicated during childhood, but it's an issue that can hound many people throughout their adult years.

Below we explore 6 reasons why children may accept responsibility for the harm which is happening to them or around them. A feature of recovery is being able to legitimately place responsibility for harm where it belongs to the best of your ability.

Children are developmentally egocentric

This area is a point in itself, but also helps to explain why children are vulnerable to falling into the five further explanations which follow. The words *egocentric* and *self-centred* usually have negative connotations, meaning something like 'selfish'. However, if we understand egocentric to mean having a tendency to see the world and experience from one's own limited perspective and needs, then ALL children are egocentric. And, the younger the child – the more egocentric they tend to be. Because children lack experience and have brains which are neurologically underdeveloped, they naturally see the world in an egocentric fashion. If you convey to a young child that they are wonderful and loved, they are wonderful and loved. Convey to a young child that they are horrible and unwanted, they are horrible and unwanted. If something good or bad happens, a young child will imagine that it's about them. This is developmentally normal.

Less cognitive and emotional development means a child has not yet developed a stable and rational sense of self or ego which can mediate between them and the rest of the world. Without an internal 'self' which can separate responsibility into *mine and yours* or *mine and the world*, everything that occurs is, from the child's perspective, about them. To say children are developmentally egocentric just means they do not have the capacity to understand when other people or events are responsible and they are not, or that something bad which is happening is not about them.

If a child is being abused, neglected or abandoned, developmental egocentricity means they will experience the harm as being *about them*. Likewise, if their family environment is one of chaos, violence and a lack of care, a child tends to see these experiences as being about them. They lack a developed sense of self which can locate responsibility with the individuals or circumstances to which it belongs. Developmental egocentricity is one reason why children absorb responsibility for the chaos or harm they experience or that's around them. As an adult, it's possible that some people still are holding responsibility for past events and having a difficult time locating it where it belongs.

Blame was directly or indirectly conveyed to the child

Emotional abuse often conveys DIRECTLY to the child that they are bad, useless, idiotic, worthless, and so on. Not only is the child's sense of self being attacked by these words, but a child can conclude that they are being emotionally abused *because* they are bad, worthless, etc... . It's a self-fulfilling prophecy. At some level of consciousness, a child decides that if people are telling me I'm bad or useless, then I must be bad or useless. *If I weren't so bad or useless, people wouldn't treat me this way. Therefore, it must be my fault that people hurt me*.

We are not suggesting that children who are harmed make these connections in such a clear fashion, but all of this can *feel true* to them. Physical abuse can convey INDIRECTLY to the child that they are bad. *If I am being physically harmed, then I must be a bad child who deserves to be hurt. If I were good or acceptable, perhaps I wouldn't get hurt. Therefore, I must be bad.* In some cases of sexual abuse, a manipulative abuser will induct the child into believing they are participating in the abuse. The child may know on some level that what is occurring is wrong, and they incorrectly accept or share blame or shame for the acts. Even when sexual abuse is completely coercive and based on threats the perpetrator makes, just being involved in these acts can leave the child feeling shame and a sense of 'badness'. One of the most common reasons children don't talk about sexual abuse is because they are afraid others will blame them or think that they are dirty or shameful. Those who sexually abuse may use this issue to their advantage.

Lacking a basis for comparison

An adult has the advantage of being able to compare their family environments or childhood experiences to other frames of reference. In this way, they can see that what was happening during their childhood was *not* normal or right. But as a child, they usually lacked a basis for comparison. The frame of reference they had was simply the childhood environment they knew. If you ask a person what they thought about childhood events, they often say something like, *that's just how it was,* or *I just thought that was normal.* So, depending on the individual, what might have been 'normal' could have been getting punched, watching your father terrify your mother, being screamed at, having your step-father put you on his knee and molest you, being left alone for three days while your parents go on a bender, and so on. We might call this *the normalisation of the pathological.* In other words, a child believes that what is pathological is normal.

How does all of this relate to the issue of blame or responsibility? Without a basis of comparison, children can become identified with all the chaos, neglect, and violence in the family environment. As a child, they cannot stand outside the family environment and say, *this is wrong, and I should not be a part of this. It's not my fault that I got born into this. I deserve to have very different experiences.* Instead, as a member of this family, they absorbed some or much of the blame for the chaos and pain that was going on.

In some instances, abusive and neglectful adults will prevent children from having experiences which would help them understand how pathological their own family is. Barbara experienced physical and emotional abuse, and she put it like this:

> **"I was never allowed to have friends visit my house. And I was rarely allowed to go to other kids' homes either, and my dad never let me join clubs after school. I thought this was happening because I was being punished for things I had done."**

"But I didn't stop the abuse from happening"

Steve is a 38-year-old man who struggles with depression and bouts of anger, which can land him in trouble at work and with friends. His step-father physically and emotionally abused him, his younger sister and his mother throughout his childhood. Steve is a big man, but he can be reduced to tears when he talks about what happened. He minimises the effect of abuse on himself, but what tears him up is the recurrent thought that he was supposed to have stopped his step-father from hurting his mother and sister. "I should have protected them," he says. He feels responsible, and it's difficult for him to appreciate how little power he had to stop what was happening.

Feeling personally responsible is also common in cases of sexual abuse. We mentioned Marie, a vulnerable girl due to years of emotional neglect. When a group of neighbourhood boys in their early 20s paid attention to her when she was thirteen, she was quickly inducted into a life of heroin use and passed around the gang as a sexual object. She didn't get off drugs and extricate herself from the gang until she was seventeen, by which time she had been badly traumatised by her experiences. What is striking, however, is how insistent Marie is that these experiences were her fault. "I was the one who took the drugs and spent time with the gang," she says. It's hard for her to appreciate how vulnerable she was at the age of thirteen.

It's really difficult for people like Steve and Marie to appreciate how powerless they were to stop the abuse. Children are physically smaller, far less experienced and often dependent on the very people who were hurting or neglecting them. Despite the facts, many can still feel guilty or ashamed that they didn't somehow stop abusers from hurting them or others they cared about.

Managing anticipatory fear

Anticipatory fear is what we feel when we are anticipating something harmful happening to us. Anticipatory fear is common with physical or sexual abuse which occurs on a regular basis. Because there is a pattern of *when* they are going to get abused, a child feels frightened in the lead-up to the abuse.

To get the experience over and done with, some children will initiate the abusive experience by approaching or antagonising the abuser. Juliet was sexually abused by an uncle.

> **"My mother would send me to my uncle's when she went out. I knew he was going to sexually abuse me, and that was really scary. But sometimes he wouldn't abuse me for a while, and that was an awful time. I just wanted to get it over with so he would leave me alone. After a while, I realised I could get him to just do it. Then he would disappear and I could watch TV."**

However, as an adult, Juliet wondered if she was at fault in some way because she had begun to initiate the abusive experiences. An important aspect of her recovery meant understanding that she was just trying to take some control and manage her anticipatory fear – she was in no way responsible for the abuse. While Juliet's experience of sexual abuse has served as an example, managing anticipatory fear can operate in much the same way concerning physical or emotional abuse which occurs on a predictable basis.

The need to protect those who harmed you

Sometimes the issue of blame is confusing for children because they feel a need to protect those who caused harm or to rationalise their behaviour. Children have a strong evolutionary need to bond with an adult, usually a parent. This desire to bond is based on our need for survival. But what if the adult you are meant to bond with is neglecting or hurting you? It's intolerable for many children to accept the reality of what is happening, so they will find ways to protect those harming them or rationalise their behaviour. Tim experienced physical and emotional neglect, and he described things as follows:

> **"When I was a kid, I didn't have a father and my mom was drunk every day. I'd get home from school and she'd be passed out or just gone somewhere and you didn't know when she'd be back. When the social workers would talk to me at school or at home I always tried to tell them what a good mom I had. I actually believed it when I told them and I was mad at them for saying bad things about my mom. I guess I just didn't want to believe I had a rubbish mom."**

For some children, locating responsibility with those who are abusing or neglecting them is too scary a proposition. You only get one biological set of parents and one family of origin. For some children, it's just intolerable to accept that these people are hurtful or neglectful and that they are responsible for it. That would mean accepting that you are not loved or cared for properly. It's too awful to imagine, so some children find ways of believing it's not true. They might rationalise the abuser's behaviour, or they might accept the blame for the abuser's behaviour. For some children, seeing themselves as bad or inadequate is a better solution than believing they have parents or family that can't care for or protect them properly. Even as adults, people we work with will often tell us they feel guilty for saying anything 'negative' about those who were hurting or neglecting them. It feels like a betrayal.

Exercise 1: Exploring the child's view of responsibility/blame

Above, we explored five ways children can accept blame or feel guilty about the historical abuse. Some of the explanations may be relevant to you. Some may not. They are:

1. *Children are developmentally egocentric*
2. *Blame was directly conveyed to you through emotional or physical abuse*
3. *You thought that what was happening was 'normal', and so the issue of blame seemed irrelevant*
4. *You accepted blame because you didn't stop the abuse or neglect*
5. *You accepted blame because of the way you managed anticipatory fear*
6. *You accepted blame because you felt a need to protect those who were causing harm*

As you think over these issues, try and access some related memories from childhood. Remember to recall how you saw the issue of blame *from your perspective as a child.* Take your time. When ready, describe below how you may have accepted blame or responsibility *as a child.*

Responsibility and vulnerability: Robert's moment of insight

At age 58, Robert struggles with significant psychological difficulties, including social anxiety, somatising (expressing trauma through the body) and very poor self-esteem. The extent of his problems are understandable given his experience of serious physical and sexual abuse, emotional neglect and abandonment. His parents paid little attention to him, he was in and out of foster care and he was sexually abused by three different perpetrators. What really stands out is his need for self-denigration. Robert frequently says:

> **"It must have been my fault because I was hurt by so many different people. I must have *given off* some sort of signal. I was so needy. I craved attention and I wanted someone to love me. I put myself in positions where people could abuse me. I invited the abuse."**

When you try and talk with Robert about how power must have worked between him as a little boy and those who abused him, it just doesn't go in. He doesn't see it and keeps insisting it was his fault.

And then there came a moment when Robert was able to make an important distinction between *being vulnerable* and *being responsible*. He *was* needy, and he did crave recognition and affection. But this was understandable because he'd never got this from his parents or anyone else. This very likely did make him more vulnerable to being abused. But it doesn't make him responsible for the fact that adults (with more power) abused him. For a child, *being vulnerable is not the same as being responsible*. When Robert was able to see this distinction, he got it: It wasn't his fault.

Keeping secrets

Some children were able to talk about abuse or neglect which was occurring with people who did not know – people who might have been in a position to help. This may have been a family member, a friend, a teacher, social services or others. However, it's *very common* for a child to keep what is happening a secret.[1] Or, they may have only hinted at what was happening in limited ways. As therapists, we frequently find ourselves speaking with people who are talking about what happened in some detail for the first time. For those who kept childhood abuse or neglect a secret, it's often helpful for them to learn how common this is. As adults, some seemed confused about why they didn't speak out as a child, or they can even blame themselves for not talking about what was happening. It's important for these individuals to appreciate that there will have been very real reasons why, as a child, they found it difficult or impossible to talk about what was happening.

Exercise 2:
During childhood, who knew the abuse or neglect was happening? Who, either in or outside the family, did not know?

Exercise 3: Why did you believe you had to keep abuse or neglect secret?
From your perspective *as a child*, did you believe you had to keep what was happening a secret from people *in* or *outside* your family? If you told someone (e.g. a friend or family member) you may still not have been able to tell others. Allow a manageable memory or two of abuse or neglect to come back to you. The memory may help you access why you had to keep the secret. Tick the relevant reasons below.

___ I was scared of telling others. Something bad would have happened.
___ If I had told others, that would have been disloyal.
___ I didn't think others would believe me.
___ I didn't know that what was happening to me was wrong.
___ I thought it was my fault, so there was no reason to tell.
___ I was ashamed of what was happening, so I didn't want others to know.
___ I did tell once and it made it worse, so I didn't want to tell again.
___ I was scared the authorities might take me away or take the abuser away.
___ Another reason? ____

Sexual abuse and secret-keeping

In certain respects, the experience of sexual abuse overlaps with physical and emotional abuse. All of these forms of abuse tend to involve distress and confusion, have a damaging effect on the child's self-concept and lead to psychological problems in later life. However, while secret-keeping can coincide with physical and emotional abuse, this issue can be especially relevant concerning sexual abuse.

In many instances of sexual abuse, there were only two people who knew that abuse was occurring: the child and the abuser. This often occurs because a perpetrator manages to groom, isolate and sexually abuse a child. Sometimes those who experience child sexual abuse can tell someone what is happening, but it is *very* common for children to keep sexual abuse secret. There are many reasons why this can occur, including:

- The abuser has threatened the child
- The child is frightened that others won't believe them
- The child is neglected and imagines that no one will care or help
- The child feels inappropriately ashamed of what is happening
- A child is taught or acquires the idea that they are participating and are frightened that others will blame them
- The child accepts gifts or other incentives and so imagines they are culpable

The unique stigma attached to childhood sexual abuse has often meant that the secret is kept well into adulthood. This can make getting help for sexual abuse especially difficult. However, the profile of historic sexual abuse has been raised substantially in the media more recently, which hopefully will reduce stigma and allow more people to seek help. The exercise below is for anyone who experienced sexual abuse.

Exercise 4: Sexual abuse and secret-keeping
If you experienced sexual abuse and felt you had to keep it secret, please describe why you believed (from the child's perspective) that you had to do this.

Indirect ways of 'telling' about abuse or neglect

You may have felt you had to keep what was happening a secret from many people, but the trauma you experienced will have expressed itself in ways other than words. We mentioned temperament earlier, the biological bit you were born with. Depending on temperament, maybe you had a tendency to express the effects of the trauma *outwardly* through your behaviour. Or, maybe you had a tendency to experience the effects of the trauma *inwardly*, i.e. through your body, emotions or thoughts. Indirect ways of telling about the abuse tend to relate to age.

Exercise 5: Indirect ways of telling

Highlight, underline or circle any *indirect ways of telling* which seem relevant to you.

As a young child (birth to 10 or 12 years), did you express the trauma as follows:

Phobias or fears, e.g. irrational fears of the dark, strangers, animals, etc…
Chronic worry or anxiety
Sleeping problems, including insomnia, nightmares, bed wetting
Going to school unkempt, smelly, or with inappropriate/shabby clothing
Social withdrawal, standing on the edge of groups
OCD or ritualistic behaviours
Trying to be perfect
Tantrums, anger, smashing things
Hiding or trying not to be noticed
Frequent illnesses
Somatising, e.g. headaches, digestive problems like constipation or stomach aches
Behaviour problems in school or the neighbourhood
Underachieving at school due to emotional or concentration issues
Problems with eating
Picking at skin, chewing fingernails, pulling hair, etc…
Other ways?____

____

As children make the transition from early childhood to their *teen years*, the above issues may continue, but indirect ways of telling can take on different forms. Circle, underline or highlight any indirect ways of telling which were relevant for you during your teenage years.

Destructive use of drugs/alcohol
Sexually promiscuous behaviour
Eating disorders such as bulimia, overeating, food restriction
Self-harming behaviours
Poor school performance, e.g. truancy, exam failure, school dropout
Unplanned pregnancy or getting a girl pregnant
Dangerous behaviour or criminality
Fighting or bullying
Getting bullied

Being abused by partners or friends
Other ways? ____

There is often a sad 'vicious cycle' which abused/neglected children find themselves in. Because it seemed impossible to talk about it, the abuse got expressed in indirect ways. But many of these indirect ways of 'telling' lead other children or adults to perceive the child as either naughty, difficult or odd. And so the child may find that adults or children are rejecting or harsh with them. This is really unfair.

Communicating with yourself as a child

This chapter may have helped you access what it was like for you as a child. You have been encouraged to see the world through the eyes of yourself as a child, to make contact with the thoughts and feelings you experienced as a child.

You may have discovered that you blamed yourself.
You may have discovered that you felt you had to keep painful secrets.
You explored the indirect and painful ways the trauma got expressed.

Along the way, you may have discovered some feelings of compassion for this kid who had such a rough time. We close this chapter with an exercise which may allow you to heal some of the hurt that you experienced as a child.

Exercise 6: Talking to yourself as a child

If you have a photo of yourself as a child, it may help you do this exercise by having a look at it. Give yourself at least 15 minutes of interrupted time to do this exercise. You may feel resistant to doing this exercise. It's not easy or natural for many. But, it can be powerful for some. If you find it is impossible, you may need support from someone you trust or a therapist.

We'd like you to sit opposite an empty chair. Please imagine that sitting in that chair opposite you is yourself as a child. You can choose how old you are, the clothes you are wearing, and the expression on your face. Imagine that this child has just had a bad experience with someone who hurt or scared them. You will need to choose a memory in which you, as a child, got hurt. Choose a memory you think you can handle – it doesn't have to be the worst memory. This bad experience has just occurred to this child you imagine sitting in the chair in front of you. What do you want to say to yourself as a child? What does this child *need* to hear? Speak to the child. You can also express care or compassion by imagining physical affection if you need to. Take your time and use your imagination as vividly as possible. When you have expressed all you need to, reflect below on your experience and what you needed to communicate to yourself as a child.

References

1. Summit, R. (1983). The child sexual abuse accommodation syndrome. *Child Abuse & Neglect*, 7, 177-193.

Chapter 10

The People Who Harmed You

"I tell myself, *they're not even worth thinking about*. But it's confusing at times because they still feel like this big presence in my life."
Kelly

"My dad abandoned me when I was two and then re-entered my life when I was 40 because he'd been thrown out of his supported accommodation. I let him stay in the guest room and he was moody, messy, and would drink all my beer. He was like the teenage son I never wanted."
Jen

This is usually an important and yet challenging chapter for many people. The extent of relationship people have today with those who harmed them can vary greatly. Some people have cut this person or people out of their lives completely. Others have no current relationship because the abusive or neglectful person is deceased, or they have no idea where they are or how to contact them. However, many people continue to have some relationship with those who harmed them. There can be many reasons for this. Some feel obligated, perhaps due to family pressure or other reasons. For others, despite everything that occurred, the person is still important, and the relationship has had a chance to heal to some extent.

Whether you have contact with the people who harmed you or not, you still have a 'relationship' with these people. If it's not an actual relationship, it's a psychological relationship, i.e. they still exist in your mind, feelings or memories. Whether you have an actual or psychological relationship, exploring this relationship in ways that supports your recovery is what this chapter is about.

Is forgiveness necessary?

This is a common question. Sometimes we are told or read that to overcome the effects of historical trauma, you have to be able to forgive those who hurt you. We do not see it as our place to say whether you should forgive these people. We have worked with people who have felt able to forgive those who hurt them and have found this to be an important part of their therapy. We have also worked with others who believe it is impossible to forgive those who hurt them. Or, they simply don't want to forgive them, or they don't see the point. Many of these individuals have also made good progress.

Our view is this: for some people forgiveness is important, but we do not think it is essential that an individual forgives in order to overcome the effects of their past. If forgiving seems possible and useful, that's fine. But if you can't or don't want to forgive, this is not something to get hung up on. The extent of the abuse can make forgiveness more difficult for some people. Also, forgiveness is much harder when the perpetrator will not acknowledge any wrongdoing, express any remorse or offer some explanation for their actions. Forgiveness is also harder if it feels very difficult to understand why they acted as they did.

Whether you forgive or not isn't the essential issue. What is vital is that those who caused harm have as little negative impact on you, your thoughts and feelings as possible. If forgiveness helps to support this, that's fine. If not, don't worry about it.

Is it important to know why someone harmed you as a child?

People who experienced childhood harm seem to largely respond to the above question in one of three ways. These responses are captured in the statements below. For the exercise below, we want you to consider *one* person who abused, neglected or abandoned you during childhood. Place a tick next to the response that *seems closest* to how you think about the question. There is no 'correct' answer – only your answer.

Exercise 1: Is it important to know why they harmed you?

___ "Yes, I do want to know why they did it. If I knew why they did it, I'd feel like it may help in some way."

___ "No, I don't want to think about why they did it."

___ "It's never really occurred to me to think about why they did it."

Some people will have chosen the first answer, **"Yes, I do want to know why they did it..."** These individuals often imagine that if they can make at least some sense of why those who harmed them acted as they did, it may help them recover.

Tom is a good example. His mother was sixteen when he was born, and the only 'father figures' he knew were the string of boyfriends his mother had throughout his childhood.

"My mom partied a lot, and there was often this collection of strange people around the house. It wasn't until I was twelve that social services finally put me and my brother and sister into foster care with this nice family. I really want to know why she had kids and why she didn't seem to care about us."

People like Tom imagine that making sense of why his mother acted as she did might help him overcome the effects of that harm. Put another way, there might be a connection between *meaning* and *healing*.

Other individuals identify more with the second statement: **"No, I don't want to think about why they did it."** Psychologists call this *suppression*, which means consciously blocking thinking about something. This was true for Martin, who was physically and sexually abused by an alcoholic father.

"What's the point of thinking about why he did it? It won't change what happened, so it's just a waste of time."

There are a few reasons we come across why people (like Martin) will want to consciously block out thinking about why they were harmed. First, some individuals find it painful or distressing to even think about the person who harmed them. And, of course, to make sense of why they may have harmed you, means thinking about them.

Second, certain people imagine that if they begin to understand why someone harmed them, they may start to feel some empathy for that person. Or, they imagine that understanding a person's harmful actions may lead to the possibility of forgiving them. Some are so angry with the person who harmed them that the idea of empathising with them or forgiving them seems unthinkable. We have a particular view on this dilemma. *Sometimes* understanding someone's action can lead to feelings of empathy or a willingness to forgive. But, in other instances, understanding *does not* lead to empathy or any wish to forgive that person's actions. For some individuals, even with understanding, the actions of those who harmed them are beyond empathy or forgiveness.

Third, for some people it seems impossible to imagine why someone would act like the person who harmed them. Figuring out why they did it feels like doing a puzzle with a million pieces, some of which are missing or torn. So, some individuals resist thinking about why they did it because it seems like an impossible quest.

If you're invested in not knowing why they did it, why might that be? Is it painful to think about? Are you worried it may in some way be connected to empathy or forgiveness? Does finding answers seem impossible? Or, is there another reason we haven't thought of?

Lastly, some people can identify with the statement, **"It's never really occurred to me to think about why they did it."** Psychologists call this *repression*, which just means unconsciously blocking thinking, i.e. blocking thinking about something without even knowing we are blocking thinking about it! For those who respond this way, it's rarely because they *don't care* or the abuse/neglect they experienced was unimportant. In fact, the opposite is often true. There is something about the harm which occurred which is **so** significant that the individual has needed to unconsciously block thinking about why it occurred. This can happen for a number of reasons, including the three reasons given in the previous paragraph.

Two final thoughts on this section: first, the purpose of this chapter is not to tell you how you should think about those who caused harm, but to allow you to explore this area to whatever extent possible. Second, what sense you have made of why people harmed you can relate to whether or not there has been a confrontation, and what happened if this occurred. We discuss confrontation later in the chapter.

Why did they do it?

If a part of you doesn't want to think about this question, here's something to consider which may make it easier: the fundamental purpose of exploring why someone harmed you is not to *excuse* their behaviour, *forgive* their behaviour or *empathise* with them.

So, what might be the point of trying to understand why people harmed you? There are a few reasons why this can be helpful. First, something awful and incomprehensible may be worse than something awful but which has become, at least to some extent, comprehensible. For some, there can be a connection between meaning and healing.

Second, energy can get tied down in suppressing or repressing what happened and the reasons behind it. When you stop pushing it away, that energy may be available to you again. If you can turn and face what you have been avoiding, what may have been worrying or disturbing can sometimes lose the sense of threat.

Third, while not true for everyone, some can feel *a lot* of anger at the people who hurt them. While anger is likely an understandable reaction, there can be a problem. The anger may churn inside, causing pain and distracting a person from life and their relationships. You could call this *stuck anger*. For some, there is a possibility that understanding why those who harmed you acted as they did can help release some of the anger.

There are at least four explanations for why someone caused harm to you during childhood. These explanations can overlap but also have unique characteristics. *Before reading the explanations below, we suggest you choose a person from childhood who caused you harm. As you read, consider to what extent each explanation sheds light on the person's behaviour*. You will have an opportunity following for further reflection through writing.

1. A person learns to be an abuser through experiences of abuse

Some people grew up in circumstances where they experienced and/or witnessed abuse. This may have been the case for the person who harmed you. As a child, this abusive environment seemed 'normal' – just the way things are. This child may *not* have experienced or witnessed mutual respect, protection and care. A child in this environment will feel fear, powerlessness and humiliation. They watch what is happening and see in-control abusers and out-of-control victims. As a child, they are one of the victims. **Most of these children will NOT grow up to be abusers themselves.**[1] However, some of these children will decide that if the world consists of abusers and victims, it's better to be an abuser. They may identify with the person doing the abusing and not identify with other victims. As they grow older and develop relationships, they may experience a sense of control and power through abusing, and it can feel better to finally have power and control rather than just being powerless and humiliated.

2. *Abuse or neglect is related to significant mental health or medical issues*

Some adults can be psychologically or medically unwell. They may have a significant problem such as psychosis, bipolar disorder or severe depression. They may have serious issues with alcohol or drug addiction. They may have issues related to a diagnosed (or undiagnosed) brain injury resulting in cognitive problems or poor impulse control.[2] They may be involved with mental health services, and some spend time in psychiatric wards. When a person struggling with significant mental health problems reaches a certain point of exhaustion or frustration, they may lash out with abuse, though they often feel distressed or regretful concerning their behaviour. If very unwell, these individuals may simply be incapable of caring for their children, and neglect or abandonment can result.

3. Abuse is a consequence of an 'empathy deficit'

The vast majority of people are sensitive to others' pain or suffering. However, there are a small number of people who have little or no capacity for empathy. Some of these people not only lack empathy, but take pleasure in seeing others in pain, i.e. they are sadistic. A lack of empathy or sadism is associated with serious characterological problems such as narcissistic, anti-social or sociopathic personality disorders. Unlike individuals from explanation number two, these people may feel little distress or regret when they harm others.

Is an empathy deficit the result of an individual's genetic makeup, or is it the result of their experiences? Research in this area is sparse, but there is at least one well-conducted study which followed twin and non-twin siblings over time.[3] The results suggest that an individual's capacity to *feel* empathy is about 52-57% due to genetics, and a person's capacity to *think* in empathetic ways is about 27% related to genetics. It's a complex area, and even these figures are based on averages. In truth, we don't have an adequate understanding of why someone is significantly empathy deficient.

In some instances, empathy deficit may result from serious and persistent historical abuse or empathy never having been shown or taught to someone. Alternatively, some people may be genetically predisposed toward extreme insensitivity. There are historical examples for both explanations. Hitler, Stalin, Mao Tse-Tung and Kim Jong-il all displayed serious empathy deficit and sadistic behaviour. Hitler and Stalin were both physically abused by alcoholic fathers whereas Mao Tse-Tung and Kim Jong-il, as far as we know, did not experience significant childhood trauma.

4. The person is not developmentally ready to be a parent or lacks support

Reason number four may overlap with any of the first three explanations. Some parents (mothers or fathers) may have had children at a time when their developmental needs were not sufficiently met.[4] In other words, they were not emotionally or socially ready to be parents. When they had children, they were a long way off in getting their basic needs met for safety, self-esteem, intimacy or belonging. As any parent knows who has had to wake up several times in the night, put their social lives on hold, or remain calm while a baby is crying for hours, it's an exasperating and selfless task. It requires a great deal of emotional maturity. Having a baby when a person is young, in circumstances where there is little support from family or a partner, or where the parent's developmental needs are unmet, can all make it difficult to provide adequate care for a baby or child.

Exercise 2: Reflection on why you were harmed

The above section suggests four possible reasons why you experienced abuse, neglect or abandonment as a child. These explanations are:

1. A person learns to be an abuser through experiences of being abused
2. Abuse or neglect is related to significant mental health or medical issues
3. Abuse is a consequence of an 'empathy deficit'
4. The person is not developmentally ready to be a parent or lacks support

Consider one person who harmed you as a child. Does one or more of the explanations above help explain why they harmed you? You can do this exercise for additional persons who harmed you if you wish, but you may need more paper.

Did you ever confront someone who harmed you?

Confrontation can happen in many ways, but it means asking someone who harmed you to explain why they acted as they did in the past. It usually means challenging this behaviour, and it often includes explaining what you thought of it or how you experienced it. In whatever form, confrontation offers the person who harmed you an opportunity to explain themselves. It is not our role to suggest that you should or should not confront. This is a very personal and sometimes complex decision.

Some individuals will have confronted those who abused or neglected them at a certain point. Others never have. We have known of cases of confrontation which were calm and helpful, cases which were downright violent, and most cases falling somewhere between.

Cynthia was emotionally neglected and abandoned by her mother. At the age of 45, Cynthia hadn't had contact with her mother for over twenty years. One day she sent her mother an email, asking to meet up. They had dinner at a restaurant, and Cynthia asked her mother why she had put her into foster care when she was nine years old. It was a difficult and emotional conversation, but it led to understanding and a restart of their relationship.

John's father was a violent alcoholic who physically abused him and other family members. We are certainly not suggesting you approach confrontation as John did, but it makes for an interesting example.

"When I was fourteen my dad was really drunk and he was ranting and throwing things around and scaring my mom and sisters. I pushed him down on the couch and I screamed at him and told him just what I thought of him. Every time he tried to get up I just pushed him down again."

Some individuals may express their anger about what they experienced *indirectly*. Rather than confronting directly and with words, the individual will 'act out' the confrontation. Michelle had little contact with her biological mother and was emotionally abused and neglected by her step-mother. And, her father never stepped in to protect her.

"I left home as soon as I could. I was 17 and I got a job and I paid for my own flat. I never told them where I was and I didn't contact them for eight years. I guess it was my way of telling them what I thought of them."

Perhaps you confronted the people who abused or neglected you. However, it's not unusual for a confrontation not to have taken place. Many felt so threatened by those who abused them that confrontation, in childhood or adulthood, evokes a lot of anxiety. In other cases, the abuser is deceased, or the person who was harmed has lost contact with them, making confrontation impossible. It's also common for people to avoid confrontation because they worry that it will divide family members, or even tear a family apart.

In some cases, people can have experiences of confrontation that are therapeutic. Those who abused or neglected may express remorse or offer an explanation which seems helpful. Maybe you have experienced this in the past. Or, if you confront someone in the future, perhaps you will have a good experience. However, it's common for confrontation to be a disappointing or frustrating experience. Many abusers feel a need to rationalise or explain away their behaviour in ways which can be confusing or infuriating. The responses below capture themes related to unhelpful confrontations. If you had a negative experience of confrontation, you can highlight or circle any themes related to that encounter.

- Denial: "That didn't happen."
- Minimisation: "Oh come on – it wasn't that bad."
- Blaming the victim: "You deserved it."
- Rationalisation: "I was trying to teach you about life."

- Excuses: "It was the alcohol, I was a single parent, we had no money, etc…."
- Red herrings: Refocusing the conversation on something irrelevant.
- Poor me: "But I was going through a bad time myself, etc…"

The responses above are different in certain ways, but they all have two things in common: the person you are confronting is not acknowledging what it was like for you, and they are not taking responsibility for their role. Some abusers find it impossible to acknowledge the impact of their behaviour on those they harmed. Some abusers actually believe that they were justified in acting the way they did – this can be a personality trait that is quite rigid.

If you never confronted the abuser, we do not have fixed ideas about whether you should. It may be important for your personal development to confront the abuser, or this may not be helpful, necessary or even possible. It's a very personal decision. Whether or not you *actually* confront the abuser, what matters is that the abuser holds as little power as possible over you, your thoughts and feelings.

Exercise 3: History of confrontation

Did you ever confront those who abused or neglected you? What happened, and was this helpful or not?

"I'm not like them"

The feelings adults have towards those who harmed them are often very negative. Anger, revulsion, fear and other painful feelings are common. Something else we find is that people can often feel a strong need *not* to be like those who harmed them. Kerry experienced emotional abuse, and she put it like this:

"My mom was insane. She would blow up with anger over nothing. A total drama queen. Me and my brothers and sisters were scared of her all the time. You never knew when she was gonna blow. I never want to be like her."

However, the person who did the harming can still seem like a big presence in one's life. As a result, some individuals feel a need to define themselves as someone who is *not like* the person who harmed them. This was true of Kerry (quoted above), who wanted to be the sort of mother for her kids she never had. She was a great mom – very caring and affectionate, and she always put her kids first. There was a problem, though. In her attempt to be completely *not like her mother* (who had been aggressive), she found it difficult to use appropriate boundaries and discipline with her children. "My kids walk all over me," she says.

Other people can find moments when they feel upset because they might see some trait in themselves which reminds them of the person who hurt them. Ralph was both physically and sexually abused by his father throughout his childhood.

"I hated him so much. He was such an angry man, and he terrified me when I was a kid. He would scream at me and punch me. He was out of control. That's why... I hate it when I get angry at my wife or friends. It makes me think I'm like him, and I hate that."

We know that most people *don't* turn out like the adults who abused or neglected them. We have research into *intergenerational patterns of child maltreatment*. This is research which explores whether people who are abused or neglected as children become parents who abuse and neglect their children. We can summarise what we seem to know, but we need to point out that research findings point to what is true 'on average', not what is true for any one individual. There is evidence suggesting that parents who experienced trauma historically are more likely, on average, to struggle with their role as parent. This is seen in the finding that parents who experience PTSD are at higher risk of raising children who also struggle with PTSD.[5] Again, this points to a higher risk on average, not what is necessarily true for any individual. And, it's important to keep in mind that the *majority* of people who were abused or neglected as children *do not* go on to abuse or neglect their children.[6]

The point being made here is that those who harmed you often cast a long shadow over your life today. This may mean you try very hard *not* to be like them. Like Kerry, this is a good idea, but it can also constrict you in some ways. Or, some individuals get upset or even scared when they see traits in themselves which remind them of the people who hurt them (like Ralph). A part of overcoming the effects of historical trauma is learning to be *yourself.* This means reducing the presence of the abuser in your head and feelings.

Exercise 4: Your letter to someone who harmed you

This exercise will help you clarify your thoughts and feelings towards someone who abused, neglected or abandoned you. If there were several people who caused harm, it will be necessary to choose one of them. If you wish, you can write additional letters, though this is optional and you may need more paper.

The purpose of writing this letter is simply to help you organise your thoughts and feelings towards a person who harmed you – to help bring these thoughts and feelings into conscious awareness. There is *no* expectation that you send the letter to this person. When a person confronts, how a person confronts, and whether a person confronts is a very personal matter.

This exercise may trigger some strong feelings, such as anger or fear. If these feelings (or impulses) start to get overwhelming, you can take a break and look after yourself, e.g. distract yourself, talk to someone, or use the strategies you acquired in the section *preparing for a safe and productive experience*. You can write your letter on your own, or you can do it with someone you trust if that helps.

Only you can write this letter to the person who hurt you, and you should do it on your terms. However, for many people it can be important to consider three areas.

1. You may want to tell them how their behaviour affected you when you were younger.
2. You may want to tell them how their behaviour has affected your life.
3. You may not need or want anything from them, but if you do, you could indicate this as well.

References

1. Child Welfare Information Gateway (2016). *Intergenerational patterns of child maltreatment: What the evidence shows*. US Department of Health and Human Services, Children's Bureau. Washington, DC.
2. Darby, R. R., Kushman, F. & Fox, M. D. Lesion network localisation of criminal behaviour (2018). *Proceedings of the National Academy of Sciences of the United States of America (PNAS),* 115 (3), 601-606.
3. Melchers, M., Montag, C., Reuter, M., Spinath, F. M. & Hahn, E. (2016). How heritable is empathy? Differential effects of measurement and subcomponents. *Motivation and Emotion*, 40, 720–730.
4. Westman, J.C. (1994). *Licensing parents: Can we prevent child abuse and neglect?* Cambridge: Perseus Publishing.
5. Lambert, J. E., Holzer, J. & Hasbun, A. (2014). *Association Between Parents' PTSD Severity and Children's Psychological Distress: A Meta-Analysis.* Journal of Traumatic Stress, 27:1, 9–17
6. Child Welfare Information Gateway (2016). *Intergenerational patterns of child maltreatment: What the evidence shows*. US Department of Health and Human Services, Children's Bureau. Washington, DC.

Chapter 11

Family

"My family? You want me to talk about my family? How much time have you got?"
Harry

Childhood abuse and neglect happen in a social context. There were people around while you were scared, hurt or lonely. These people may have known a lot about what was happening to you, had only a partial picture or knew very little. Whatever the case, these people normally *matter*. In the previous chapter, you explored your relationship with people who harmed you. In this chapter, we explore the family as a whole. Even if the primary person who harmed you was someone outside the family, your family relationships normally matter concerning what happened.

As you read and work on this chapter, you may need to define 'family' in whatever way works. For some, family will be quite conventional – a mother, a father, some siblings and certain extended family members. For others, 'family' may have been a shifting kaleidoscope of people – biological parents, step-parents, partners of parents, step-siblings, foster parents, or even people you identified as carers in a residential setting or elsewhere. You should consider 'family' as the significant people who were around you as you were growing up. This chapter represents an opportunity to explore your relationships with these people. This exploration mainly looks back into your past, but also looks at the future.

Clarifying roles

The roles that people played in your family are not always straight forward. However, it's possible to consider family roles in terms of perpetrators, victims, protectors, bystanders and collaborators.

- *Perpetrators* have power and are the ones causing emotional and physical suffering, or neglect.
- *Victims* have less power and are the ones on the receiving end of abuse or neglect.
- *Protectors* will try to shield or defend victims. Sometimes protectors are successful, but sometimes the protector is not strong enough.

- *Bystanders* have some power and might be able to intervene and help victims, but they mainly don't. To be a bystander, you have enough power to help, but don't.
- *Collaborators* have some power. They don't directly cause the harm, but in some way assist the perpetrator.

Now for the complicated part. Family members, including yourself, don't always fit neatly into one role. Sometimes a parent can be both a victim and a perpetrator. Sometimes a sibling can be both a victim and a collaborator. A protector can also be a victim. There are many permutations. Maureen was physically and sexually abused by her mother's partner. But so was her older sister Janet.

> **"If anything, I think he hurt my sister Janet even worse than me. She would fight back, so it was worse for her. What I can't understand is why Janet would *hurt me*. She broke my things and punched me when she had the chance. She was horrible to me. He beat my mother too, and most of the time she was too drunk to care about what was happening to us."**

Step-father was a perpetrator. Maureen was a victim. Janet was both a victim and a perpetrator. Maureen's mother was both a victim and a bystander. Family roles are often complicated like this.

Exercise 1: Clarifying your family roles

Write the names below of *all* important family members, as you construe your 'family'. Near each name, indicate the role or roles each person played. You can refer to the five roles and descriptions above for help. Don't forget to include yourself (oddly, people we work with sometimes do this). If a significant person (such as an abuser or protector) was not technically a family member, add them too. When you finish your diagram, answer these questions: What did it feel like to do this? Was anything interesting about this exercise?

Who might have protected you?

By definition, people who experienced childhood trauma did not receive the protection they needed. The intensity of anger or disappointment some people feel towards those who might have protected them can rival feelings directed at the people who directly hurt them. Gavin was emotionally and physically abused by his step-mother.

> **"I hated what she did to me, but she was a lunatic and an alcoholic. My dad knew what was happening. He didn't stop her. In a way, I blame him even more."**

If the main abuser was a parent or partner of a parent, most often the child will have looked to the other adult for protection. But a child who is vulnerable and frightened will look to anyone they imagine can protect them. It might be another family member, like an older sibling, an aunt, an uncle or a grandparent. Depending on the circumstances, it might even have been someone who was not a family member.

We usually find that there were people who might have protected you. Maybe this person tried to protect you and failed. Maybe they didn't try. Juliet was emotionally neglected by her mother and sexually abused by an uncle.

> **"My father left the family when I was a baby. He lived overseas, and I only spoke with him infrequently. I didn't know my mom was on drugs until I was about 9, but I knew she was never well. My uncle babysat for me, and I was sent to his house a few times a month, and he would sexually abuse me. I hoped my mom could see what was happening from just looking at me, but she didn't seem to. I tried to tell her a couple of times when I was a bit older, but she seemed not to understand. I could never tell my dad, because I just didn't know him. It's strange, but I was 18 before it occurred to me that my uncle had been supplying my mom with drugs."**

Juliet's mother was responsible for protecting her but failed to do so. She also appears to have collaborated in the abuse perpetrated by the uncle. Juliet's father also failed to protect her. He had no idea of what was going on, but he had failed to develop a relationship with Juliet in which she might have been able to confide in him.

Exercise 2: A lack of protection:

Who might have protected you but didn't? ________________________________

There are many possible reasons a child may not have got protected. Tick any that apply to you. After ticking those that apply there is space for you to journal any additional thoughts of feelings you see as important.

___ The abuser isolated me and the abuse happened in private.
___ I told them what was happening, but they didn't believe me.
___ They took the abuser's side.
___ They were too ill psychologically or physically to protect me.
___ They moved away. They were too far away to help.
___ They loved the abuser and so they just closed their eyes to it.
___ They ignored the signs of abuse.
___ They were getting something out of it, like drugs or money.
___ They couldn't bear to leave the abuser.
___ If I was getting abused, they weren't.
___ They blamed me for the abuse.
___ They were just a weak person. They couldn't stand up to them.
___ They just couldn't bear to acknowledge it was happening. They were in denial.
___ They were too afraid of the abuser to try and help.
___ They were too wrapped up in themselves to care.
___ They were scared the abuser would get into trouble.
___ They were worried about their reputation and didn't want it getting out.
___ They were financially dependent on the abuser and didn't want to risk that.
___ The abuser convinced them that I deserved it.
___ Other reason ____

Exercise 3: A letter to those who didn't provide adequate protection

Below we would like you to write a letter to a person who didn't protect you as they should have. This person may have known what was happening or perhaps didn't. It may help to tell them what happened, how it affected you, and what you needed from them. Tell them your thoughts and feelings about not getting protected. If it helps to imagine them in an empty chair and speak to them first, you can do this to help you know what to say in your letter. As in the previous chapter, the purpose of writing this letter is to help you organise your thoughts and feelings towards someone who did not protect you. There is *no* expectation that you actually send this letter.

Your relationship with a person who might have protected you

We find that some people have been able to repair a relationship with the person who failed to protect them. Others have not, but are open to the idea of repair. Some have no interest in ever speaking with or seeing this person again. A lot depends on the circumstances of the abuse and how much this person knew about what was happening. A lot also depends on the sense the person who was harmed makes out of *why* this person did not protect them. Perhaps most important is whether the person who was harmed and the person who might have protected them ever really talked about what happened. What can make things easier is if the person who did not protect can offer an honest explanation and express remorse or regret. Repair is much more difficult if this conversation never occurs or if the person denies or minimises their role in bystanding, or even colluding.

What are your thoughts about your relationship now with someone who did not protect you? Is there something you want to discuss with them to attempt a repair, or do you think this is impossible or simply not necessary at this point? An exercise at the end of this chapter allows you to explore if you want to repair any family relationships, so you can come back to these questions.

The other children

Some individuals may have lived isolated childhoods with no siblings. For most, there were other children around as the abuse or neglect was occurring. Many don't come from a conventional family situation. Those experiencing childhood harm may have come from unstable and messy family circumstances, and the children they are in contact with can reflect this. The other children you formed relationships with may have been biological brothers and sisters, cousins, step-brothers or step-sisters, foster brothers or sisters or children you knew in a residential setting.

The relationships with these other children can vary greatly, but are normally significant in one manner or another. The age difference between you and these other children is often a significant factor in the roles you played. Making sense of the abuse or neglect you experienced happens by comparing your experience to the children around you and the way you and they coped.

Like Marie, some were 'the black sheep' of the family.

> **"I don't know why they hated me so much. My parents ignored me or shouted at me, especially my mom. My brother was the golden child. If something went wrong, I was always the one who got punished. I haven't spoken to my brother in three years."**

There can be several variations on who gets hurt, who doesn't, and how other children respond. Tick what applies below. If there isn't a scenario which applies, write your own at the bottom.

Exercise 4: Variations on children's roles

___ I was the black sheep of the family. The other child/children got love and safety, but I was singled out and hurt.

___ We all got abused and neglected. They didn't care who got hurt.

___ We all got hurt, but I was the oldest (or most capable), so I was responsible for protecting the others.

___ We all got hurt, but I was the youngest (or most vulnerable), so the older children tried to protect me.

___ I sometimes took the hurt so some other child wouldn't.

___ Some other child took the hurt so I wouldn't have to.

___ I wasn't hurt the most. Another child was, and this was hard to deal with.

Another variation:

____

____

____

Children in the trenches

Marcus described his family in a way which has always stuck with us.

> **"There were five of us children, and I was right in the middle. My mom and step-dad were always shouting at each other or us. Sometimes crockery or chairs would go flying, the dog would be howling and we would either be hiding or trying to fight back. It was like the five of us had been conscripted into a war we didn't want to be in, and we spent most of our time trying to figure out how to survive."**

Some people we work with can relate to the analogy between conscripted soldiers and children in a chaotic, unsafe home. However, the important point is that you and the other children around you had to figure out how to cope with whatever was happening. Sometimes children in unsafe circumstances will bond together and form a united front against those who are doing the harming. They might look out for and protect one another, even taking the blame sometimes. But in times of threat and chaos, it's also common for children to turn on one another or identify with those who are doing the abusing. Sometimes an older child, rather than protecting others, will become abusive themselves. So perhaps Marcus' analogy to war is appropriate. Soldiers can bond closely when under great stress, but the opposite might also be true.

What is almost always the case is that the 'other children', for good or ill, were important in some way. This is why there is usually a need to talk about the other children in therapy.

Exercise 5: Your relationship with the other children
How did you and other child/children cope together back then? Did you confide in each other and bond together? Or, did your childhood circumstances push you apart?

Why family members can avoid speaking about the past

There is nothing commonplace or mediocre about trauma which happens in families. Sometimes when family members are exposed to trauma, it brings people closer together, and strong bonds and loyalties develop. However, it's not unusual for trauma to push family members away from each other or even blow a family completely apart. Sometimes this is just as it has to be. Perhaps what occurred means that these relationships cannot be repaired. But sometimes it's sad that trauma has put distance between some family members, and repairing a relationship is a part of the individual's recovery. You will probably know what is right for you. Below are explanations of why family members can end up feeling distant from one another as adults. Perhaps you will recognise something.

Too risky to speak about

If something really important can't be spoken of, then all that can be spoken about is rather trivial. Sometimes there is distance between certain family members because they were involved in events they feel they can't discuss. The thought of bringing up what happened can elicit anxiety.

Martha and her brother were sexually abused by an older cousin.

> **"I was about seven when it happened, and my brother was five. He's never mentioned it to me and I've never brought it up either. Sometimes I want to speak with him about it because I know it messed me up and I wonder if that happened to him as well. I'm not sure he even remembers it, and I'm worried it will upset him if I bring it up. But there has always been this distance between us, and I wonder if that's what it's about."**

There are many reasons why a person might find it difficult to talk about what happened with a family member who was also affected. Sometimes family members dodge each other or keep things superficial as a way of avoiding the subject.

Guilt

Complicated and unexpressed guilt can create distance within relationships. When people find themselves sharing disturbing circumstances, guilt is a common emotional artefact. Sometimes people feel guilty because they believe they should have done more. Steve's father physically abused him, his younger sister and his mother.

> **"I should have stopped him from hurting my sister and mother. But I didn't. I hate that they got hurt the way they did. Every time I look at them I think about that. It can be hard to spend time with them."**

We pointed out to Steve that he was smaller and much weaker than his father, but that didn't make him feel much better. When we asked Steve why he doesn't tell his mother and sister how he feels, the blood runs from his face. "What if they say that I should have helped?" he says.

Like Steve, some people feel inappropriately guilty that they didn't stop the abuse. Others can experience 'survivor's guilt'. They feel bad because they didn't get abused or didn't get abused as badly as another family member. They might have a difficult time discussing it. Whether the other person feels the same way or not, it can feel like an invisible barrier.

Family members can trigger traumatic memories
If an individual struggles with intrusive memories, flashbacks, or nightmares related to what happened, it's common for them to cope by avoiding whatever might trigger these experiences. For some, seeing or talking with family members who were there when it happened can trigger such memories. Some people will feel they need to avoid family as a way of avoiding the memories. This can be sad in some cases, as these relationships may be important.

Different perspectives or denial
Sometimes what happened does get talked about, but family members discover they have very different perspectives, or someone even denies what the other believed happened. Different views about something so incredibly important can push people away from one another. However, people can remember events differently, especially when the events occurred many years ago. And, as we mentioned previously, children can have very different biological temperaments. This can mean that if two children experienced similar events, for one it may have been 'bad', while for the other it was truly traumatising. Whatever the case, different memories and views can create distance as well.

Unfair treatment
The feeling of anger is a normal response to a perception of unfairness. If you were abused and someone else was treated fairly well, anger is an understandable emotion. However, it might not feel possible to talk through perceptions of unfairness with someone. It might be really difficult for the other person as well, as they might not feel good about the unfair treatment either, or they may need to suppress it. If anger goes unexpressed and unresolved, it transforms into resentment. It's very difficult to feel close to someone you resent.

Exercise 6: Why your family can't speak about what happened
Tick any reasons why you and other family members may find it difficult to speak about what happened in the past.

___ It feels too risky to speak about
___ Guilt that people feel gets in the way

___ Speaking about it may trigger traumatic memories
___ There are different perspectives on what happened or someone needs to deny it altogether
___ Some of us were treated better than others, and that's hard to acknowledge

Below you can add any further thoughts about why it's been hard to discuss the past.

The future

Trauma involves extreme circumstances, and extreme circumstances usually elicit extreme results. In this respect, shared traumatic circumstances can bring people together and build strong bonds and loyalties, or they can push people apart. It often goes one way or the other. If you shared traumatic circumstances with family members, are close to them, and can occasionally talk about what happened in a helpful way, we are pleased. These people may be able to understand what you went through, perhaps better than anyone else.

However, your relationships with people you experienced trauma with may be conflictual, distant or shallow. This is common and one of the effects of historical trauma in families. If you have grown distant from people you shared traumatic circumstances with, there is no specific advice anyone can give you. Your situation is unique. Perhaps you are managing these relationships as you need to for the sake of your recovery. Or, perhaps talking to someone you grew up with about what happened will allow you to feel closer to them and support your recovery. Sometimes this really helps, as was the case for Marie, who we mentioned earlier in this chapter. She was emotionally and physically abused by both parents, though her older brother wasn't. They hadn't spoken for over three years when he called her out of the blue.

> **"I never liked my brother, maybe because I resented that they seemed to love him and hate me. We had never spoken about what happened when we were young. Sometimes I doubt my memory, so I asked him what he remembered. I was really nervous, but he remembered everything just like I did. The times I got screamed at and locked in my room. It made me feel a lot better just knowing that he accepted that it all happened. I hope we will stay in touch now."**

Perhaps the relationships you have today with other family members are good, and there is nothing that needs developing. Or, perhaps these relationships today seem too complex or broken to deal with at this point in your recovery. But perhaps you think it would be useful to try and develop these relationships and even speak about what happened. It's a very personal decision.

Exercise 7: Repair concerning a family relationship

Some people feel there is no need to develop or repair a relationship with another family member. However, for others, childhood events had the effect of damaging relationships with people who were and still are important to them. If this is the case, do you want to develop or repair a relationship with a family member who is still important to you? What might you wish to do about this?

A SESSION ON PERSONAL DEVELOPMENT

The following chapter asks you to consider what personal development and the future might look like for you. You are approximately halfway through this programme. The beginning of this programme seemed too early to properly consider this area, and the end seemed too late. Right here seemed about right. You will get a break from thinking about past harm, so you might imagine considering the future will be much easier. It can be for some, but in our experience, it's not unusual for those who experienced childhood harm to feel uncomfortable with or even resistant to thinking about their future. If this occurs, it's quite common.

Chapter 12

What Does Recovery Mean to You?

"Sometimes I have this fantasy where I have a great life and the people who hurt me show up, and they're like, 'wow, look at her'. I deserve to have a life. But sometimes I want to have a life just to piss them all off."
Abby

Thus far, it's been important to spend quite a lot of time reflecting on how the past has impacted your present life. For example, you have explored how childhood trauma relates to painful psychological symptoms, your sense of self, relationship patterns and post-traumatic memories. This chapter focuses less on the effect of trauma or *post-traumatic reactions* and more on *post-traumatic growth.* The focus here is on really understanding your needs and imagining the future you want to create.

Cell regeneration as a model of hope

When an individual has lived with the painful effects of past trauma for many years, they can sometimes lose hope that change is possible. But, this can become a self-fulfilling prophecy. Pessimism concerning the possibility of change can itself get in the way of changing! Alternatively, belief or hope in the possibility of change supports and encourages change.

The human body can act as a source of inspiration concerning the possibility of change. Our entire body is built out of highly specialised cells. These cells are constantly regenerating or renewing themselves. Taste bud cells renew themselves every 10 days, stomach cells every 2-9 days, skin cells every 10-30 days, red blood cells every 4 months, liver cells every 6-12 months, and so on.[1] And, there is evidence that parts of our brain can regenerate as well, including the hippocampus, where memories are stored.[2] On a biological level, we are hardly the same person we were just a while ago. Regrowth or regeneration isn't just a possibility. Concerning our physiology, it's who we are right down to the cellular level. And, if we take reasonably good care of our bodies, we can aid this constant process of regrowth. That's what this chapter is about – the idea that change and regrowth are possible and that by taking care of ourselves, we can aid this process.

Michelle never knew her dad, was neglected by her mother, and was sexually abused by several men as a young teen. During a group therapy session, she shared a fascinating thought concerning cell regeneration.

> **"I like the idea that my skin cells regenerate at least every month. Those disgusting men that abused me all those years ago – they touched me then, but this means that they never touched the skin I have today. Sometimes I look at my skin or touch my skin, and I think, *this is my skin now*."**

Objects and subjects

Jean-Paul Sartre made what he felt was a critical distinction between *objects* and *subjects* in a 1943 publication entitled *Being and Nothingness*.[3] Sartre was a 20th-century existential philosopher, meaning he felt compelled to write about these ideas in a way which is incomprehensible to normal human beings. Reading the fine-print 688 pages of *Being and Nothingness* is not a lot of fun for most people. Nevertheless, Sartre's discussion of objects and subjects can have genuine relevance to those who experienced childhood harm.

In brief, Sartre said that the world is filled with objects and subjects, and he defines these terms. Objects, for example, are rocks, trees and very basic animal life. Objects are inanimate or simply react to the environment. If an object changes, this results from processes the object does not direct. As human beings, we are *not* objects – we are subjects. The critical difference is that human beings possess free will and are capable of envisioning and directing their futures. In other words, we can make genuine choices. But Sartre also made the point that human beings are capable of treating other people *as if* they were an object. Many people we have worked with, to a greater or lesser extent, got treated as if they were objects. The message they received may have been *you are not free to create your life and determine your future. Other people or circumstances will control you and determine your existence*. If a child is treated as an object, they can begin to see themselves as an object. They may begin to imagine they have little capacity to direct their lives.

This chapter is an opportunity for you to explore your subjectivity – that especially human part of you that is capable of determining your needs and directing your future.

Complex trauma and learned helplessness

Some of the most extraordinary discoveries happen by accident. This was true of *learned helplessness*, one of the most established and significant concepts in all of psychology. In the 1960s, a young psychologist named Martin Seligman was helping out with some experiments concerning principles of learning.[4] If the idea of using electric shocks on animals is upsetting for you, we are sorry, but it's part of the story.

Seligman was involved in experiments where dogs were taught to associate a sound with electric shocks. The dogs were placed on a metal grid next to a short barrier they could easily jump over to escape the shocks. But when these dogs were shocked, they just lay there and suffered rather than trying to escape. This didn't make any sense because the dogs should have quickly figured out that they could escape the shocks by jumping over the barrier. Seligman was confused until he learned that *these particular dogs* had been used in an earlier experiment where they were repeatedly shocked but had *no* means of escaping. These dogs had acquired the idea that they were helpless to escape shocks. In the present experiment, they were capable of escaping the shocks, but it didn't occur to them to try because their past experiences had taught them that escaping shocks was impossible. Their past experiences had taught them that they are helpless to control their present circumstances (this is *learned helplessness*).

This experiment was replicated with dogs and other animals many times and showed the same results. More humane research on learned helplessness has been done with children and adults, and the same results were found.[5] People who have been exposed to repeated harmful circumstances tend to develop a pessimistic or depressive view which leads them to believe that there isn't much they can do to control their lives.

Through repeated experiences of childhood abuse and neglect, individuals acquire the idea that they aren't in control of their feelings and lives. Many acquire the idea they should not bother hoping that change is possible. But this pessimistic perspective is just that: *a perspective*. It's not necessarily 'the truth'.

If the principle of learned helplessness leaves you feeling angry, perhaps that's a good thing. You can use that anger in a healthy and constructive way by deciding that it's up to you to determine how you will see yourself, your life and the future. As Sartre would say, you're not an object – you're a person who, despite what happened, is still free to determine how you will view yourself, others and the world.

Complex trauma and barriers to personal development

There can be a variety of reasons why change can seem difficult or even impossible for those who experienced childhood harm. Some of the most common reasons we come across are described briefly below. See what you can identify with.

Not feeling you deserve to have a good life
The experience of repeated childhood abuse or neglect can impart the message that *you don't deserve to have good and intimate relationships, positive feelings about yourself or personal success.* It's difficult for impressionable children to resist such messages, which may endure through their thoughts, feelings and behaviours in adulthood. In order to access needs and act to get them met, a person has to believe that they deserve to have needs and to get such needs met. Do you believe you deserve to have good feelings about yourself, good relationships, and a good life?

Time spent experiencing threats and worry
As we explored earlier, those who experienced childhood harm tend to spend more time in states of *fight or flight* or *shut-down*, even when threats are minimal or non-existent. Such states are distracting. It's difficult to build a house if you are always focused on preventing one from burning down. Is it hard to focus on your needs and personal development because you spend a lot of time experiencing threats and worrying?

Confidence
In a word, what is it that people who experienced childhood harm need most? Of course, there is no single answer – individuals are too complex for that. However, a good answer for many is *confidence*. Repeated noxious childhood experiences tend to knock the confidence out of a person – confidence that they are good and capable, that they are lovable, that they can make a significant contribution, and that they can create change. Confidence means you are willing to experiment with change – make mistakes, learn and adjust, and put yourself in new situations. Childhood trauma can sap confidence, leaving people stuck in fear and avoidance. Difficulties with self-confidence can be associated with Seligman's idea of learned helplessness explored above. Does a lack of confidence get in the way of experimenting with change?

Other people in your life
You may be in supportive relationships at this time in your life. However, some people who experienced childhood harm are currently in relationships with people who are not supportive of their personal development. The idea that you will develop yourself and your life may feel threatening to them. Rather than supporting you to heal issues associated with past harm, they may exacerbate such issues. This can make it harder for you to focus on change which is important. Is this issue relevant to you?

Change evokes anxiety

The very idea of change can evoke anxiety. Some can worry that if they start accessing their needs for love, self-expression and meaning, and create change concerning those needs, they might lose something. For example, some worry they will lose a relationship or financial support. Or, some fear that stepping out of the daily pattern means something bad will happen. Bad things *did* happen in the past, so they can be quicker to imagine that new relationships or circumstances will 'go wrong'. Not changing may seem like a way of 'playing it safe'. Does the very idea of changing evoke anxiety for you?

Exercise 1: Barriers to change

To what extent are the barriers to change described above relevant to you? Place a number between 1 and 5 next to the barriers below (1 meaning *no problem* and 5 meaning *a serious problem*).

I don't feel I deserve to have good feelings about myself, good relationships, and a good life ___

Spending time in 'survival brain' and coping with threats distracts me from focusing on my personal development ___

I lack confidence that change is possible ___

There are people in my life who would not like it if I were to change ___

I'm anxious about changing. I might lose something/something bad might happen ___

Are there any further reflections you have about what seems to get in the way of change?

Ambivalence concerning change is normal

Before offering you an opportunity to explore what personal development or change means for you, we want to make what we see as an important point. It's normal to feel *ambivalent* about making important changes in how you think, cope or meet your needs. But what is meant by ambivalence? Ambivalence means the coexistence of positive and negative feelings towards a situation or action, which simultaneously draws a person in opposite directions. It means having 'mixed feelings' about change.

In other words, it's very likely that there is a part of you that wants to change, and another part of you that wants things to remain the same. We can characterise these different parts of you in any number of ways. For some people, the insight they make into how they were impacted by past trauma is a strong force propelling them towards personal change. Or, some people come to see that their thoughts about themselves, others or life are simply *ideas* driven by past experience, and they can decide to see things differently. But there will be parts of you or aspects of your relationships that will also resist change. For example, traumatic core beliefs, discussed in later chapters, are deep-rooted, and they do not want to change. And, some people find the notion of change very difficult because they don't feel they deserve to have something better or different. Change can be exciting. It is also normally uncomfortable or scary.

Perhaps the simplest and most compelling way to understand the experience of ambivalence is to consider how pain works. There was a moment during a Louis Theroux documentary called *Heroin Town* in which Louis is speaking to a recovering heroin addict named Mickey Watson. Mickey has been clean from heroin for many months and spends time trying to help addicts who are still using. At one point, Louis says something like, it must be frustrating – how do you go about convincing people to stop using heroin? Mickey shrugs and says *when the pain of changing seems less than the pain of remaining the same, that's when you'll change*. Even though this conversation centred on the issue of heroin addiction, this point of view seems to capture the experience of ambivalence as applied to all manner of issues.

We do not mention the complexities of ambivalence to illicit pessimism. Despite the experience of ambivalence, we have seen many people change their relationship with themselves, others or life. And these changes do not have to be objectively large to be important or positive. We mention the issue of ambivalence because it's essential for individuals to be realistic and compassionate with themselves about the very real challenges of creating change. The impact of complex childhood trauma is normally profound, and recovery is best thought of as a progressive, ongoing and life-long process – not something you do in a few months.

What does 'recovery' mean to you?

As mentioned in the introduction, the historical trauma programme supports the principles of 'mental health recovery'. The idea of 'recovery' for individuals experiencing mental health difficulties began to gain ground in the 1980s. This was a 'movement' that developed in part as a reaction to so-called 'medical models' of mental health provision. The recovery model was not just advanced by certain clinicians, but was in many ways driven by consumers of mental health services who had their own views about the sort of help and collaboration that was needed.

The recovery approach sees people with mental health difficulties as *active participants* in the process of change and development, rather than 'patients' who simply get 'treated' by experts. Also, recovery from mental health difficulties is seen as *a personal journey* rather than a set of outcomes determined by a particular time frame, diagnosis or prognosis. Recovery is not about finding a 'cure'. Recovery emphasises the ongoing personal development of an individual.

The recovery model also emphasises the *social nature* of the individual's mental health difficulties. Such difficulties must be seen in the context of the individual's relationships and the lives they are trying to develop. This will have to take into account the individual's needs, sense of identity, aspirations, unique talents and personal projects.

If notions of cure and treatments by experts are de-emphasised within the recovery model, what is emphasised? Several themes and principles have been highlighted as important to supporting recovery. In 2004, over 110 panellists participated in developing mental health recovery principles, including clinicians, mental health consumers, family members, providers, advocates, researchers, academicians and others.[6] This group suggested that recovery principles include hope, empowerment, respect, peer support and self-direction. In addition, support to the individual seeking help must be individualised and person-centred, holistic, non-linear and strengths-based.

The recovery model also emphasises the individual's capacity to know what is needed for their development. With this in mind, recovery will mean different things to each individual. People we have worked with have answered the question, *what does recovery mean to you?* in a variety of ways:

"It means that I can focus on my work and my family without feeling so angry or getting messed up in my head about the past." Pete

"Recovery means not hurting myself and not letting other people hurt me either. It means liking myself." Molly

"It means being able to do what I want without feeling anxious or worrying about getting a panic attack." Brandon

"It means that I wouldn't hate the world. It would mean that I could see life as being good or having beauty." Ryan

"Recovery would mean that I can have a relationship with someone who I feel close to and who doesn't hurt me." Shelly

Exercise 2: What does recovery mean to you?
Below is an opportunity for you to answer this question. Some individuals discover an answer that comes straight to mind and that they feel confident about. Others are unsure and perhaps need time to let the question percolate, like a pot of coffee being brewed. One individual said, "I came up with an answer straight away, but I wasn't too sure about it. I found myself thinking about the question over the next few days. One morning I woke up and a different answer came to my mind, and I thought, *that's it. That's what recovery means to me*."

So, what does recovery mean to you?

The very personal and relative meaning of change

The commitment in time and emotion you are making to this programme is substantial. Most people doing this programme have to encounter *more* anxiety to get themselves through it. We assume you are doing this because you are 'fed-up' with the difficulties you struggle with, and you want a better relationship with yourself and a more fulfilling life. In short, you are here because you want change. In a moment, you will have another opportunity to explore what change means to you in more detail. However, we want to make a couple of points for your consideration.

First, what constitutes 'change' is very *personal*. Recall for a moment the discussion on Abraham Maslow's hierarchy of needs from a previous chapter. The change you want in your life will relate to your needs for safety and security, love and belonging, self-esteem, and self-expression and meaning. However, the way you relate to these universal needs will be unique.

Second, what constitutes 'important' change is *relative*. There is no 'correct' amount of change. We have seen individuals make what would appear to be *big changes*, such as leaving a destructive relationship, falling in love and beginning a healthy relationship for the first time, making allegations to the authorities about past abuse, being accepted onto further education, interviewing and landing an important job, and so on. However, we have seen others make changes that may not appear 'big', but are in fact giant, for *those* individuals. It all depends on where you are starting from concerning your confidence and how disturbing your past is to you. Staying off drugs, going to a social event or just learning to talk to yourself in a caring way can feel very significant for some.

Mary Ann is a good example. Physically and emotionally abused by her mother and father, and then sexually assaulted on more than one occasion as an adult, she entered therapy in a very bad state. She was socially isolated, clinically depressed, socially phobic, and unemployed for the past five years… and her confidence was near zero. As therapy progressed, she formed an idea of something that was important to her. She wanted to go bodyboarding. Going bodyboarding with a friend was one of the few happy memories she had from childhood, and doing that on her own just seemed important. She was terrified. It meant being in the public eye and doing something she wasn't confident about. She also decided she was going to wear a bathing suit. This worried her because past abuse left her with a very poor body image, and she imagined she would feel exposed and vulnerable. So, for Mary Ann, going bodyboarding was about a lot more than going bodyboarding – it represented much that was important concerning her needs and recovering from the impact of past events. After several weeks of group therapy, she finally managed to do it.

> **"It was about as bad as I thought it was going to be. I only slept for about an hour the night before and I had a nightmare as well. When I got into the water there were a lot of people around and my heart was going so fast I thought I might have a panic attack. But I forced myself to do it. My target was to stay in for ten minutes, but when I got to ten minutes I was starting to calm down and I was focusing more on bodyboarding than the other people. I don't know how long I was in the water for but I only came out because I got so cold my hands were starting to turn blue" (said with a big grin).**

To most people who don't understand the effects of historical trauma, going bodyboarding may not seem like much of an achievement. For Mary Ann, it was. Where does confidence come from? Well, it can come from the positives and encouragement we get from others, something that was deficient for many who experienced childhood harm. But confidence is also a product of having some success. Even smaller successes can build confidence, which sets you up for further success. This is a 'positive cycle' – quite the opposite of a vicious cycle.

Below you have an opportunity to write about what might constitute change for you. We will rely on Abraham Maslow and core human needs to guide this exercise. The principles to keep in mind are:

1. You are not an object – you are a subject, and so you are free to determine your life in some manner. Thank you, Sartre.
2. If past abuse or neglect gave you the idea that you can't control your circumstances or direct your future (learned helplessness), you can stick two fingers (British) or one finger (North Americans) up to that notion. Thank you, Seligman.
3. Change is personal and relative to your starting point today. It's up to you and no one else to decide. Thank you, Mary Ann.

Exercise 3: Exploring what change means for you

One way to explore change is to think about it relative to the core human needs Maslow described. You have an opportunity to do this below. However, don't feel you need to be limited to this approach – you can explore how you want to create change in your life in whatever way works for you.

Safety

Are there threats you are facing? Do you need to sort out your circumstances or relationships so you can feel more secure? E.g. financial, legal, housing, relationships which are threatening?

Belonging and intimacy

Is past trauma expressing itself through feelings of loneliness or unrewarding relationships? Do you want to repair or develop current relationships? Do you want to develop *new* friendships or a sense of belonging to a group?

Relationship to self
Your relationship with yourself is experienced through how you typically think about yourself, feel about yourself and talk to yourself. And, the way you care about yourself (self-care). Are there ways in which you want to develop a healthier relationship with yourself?

Self-expression and meaning
Do you know what your natural skills and interests are? In what way do you want to develop and express your abilities and interests, e.g. education, career, parenting, roles in supporting other people, being creative, etc...?

Other
Are there any other needs or goals you want to work at?

Three encouraging thoughts

We leave you with a few encouraging thoughts. First – here's an interesting question. How should you evaluate your progress in creating change in yourself and life? Many believe the only way to evaluate progress is by looking at *outcomes*. Did you achieve what you set out to achieve? Of course, this is one way to think about it. However, we think it's often more important to consider the *process* of attempting to change. It's what you did along the way, not the result.

We remember Mark, a young man who was very socially anxious and had a poor sense of self. He had wanted to ask a girl out, something he had never done before, and we encouraged him to try. He arrived at one session dejected and depressed. He'd asked a girl out, and he'd been shot down. The outcome was not good (no getting around that). However, the process (asking her out) was amazing for a guy who had been abandoned by both parents and suffered abuse and neglect in a series of foster homes. No matter what the *outcomes* of your efforts to create a better life for yourself, there is real value in giving credit for the *process* or attempts made at getting your needs met.

One feature of the programme's final chapter is the opportunity to reflect on the change you may experience while doing this programme. As you work your way through this programme, we suggest keeping your eye on the process of trying to make changes at least as much as outcomes. Your efforts are important, no matter what they lead to.

Second, you don't need to wait for anyone else to tell you how or when you should begin working at change. You don't need anybody's permission to start creating changes in your life.

Third, some individuals can feel worried about stepping out of the pattern they know so well, no matter how painful or unrewarding that pattern might be. However, most attempts at change are not an 'all or nothing deal'. Thinking or acting differently or making a decision can be thought of as a way of 'experimenting' with change. See what happens. If it clearly doesn't work or makes things worse, you can stop and experiment in another way. For some, it's a process of experimenting with change and all the miss-fires that lead to important discoveries.

References

1. Pantaleo, A., Giribaldi, G., Mannu, F. Arese, P. & Turrini, F. Naturally occurring anti-band 3 antibodies and red blood cell removal under physiological and pathological conditions. *Autoimmun Rev*. 2008 Jun7 (6):p. 458.
2. Spalding, K.L., Bergmann, O. Alkass, K. Mash, D.C. Druid, H. & Frisen J.. Dynamics of Hippocampal Neurogenesis in Adult Humans *Cell*. Volume 153, ISSUE 6, P1219-1227, June 06, 2013.
3. Sartre, J. (1993). *Being and Nothingness*. New York: Washington Square Press.
4. Seligman, M. E. P. (1990). *Learned optimism: How to change your mind and your life*. New York: Vintage.
5. Nolen-Hoeksema, S., Girgus, J. & Seligman, M. E. (1986). Learned helplessness in children: A longitudinal study of depression, achievement and explanatory style. *Journal of Personality and Social Psychology*, 51, 435-42.
6. National Consensus Statement on Mental Health Recovery (2004). U.S. Department of Health and Human Services Substance Abuse and Mental Health Services Administration.

PART III

A FOCUS ON RECOVERY

We want to introduce part III by mentioning something we really liked that a client named Darrel said. Darrel was a 45-year-old builder and a person with a very good analytical mind. As a child, he had been badly neglected within his home and then sexually abused during a placement in foster care. As an adult, he had struggled with alcohol until a few years before we met him. During a group session, he said something which rang true about recovery.

> **"Insight is really important, but it's not enough. I had some fairly good insight many years ago, but it didn't do the job on its own. You have to live the solution."**

Darrel's point makes intuitive sense to most anyone who struggles with trauma. Insight really *is* essential, and it's a form of inner change. Without being able to connect the dots, many people will unconsciously recreate distress that reflects the disturbance of their childhood experiences (recall the earlier chapter on retraumatisation). However, as Darrel suggests, *insight doesn't do the job on its own.* Many people with good insight will continue to traverse well-worn painful patterns. In addition to insight, it's also necessary to experiment concerning your life and relationships, and there are countless ways to do this. Insight can be thought of as a trustworthy base from which to experiment further.

Much of what follows will continue to encourage insight, but the emphasis will shift towards, as Darrell eloquently put it, *living the solution.* The very mention of experimentation or change can elicit anxiety in some who experienced childhood harm. If this is the case, keep in mind that you are in control of how you use the Guidebook and can go at a pace which is manageable.

Group Session 14

Being Present and Connected

If paying attention is a train, then trauma is the cow standing on the tracks.
A line from Gary's journaling

"My friend took me to this meditation group once. Oh my god, I wanted to shoot myself after about three minutes. I don't think I was meditating, unless meditating means trying to figure out how to escape from a room full of people without anyone noticing."
Janine

Past trauma has a way of interfering with our capacity to attend and feel connected to life, others, and ourselves. Trauma does this by controlling our mental lives (thoughts, images, memories) and our body-based experiences. This chapter is going to explore what for some people can seem like a strangely unfamiliar question: What thoughts or images do you actually want to have in your mind and how do you want to feel within your own body? If you have thoughts or body-based sensations which are undermining attention and connection, can you notice them and exert some sense of control?

You may be familiar with this topic, but the idea that we can notice and exert control over trauma-based thoughts and body-based experiences can be a strangely new idea to some people we work with. Or, others may be familiar with this idea but really lack confidence that control is possible. For many, it has always been others who seemed to control their thoughts, emotions, and body-based experiences, so it may be difficult to imagine they can have control or even a sense of permission to exert control. Our view is that your mental and body-based experiences *belong to you.* To whatever extent you lack confidence to manage them, this chapter is an invitation to see if you can move things in the direction of recovery. Some will have experience with this topic and perhaps some confidence, but for others it can seem new. If it feels like a beginning or you really lack confidence, that's okay – to be fair, it's a really difficult topic for many, and much of the remainder of the Guidebook will build on ideas found here from a number of perspectives.

We also explore the practice of mindfulness and what is referred to as 'the observing self'. It would not be surprising if you were familiar with mindfulness as it has become incredibly popular through book publications and social media over the past 30 years.

You may have positive associations with mindfulness. However, a number of people we have worked with dislike the idea of mindfulness, and some have had negative experiences with it. Here are some actual quotes: "I hate mindfulness"... "I stopped reading"... and "this stuff is patronising."

If you have developed negative ideas about mindfulness, we encourage you to continue. We have looked very closely at any available research and clinical observations which help us understand how mindfulness can be safe and helpful and why it can go wrong for people struggling with trauma symptoms. We have also listened very closely to clients we have worked with and have rewritten this chapter a number of times to get it as right as possible. There are both risks and opportunities in recommending mindfulness for people with a trauma history, and we have been careful to explore mindfulness in what we believe is a *trauma-sensitive way*. Any discussion of mindfulness is explored from an entirely non-religious perspective, so it should not conflict with religious beliefs the reader may hold.

The important role of attention

Paying attention can include a sense of concentration, being absorbed in what you are doing, feeling in control, and a loss of self-consciousness. When an individual is truly absorbed in what they are doing, this has been described as a 'state of flow'.[1] The capacity for attending or concentrating has been connected to being able to learn, feelings of competence, well-being and happiness,[2] as well as self-esteem.[3]

Being absorbed in what has meaning, importance, or value is a powerful symptom of well-being. The ability to pay attention can be considered both a cause and a symptom of well-being. We might say that a feature of recovery is to become so focused on what has value that the traumas from the past begin to lose their hold over you.

Everyone who has experienced childhood trauma is unique, and yet one of the issues they tend to share in common is a difficulty with attention. This is reflected within the historically proposed diagnosis of Developmental Trauma Disorder, which indicates problems with 'attentional dysregulation'.[4] Attentional difficulties can express themselves in many ways: problems with concentration, difficulties staying connected to people and events around you, not being aware of the signals coming from your body, accident proneness, going into a room and not remembering why you went in there, losing personal items, brain fog, forgetting appointments or being late, etc....

Individuals who experienced childhood trauma are far more likely to be given a diagnosis of Attention Deficit Hyperactivity Disorder (ADHD).[5] Symptoms of ADHD, such as inattentiveness (difficulty concentrating and focusing), hyperactivity, and impulsivity, are often seen to result from a 'brain chemistry imbalance'. It might be the case that an individual with a trauma history currently has a brain chemistry imbalance, but what's the underlying cause? Is it simply a matter of biology, or does past trauma and associated PTSD issues play a role? And, was a trauma history properly assessed and considered when a diagnosis of ADHD was made? If we don't know the answers to these questions for a particular individual, we can't understand the nature of their attentional issues.

Problems with attention associated with abuse or neglect are often first seen in school performance. In the classroom, such children are more likely to struggle with concentration, can be either passive or blow up with anger, or appear to be 'spaced out'.[6] The result is often impaired reading ability, lower grades, and more days of school absence.[7] Difficulties with school performance can then do further harm to an already compromised self-image.

Problems with attention don't evaporate when an individual becomes an adult at the age of eighteen. We mentioned Robin before, a woman who experienced neglect and deprivation within the family home and was sent to live with an aunt at eight, where things did not improve much. While the expression of attentional difficulties varies between individuals, Robin's description is familiar.

> **"Sometimes my kids are talking to me and I realise I have no idea what they're saying, or I'm listening to a podcast and I'm suddenly aware that I don't know what's going on. It's like I'm in two places at the same time."**

In a sense, Robin *is* in two places at the same time. She's in the world at this moment, wanting to listen to her children or a podcast, *and* she is experiencing the effects of childhood harm. Trauma is interfering with her capacity to be present in the moment and connected to the world around her. Being connected to the present moment while suffering the effects of trauma is like trying to listen to the radio through a lot of static.

Understanding how past abuse or neglect has contributed to difficulties with attention can help some people look at problems concerning achievement and relationships with more insight and self-compassion. George is a man in his 40s who experienced childhood sexual abuse and substantial bullying from peers and teachers at school.

> **"At school I always just thought I was stupid. When I was older I lost a couple of jobs and it felt like I was in school all over again. But I was scared and worrying all the time."**

George had decided that his problems at school and work were because he was 'stupid'. But George was not able to pay attention at school or work because you have to feel safe in order to pay attention (more about this later). This insight opened the door for self-compassion, rather than self-blame.

We mentioned Bob in a previous chapter, an individual who was neglected by his mother and abused by a stepfather. He laughed when he described his experience, but his problems connecting to the world were very real.

> **"My head is like a movie which has no plot and a bad soundtrack. Songs get stuck, all sorts of random thoughts, ridiculous scenarios playing out. It's like having a room where so much rubbish has been piled up that you can't really do much in there."**

If you can identify with having attentional problems, it's useful to point out that attention is like any other skill – it can be worked on and developed. This chapter will support you in this manner, but first, let's look in more detail at *why* those who experienced childhood harm are more likely to experience problems with attention.

Attention and the need for safety

What's different about individuals with a traumatic history and those who largely felt cared for and protected? Certainly one difference relates to a core feature of PTSD – a *heightened sense of threat.* Individuals who experienced circumstances of childhood harm and often further trauma in adulthood tend to feel less safe in the world and in their bodies. Being able to attend and feel connected requires that you feel reasonably safe.

When anyone feels a sense of threat, they will try to find ways of responding – of trying to get to safety. Over the years we have noticed certain ways individuals respond to a sense of threat. These all are genuine attempts to seek safety, but especially when there is a background of trauma, they can each disrupt attention and connection. They can be sneaky, powerful, and compelling. There can be a part of you that feels you *must* respond in the ways indicated below, which is one of the reasons recovery can feel so challenging.

Ruminating over social encounters

Childhood harm was interpersonal – it was other people who were scaring, hurting, or neglecting you. So it's understandable that today it's relational experiences that can seem threatening. In her 60s, Diane felt lonely and wanted a sense of community and connection, but this was scary.

"Sometimes I can go to the coffee morning at our village hall, but I worry so much that it's hard for me to focus on what people are saying and my mind goes blank."

And, it's not just spending time worrying about present or future events, but also past events. Shelly was emotionally neglected and spent the latter part of childhood in care.

"After I've been with people I can spend ages pulling it all apart. Did I make a joke that offended someone? Did someone think I was bragging because I mentioned the holiday we went on? I complimented someone, but did they take it the wrong way? This is why I sometimes don't even want to be with people."

Social fears are understandable for those with a history of being harmed by others. Mental worry is a way of trying to seek safety and protection. At some level of consciousness people imagine *if I worry enough, perhaps I can find safety*. However, for those with a trauma history, mental worry is more often a problem than a solution. And, ruminating about future or past social encounters drags a person out of the present moment. In this way, worry and social anxiety can hijack our attention.

Shame

We will be exploring this feeling in detail in chapter 15, but trauma-based shame is a feeling of 'badness' with respect to ourselves. It's a sense of inadequacy or defectiveness which I feel about myself. When trauma-based shame is triggered, it can seem like it's fundamentally about a current event – some mistake we made (real or imagined) – but shame is this old feeling that has been around since it was generated all those years ago through abusive experiences. When trauma-based shame gets activated in the here and now, punitive self-talk can cloud over the world happening right in front of us. We are not paying attention or connected to life or others because we are in our heads with this feeling of shame and punitive self-talk taking centre stage.

For those who have abusive histories, shame can seem like a necessary punishing feeling which can protect a person from making mistakes in the future. But, as we explore in a later chapter, trauma-based shame is a fundamentally unhelpful and unnecessary feeling. If possible, you may need to take this on trust at the moment.

Stuck anger

It's important to acknowledge that individuals who experience childhood harm (and often further harm in later life) can have very genuine reasons to feel anger. Trauma occurring in relationships that were supposed to be safe is fundamentally wrong and unjust, and anger is a normal and understandable reaction. However, the way that anger can be experienced by some people who have experienced trauma can interfere with attention and connection.

In his late 50s, Adam experienced abusive parents, years of school bullying, and an abusive partnership of more than 20 years. He seemed to need the first 15 minutes of every therapy session to vent anger about the government, the other drivers on the road, the utility company, his neighbour's dog, etc… . At one point his therapist suggested he journal any angry scenarios which start running in his mind. His response was interesting.

> **"I spend a huge amount of time with these angry fantasies running around in my head. It's things from the past, things going on at the moment – but there are also these angry scenarios where I'm getting some sort of revenge. I don't plan to do it, but it just goes on. It's exhausting."**

The angry mental scenarios Adam experiences are not unusual for many people who were traumatised. For Adam, his anger was often directed outward at others or the world. For others, stuck anger can be directed inwards, at themselves, for real or imagined mistakes. Anger is an emotion designed to protect us or others. Anger is the emotional counterpart to the 'fight' aspect of the 'fight or flight' response. The problem for many who were traumatised can be that they are feeling anger about past or present events which they can't or don't feel able to 'fight' against. So, the images and thoughts driving anger circulate inside the individual's head and body. Anger was designed to be a short-acting emotion which motivates us to protect ourselves, get a need met, or set something right. But if anger is an emotion we are *living with* that is based in past trauma, it can seem like the one getting hurt is ourselves. Part of the hurt is that stuck anger interferes with our ability to pay attention and connect to what is important in the present moment.

Intrusive unwanted memories

Another understandable symptom of PTSD is re-experiencing. These are memories of events which have not been 'processed' or 'put to bed'. These memories can be triggered by associated events or come 'out of the blue', and they usually arrive with difficult physical sensations, emotions, and thoughts. Typically, they are memories of experiences where we were harmed and frightened. Or, they may be upsetting memories of times we imagine we did not cope well or made mistakes we regret. Like social worry and stuck anger, intrusive unwanted memories are designed to protect us. The body and brain seem to be saying *if you keep in mind what was disturbing from your past, then maybe you can avoid harm in the future*. Continuing to remember distressing experiences has been a part of trying to remain safe for most of human history. If I went into a cave last week and there was a sabre-toothed tiger in there, I will have reoccurring memories of feeling frightened by the tiger. These memories encourage me to avoid going back into that cave.

However, if the danger of the past is now over, associated distressing memories are not serving the purpose they were designed for. Rather than keeping us safe, these memories have become a problem. And, within our daily life, intrusive unwanted memories wrench us out of the present moment and into the past. When this happens, it's very difficult to pay attention or stay connected to the world in front of us.

Frantic mind

Earlier in the chapter, we mentioned Bob, who told us that his head was "like a movie with no plot and a bad soundtrack." It's a good example of what might be called *frantic mind*. What we are suggesting is that feeling unsafe is what compromises attention and connection. Sometimes, the sense of threat has an obvious source, like being in a crowded superstore. However, some people tell us they feel this sense of threat in their bodies. They can just wake up with a sense of something bad happening or it catches up with them at certain times. So, their minds may go at a frantic pace to avoid anything upsetting. The mind leaps from one thing to another without being able to focus for any period of time. Slowing down mentally, sitting quietly, or listening attentively may not seem like something they can afford to do. The mind may fill up with random thoughts, stuck music, repetitive phrases, etc… It's like 'mental filler'. Frantic mind is a way of trying to protect yourself from something scary or upsetting – it's a means of pushing away (or suppressing) memories or other effects of trauma. Even though a frantic mind is trying to protect you, it can be very tiring and get in the way of paying attention or connecting to what is in front of you.

If you struggle with attention for any of the above reasons, it's important not to punish yourself—trauma results in an individual feeling less safe in the world. Social worry, shame, stuck anger, unwanted memories, and frantic mind are all attempts to seek safety. They may compromise attention and connection in the moment, but they are not 'irrational', and no one is 'failing' for falling into these difficulties. As mentioned, an individual can feel compelled to respond in these ways, but this is not necessarily the case. You can have some control if you can see what is happening.

Exercise 1:
We described five consequences of historical trauma which can interfere with your ability to pay attention and connect with the world. They are:

- Ruminating over social encounters
- Shame
- Stuck anger
- Intrusive unwanted memories
- Frantic mind

Everyone is different, so you may recognise that some of these issues are more problematic than others. How do they affect you and your ability to attend and connect?

Paying attention and mindfulness

By paying attention, we are referring to our ability to focus on what we need to. It means having a sense of connection to our immediate experience: taking in what your friend is saying, concentrating on doing the dishes or making a repair, being aware that you are cold, noticing that your heart is beating harder, being aware of thoughts and images that are generating anger. However, our capacity for attention should also allow us to decide on what we *do not* want to pay attention to. We should not only be able to *focus* our attention on what makes sense, but we should also be able to shift our attention away from what we do not wish to experience. Focusing attention *and* being able to shift focus are equally important attentional skills.

The human brain has changed very little over tens of thousands of years, so it's not surprising that there has been an interest in the relationship between paying attention and well-being for most of recorded history. Traditions such as Buddhism have explored the role of attention for 2,500 years, and the Sanskrit word *sati* was used to refer to remembering, or with respect to personal development, remembering to attend to the present moment. The word *mindfulness* was an English translation of sati used in 1910 by a Buddhist scholar named Rhys Davids,[8] and the popularisation of the term and practice of mindfulness really began in earnest in the 1980s and 1990s with teachers such as Jon Kabit-Zinn.[9]

So, what is mindfulness? Most definitions of mindfulness emphasise paying attention to experience in the present moment. This can mean paying attention to the world in front to you – your book, someone speaking, the feel of the soapy water as you do the dishes. Or, paying attention to your inner world – thoughts, feelings, or body sensations. Many definitions of mindfulness add the idea of paying attention to present experience *without judgement*. Not leaping to judge or place value on your experience can sometimes allow an individual to see what's happening with more clarity. However, in respect to people with a trauma history, it's important not to take the idea of being non-judgemental too far. Mindfulness should allow for *all* experiences, and there are times when making a judgement is part of your authentic and acceptable experience. "*What happened was wrong and it should not have occurred.*" Judgements like this are part of mindfulness too. Being non-judgemental simply means accepting that it's okay to have whatever thoughts come up.

Can mindfulness be helpful to those with a trauma history and trauma symptoms, or does it come with risks? This is worth exploring before we go any further. As we have said all along, safety and stability are the fundamental basis for recovery. Let's look at the potential benefits of mindfulness and then explore some concerns.

In one way or another, mindfulness exercises are designed to help an individual focus on the present moment and connect to others and life. Childhood trauma can drag an individual out of the present moment and into a past laden with distressing memories and associated feelings. Or, a history of past harm can pull a person out of the present moment as they worry excessively about imagined future threats. So, if mindfulness can help a person stay connected to the present, it would seem to be an especially good fit for those who experienced trauma.

It also needs to be said that mindfulness is evidence-based, and studies have shown that it can help with many problems which often coincide with trauma, including anxiety,[10] depression,[11] and substance misuse.[12] A review of 18 studies found that mindfulness for adults can be helpful in reducing symptoms of PTSD, including reductions in avoidance and shame-based self-appraisals.[13] Another review of 17 studies suggests that mindfulness can be helpful specifically for adults who experienced childhood harm, but there were concerns raised about potential negative effects and the need for mindfulness to be adapted for this group of individuals.[14]

Despite the positive indications, it's very difficult to know whether mindfulness will be helpful (and safe) for any individual who is struggling with the effects of childhood trauma. For one thing, there is no such thing as 'mindfulness practice' – there are many different mindfulness practices or exercises. As we will discuss, our experience is that certain mindfulness exercises may be safer, gentler, and more helpful than others for those who have experienced childhood harm.

For those with a trauma history, a second concern is that some mindfulness practices may cause these individuals to be *more* exposed to symptoms of trauma.[15,16] What many mindfulness exercises have in common is that they ask an individual to *slow down* and attend to present experience. For those not struggling with trauma reactions, the individual might experience a heightened connection with thoughts, emotions, and life. For those who struggle with unresolved symptoms of trauma, the experience of slowing down and paying attention may result in a heightened experience of… trauma symptoms! An important feature of recovery is about slowing down so you can pay attention and get connected with your experience – the life in front of you, your relationships, your body sensations, your feelings, and your thoughts – but when you slow down and pay attention, there is a possibility you will be more exposed to trauma symptoms. This 'catch 22' scenario is just another reason why childhood trauma is so damn unfair.

So, what are we to do? Over some years of trying out different versions of this chapter with clients, we believe we have found a balanced approach to mindfulness that is helpful and less likely to lead to destabilisation. While there are many different mindfulness exercises, there are two broad ways that mindfulness is done. First, there is *mindfulness meditation*. This most often involves sitting or lying down while doing a formal mindfulness exercise. There are many ways of doing this, but an example is focusing your attention on the intake and exhalation of the breath. Second, there is *mindfulness living*. With mindfulness living, you continue to go about your daily life but you apply mindfulness to whatever you are doing.

For those struggling with trauma symptoms, our experience is that *mindfulness meditation* can be more likely to exacerbate trauma symptoms for some people, whereas *mindfulness living* exercises can be safer. This is a point made by David A. Treleaven in his excellent book *Trauma-Sensitive Mindfulness*: "I'm sometimes asked whether it's mindfulness that's problematic for survivors, or whether it's mindfulness meditation that causes issues. As you will see, I lean toward the latter."[15]

We agree with Treleaven. The reason more formal mindfulness meditation exercises can cause problems for certain traumatised people is that they ask you to *slow down,* shut out the rest of the world, and focus attention in a narrow manner. This can leave some more exposed to trauma symptoms. It's possible that mindfulness meditation may be very helpful to you and it would be patronising to suggest you should not attempt it, but we are saying approach it with thoughtfulness. In this chapter we will introduce you to three exercises for mindful living. For those who are interested, we will briefly say more about mindfulness meditation at the end of the chapter.

The observing self: the key to making mindfulness work

Mindfulness is not mysterious or mystical. It just means paying attention to experience in the present moment, whether we are attending to the world and people in front of us or the inner world of thoughts, feelings, or sensations. In mindfulness, our attention has a quality of concentration and focus. We feel a sense of connection, whether we are aware of the soapy dishwater as we do the washing up, the words our friend is speaking, the mental planning we are doing as we think about the grocery shopping, or the awareness that we are cold.

However, as we explored earlier, when the effects of past trauma show up, they disrupt our attention and connection to present experience. Here's an analogy which may help. Suppose you planned a really nice dinner party and it's going well. People are enjoying the food, drink, and each other's company. Suddenly an uninvited guest arrives who tells offensive jokes, spills beer all over the carpet, and starts an argument. The uninvited guest – that's trauma symptoms.

So, what is *the observing self* and how does it support mindfulness? The part of us that can step back from our immediate experiencing and notice or observe what we are experiencing – that's what we call the observing self. It sometimes goes by other names such as dual-awareness or meta-perception. The observing self is a natural cognitive ability, so you probably have a sense of it.

For our purposes, if we are engaged in life in some manner and then trauma symptoms start interfering and distracting, the observing self is that part of us that can notice that trauma symptoms are occurring. You might think, *wait a minute, if I'm experiencing trauma symptoms, I must be aware that I am experiencing trauma symptoms!* Actually, we can sometimes be *so close* to our experience that we don't have the necessary distance to really notice the experience. We can get 'fused' with the experience, meaning we are on autopilot. If this seems complicated, here is an example.

We mentioned Daniel previously, a military veteran who had been raised by an unstable and rejecting single mother. His darts club had organised an outing at a time when he had to work.

> **"All these angry thoughts kept going through my head. They know I have to work, so why plan it then? None of them really care if I'm in the club or not. Most of them are insensitive assholes..."**

Daniel had fantasies of writing an angry resignation email. Then, Daniel had a moment when he was able to access his observing self. He wasn't *just* having those angry thoughts and images; he could step back and observe what was happening. He stopped in the middle of his kitchen and thought, *oh wow – I have been walking around the house getting almost nothing done for the past two hours, my head full of all these angry thoughts and fantasies.* He was no longer 'fused' with the angry thoughts and images because he was observing what was happening with some distance. Trauma reactions get 'baked into' our psychology through frightening experiences, so when triggered, we experience them automatically. Your observing self is your cognitive ability to have awareness that trauma symptoms are occurring.

People who experience trauma can feel overwhelmed by body-based and emotional reactions. Especially when triggered and emotionally dysregulated, it can seem like they just *are* the reactions. They are so *close* to the reactions that it may not occur to them that they can have some control over what is occurring. The observing self allows you to get some distance. Imagine a washing machine that has a glass window.[17] It's running, and clothing and suds are flying around in there. A trauma-based reaction can feel like you are inside the washing machine. Accessing the observing self is more like you are outside the washing machine and looking through the window as you watch the churning suds and clothing. You're paying attention, but you are not getting thrown about. Because you have some distance, you can bring curiosity or reflection to the experience. You can then have more control over how you want to react.

Direct or spontaneous experience can be great and we don't want to go through life seeing everything from the perspective of the observing self. But, if trauma symptoms are hijacking our ability to pay attention and feel a sense of connection, having enough distance to observe that this is occurring can allow us to redirect our attention. If you are anxious and worrying, the observing self can notice this, and you may think, *oh wow, I've been worrying for 20 minutes now and really upsetting myself.* If you have been mentally reliving a disturbing experience, the observing self can notice this, and you may think, *wow, I've spent the last 15 minutes remembering what happened 10 years ago, and the muscles in my shoulders are all tense.* There are countless ways the observing self can step in and allow you more awareness of your experiences. Direct experience of trauma symptoms can be like walking around in a storm, exposed to the cold wind and rain. Accessing the observer self can create a moment where you now experience the storm from behind a window.

So, how can mindfulness and the observing self work together? Mindfulness just means paying attention to experience in the present moment. The observing self can support mindfulness in the following way: if paying attention in the present moment (or being mindful) is disturbed by trauma symptoms, the observing self can notice this is happening. By having awareness of the trauma symptoms, you can choose to redirect your attention, if this is what you wish to do. It's important to point out that being mindful and using the observing self are not means of suppression, distraction, or avoidance. Through the observing self you *are* noticing trauma symptoms. You pay attention to it for a moment. But you are also aware of how it is compromising your attention or ability to feel connected to life and others, as well as what is important for you at *this* moment. And, if you wish, you are now able to redirect your attention.

Mindful living: Noticing thoughts and images

This exercise is designed to help you get a sense of using mindfulness and the observing self together. First, you need to select some task that will take anywhere from 3 to 20 minutes. It can be making a cup of tea or coffee, doing laundry, cleaning the kitchen or bathroom, doing the dishes, mopping or vacuuming, gardening, washing a car, grooming a pet, etc… . To make this easier, try to avoid complex tasks that require hard thinking, like cooking a difficult meal or making a challenging repair.

See if you can do the task mindfully. If you are folding laundry, *simply* pay attention to folding the laundry. If you are loading the dishwasher, *merely* pay attention to loading the dishwasher. If you are vacuuming, *just* pay attention to vacuuming. What is likely to happen is that while you are doing the task, you will have verbal thoughts or visual images come into your mind. If the thoughts or images are about your task, that's fine – you are all in one place. However, if the thoughts or images have nothing to do with your task, your mind is elsewhere. If you can notice these thoughts or images, you are using your observing self. You may say to yourself, *ah, I'm thinking about…* . Now, see if you can return your full attention to the task.

It will be interesting to see if the thoughts or images that come into your mind are quite ordinary or whether they are trauma symptoms, e.g., social worry, angry scenarios, frantic mind material, or intrusive unwanted memories. If this is the case, you can respond in the same way—the observing self notices the thoughts or images, and then you return your attention to your task.

Exercise 2: Noticing thoughts and images

When you have completed this exercise, see if you can describe the experience below. How easy or difficult was it to mindfully attend to the task? Were you able to bring your observing self to your experience which helped you have awareness of thoughts or images which interfered with mindful attention on your task? Were thoughts or images of a harmless and ordinary form, or were they trauma-based?

What was the point of the previous exercise? If trauma symptoms are interfering with attention and connection, mindfulness and the observing self can help you *see* the trauma symptoms rather than just *be* the trauma symptoms. When you see that symptoms interfere with attending and connecting, there can be a moment in which you decide to take control and direct your attention. Traumatic events share one thing in common: you did not feel safe or in control. Even small moments where you can feel a sense of control in respect to trauma symptoms can feel important.

Trying to be mindful all the time is probably too much for most of us, and allowing for spontaneity and mental slack is healthy too. However, as Jon Kabit-Zin likes to say, you can 'drop into mindfulness' whenever you want.[18] The exercise you just did – it's not designed to be done once. You can literally 'drop into' this way of living whenever you need to. If you are feeling mentally scattered or disconnected from life, you can decide to 'drop into mindfulness' and consciously pay attention to life as you are experiencing it. And, as you pay attention to your direct experience, the observing self can be there like a good friend, keeping an eye on things and allowing you to redirect attention as you wish.

Mindful living: Noticing body sensations

As clinicians such as Bessel Van der Kolk[19] and Peter Levine[20] have convincingly pointed out, traumatic experience is stored away in our bodies. Clients who experienced childhood abuse and neglect seem to understand this intuitively. If past experiences of childhood harm get triggered in the moment, it's not just thoughts or memories which begin to play through an individual's mind. The body itself 'remembers' these events and will react. Muscles constrict, breathing accelerates, and other physiological reactions occur that we are not even aware of – hormones such as adrenalin and cortisol entering the blood steam. It's even possible that whatever is triggering a reaction is outside our conscious awareness, but our brains and bodies are picking up on it anyway. Most traumatised individuals have had experiences where they are in objectively safe situations but their bodies are reacting as if there was a threat. Have you ever had thoughts like, "I'm just sitting in a café with a friend – why is my heart pounding?"

If the effects of trauma are living on in our bodies, it makes sense that a lot of traumatised people do *not* want to pay attention to what is going on in their bodies. Drugs and alcohol, OCD, deliberate self-harm, or obsessions with food can all be ways of trying to get rid of body sensations, or at least distract ourselves from them. But all of this comes with a cost. If we are not able to have some awareness of what's happening in our bodies, it's hard to respond to body distress.

So, how might trauma show up in our bodies? There are many ways, but three are common: muscle constriction, shallow/quick breathing, or a general shaking or trembling. Let's look at these briefly. *Muscles* constrict to prepare us to run, fight, or protect our organs from attack. This is very useful if we are genuinely threatened by physical assault, but problematic if we are physically safe. If past trauma means we are unconsciously constricting muscles for periods of time, this can contribute to headaches, jaw pain, back and neck pain, frozen joints, loss of movement, or pinched nerves.

Breathing which is shallow and quick is a natural nervous system response to a perception of threat, whether or not we are consciously aware of the threat. There may be times when you are aware you are breathing in a shallow or quick manner despite being in reasonably safe circumstances.

Shaking or trembling is a normal response when adrenalin is released in response to a real or imagined threat. Also, following a traumatic experience, most mammals will shake as a way of discharging excess energy and 'coming down' from a frightening experience. So, some people who have a trauma history and who continue to experience a perception of threat (real or imagined) can find they shake or tremble. For some, shaking or a tremor comes and goes. For others it's often there in a low grade way and can be more pronounced in times of stress.

Exercise two is similar to exercise one, but with a couple of differences. Rather than being aware of thoughts and images, you will use the observing self to notice body-based reactions or sensations. You can choose a task as you did in exercise one and use the observing self to notice body-based reactions while being mindful of the task. Or, you can do this with a bit more flexibility. Just keep the practices of mindfulness and the observing self in mind. When you are working around the house or are out and about –

maybe driving or at the store or work – you can access mindfulness and the observing self and check in on what's happening in your body.

The observing self can notice muscles that are constricting. Common locations are:

Shoulders riding high
Abdominal muscles constricted
Jaw or teeth clenched
Area around the eyes tight
Buttock or legs constricted

The observing self may notice times when breathing is quick and shallow with no obvious threat. Or, the observing self may notice shaking or a tremor.

If you are doing exercise two, notice constricted muscles, and you are safe, an obvious response is to let the constriction go. If you notice quick and shallow breathing, the breathing exercise you learned towards the start of the programme can be a helpful response. Or, just take a large breath, hold it for as long as comfortable and blow out slowly. That can discharge a surprising amount of trauma-based tension. Trembling can be a bit trickier, but relaxing muscles, breathing, and aerobic exercise can all help.

Exercise 3: Noticing body sensations

If you are able to bring your observing self to certain experiences and notice muscle constriction, shallow/quick breathing, or shaking, you are welcome to journal below your experience and any means you tried to respond. What was this like?

Mindfulness of present experience when it's really difficult!

You may have found the previous ideas interesting and helpful. Perhaps mindfulness has helped you be more consciously connected to immediate experience. Perhaps the idea of the observing self is creating a bit of space which allows you to *see* rather than just *be* a trauma response. However, we are realistic with respect to how tricky and powerful trauma symptoms can be. It's not unusual for people to say things like, *this mindfulness stuff... this observing self stuff...it may help other people, but if I am really struggling, I just can't make it work.* This is understandable.

You know how certain products are sold as 'extra strength'? There is a way of being mindful which is a bit like that. In exercise one you were being mindful of some task – *just* paying attention to whatever the task was. The mindfulness skill we are suggesting here works as follows: in addition to bringing your attention to present experience, you literally describe your experience in real time. You might call this skill *mindfulness of present experience with narration.*

We mentioned Donald earlier. He was the guy who gave us that fantastic metaphor to describe the way he struggles with traumatic memories. This was the metaphor about how he's standing in a pool trying to hold a ball underwater. He was due to pick up his daughter from primary school when he got triggered and began experiencing unwanted childhood memories. He needed to walk to his daughter's school, but he felt scared and confused. As he did what was necessary, he was mindful of present experience with narration.

> **"Okay, I'm checking to make sure the dog is in the house. Now I'm putting my sunglasses on. I'm opening the front door and now I'm closing it behind me. I'm walking down the path to the front gate and I can feel the sun on my face and it's warm. I can hear someone cutting the grass. I'm opening the gate and now I'm closing it behind me. I'm walking down our street and I can hear birds and my neighbour is putting out their rubbish..."**

Donald narrated his way mindfully all the way to school. His narration brings him back to the now, and the intrusive traumatic memories lose a grip on him. Recovery from trauma is not about suppressing memories or future worries, but about choosing when and how to deal with it all. Donald used mindfulness of present experience with narration because it was important for him to remain present and connected for his daughter.

Exercise 4: Mindfulness of present experience with narration

If you are really struggling and require an 'extra strength' application of mindfulness, you can try mindfulness of present experience with narration. You are welcome to journal any experiences below. How did it go? Was it useful?

Information on mindfulness meditation for those who are interested

We mentioned previously that there are two ways to apply mindfulness: mindfulness living and mindfulness meditation. Mindfulness living is where you apply mindfulness to life as you are directly living it. Mindfulness meditation involves a number of practices where you are focusing attention in a specific way, most often when sitting, lying down or walking. We have explored a few mindfulness living exercises in this chapter, paying special attention to the observing self, but have said little about mindfulness meditation.

In our experience, mindfulness meditation exercises may be more challenging as they require the individual to really slow down and let go of certain defences. Some of the individuals working with this Guidebook may be able to benefit from mindfulness meditation now, but for others, it may not be the right time in their recovery. The reason we do not specifically describe and encourage mindfulness meditation exercises in this Guidebook is we can't know who it's likely to be safe and beneficial for and who may be left more exposed to trauma symptoms.

If mindfulness meditation is something you are quite interested in and you want to learn more, there are numerous books and resources available. Jon Kabit-Zinn's *Wherever you go, there you are*[21] is a well-rounded introduction to mindfulness and a good starting place for many.

Joining a meditation or mindfulness group or class can be useful for some as you can be supported and guided by a teacher. However, if you are considering this, it can be a good idea to speak with the teacher first and make them aware that you have a trauma history and may be struggling with certain trauma symptoms. Explore whether the group is right for you. If in doubt, perhaps error on the side of caution. Extended meditation retreats are unlikely to be a good idea for those experiencing trauma symptoms.

If using mindfulness to support recovery from trauma is something you really want to go farther with, the safest approach can be to work with a clinician who has training and experience in mindfulness *and* working clinically with those who experienced trauma.

References

1. Csikszentmihályi, M. (1990). *Flow: The Psychology of Optimal Experience*. New York City: Harper and Row.
2. Csikszentmihályi, M. Abuhamdeh, S. & Nakamura, J. (2005). Flow. In Elliot, A. (ed.). *Handbook of Competence and Motivation*. New York: The Guilford Press. pp. 598–698.
3. Nakamura J. & Csikszentmihályi, M. (2005). The concept of flow. In Snyder, C. R. & Lopez,S. J. (Eds) *Handbook of Positive Psychology*. Oxford, UK: Oxford University Press, pp. 89–105.
4. van der Kolk, B. A. (2005). Developmental Trauma Disorder: Toward a rational diagnosis for children with complex trauma histories. *Psychiatric Annals*, 35(5), 401-408.
5. Boodoo, R., Lagman, J.G., Jairath, B. et al. (2022). A Review of ADHD and Childhood Trauma: Treatment Challenges and Clinical Guidance. *Current Developmental Disorders Reports*. 9, 137–145
6. Sitler, H. C. (2009). Teaching with awareness: The hidden effects of trauma on learning. *Clearing House: A Journal of Education Strategies, Issues, and Ideas,* 82(3), 119-124.
7. Kuban, C., & Steele, W. (2011). Restoring safety and hope: From victim to survivor. *Reclaiming Children and Youth*, 20(1), 41-44.
8. Rhys Davids, T. W. (1910). Dialogues of the Buddha (Vol. 2). London: Henry Frowde.
9. Kabat-Zinn, J. (1991). *Full catastrophe living: using the wisdom of your body and mind to face stress, pain, and illness*. Delta Trade Paperbacks.
10. Khoury B., Sharma, M., Rush, S. E. & Fournier, C. (June 2015). Mindfulness-based stress reduction for healthy individuals: A meta-analysis. Journal of Psychosomatic Research. 78 (6): 519–528.

11. Blanck, P., Perleth, S., Heidenreich. T., Kröger, P., Ditzen, B., Bents, H. & Mander, J. (March, 2018). Effects of mindfulness exercises as stand-alone intervention on symptoms of anxiety and depression: Systematic review and meta-analysis. Behaviour Research and Therapy. 102: 25–35.
12. Sancho, M., De Gracia, M., Rodríguez, R. C., Mallorquí-Bagué, N., Sánchez-González, J., & Trujols, J., et al. (2018). Mindfulness-Based Interventions for the Treatment of Substance and Behavioral Addictions: A Systematic Review. Frontiers in Psychiatry. 9 (95): 95.
13. Hopwood, T. L. & Schutte, N. S. (2017). A meta-analytic investigation of the impact of mindfulness-based interventions on post traumatic stress. Clinical Psychology Review. Volume 57, November 2017, Pages 12-20.
14. Joss, D. & Teicher, M. H. (2021). Clinical Effects of Mindfulness-Based Interventions for Adults with a History of Childhood Maltreatment: a Scoping Review. Current Treatment Options in Psychiatry. Volume 8, pages 31–46.
15. Treleaven, D. A. (2018). *Trauma-sensitive Mindfulness: Practices for Safe and Transformative Healing*. New York: Norton.
16. Lindahl, J. R., Fisher, N. E., Cooper, D. J., Rosen, R. K., & Britton, W. B. (2017). *The varieties of contemplative experience: A mixed-methods study of meditation-related challenges in Western Buddhists*. PLoS One:12 (5).
17. Ferris, T. (2017). *Science VS Podcast.* The podcast edition is entitled *Meditation*, in which the 'washing machine metaphor' is described.
18. Kabit-Zinn, J. (1994). *Whereever you go, there you are*. London: Piatkus.
19. Van Der kolk, B. (2015). *The body keeps the score: Mind, brain and body in the transformation of trauma*. London: Penguin Books.
20. Levine, P. A. *Healing Trauma: A Pioneering Program for Restoring the Wisdom of Your Body.* Colorado: Sounds True Adult.
21. Kabit-Zinn, J. (1994). *Whereever you go, there you are*. London: Piatkus.

Chapter 14

Getting Emotions on Your Side

"I can feel so angry about the dumbest things. Something will set me off,
and then my mind goes around and around, and after a while
I can't even remember what made me angry in the first place."
Marjorie

Childhood trauma is an emotional problem. If childhood abuse, neglect or abandonment had no impact on an individual's emotional experience, it simply wouldn't be the problem it is. In this chapter we will explore why people who experienced childhood harm often struggle with emotions.

So, what are emotions? In one respect, this may seem like a ridiculous question. Everyone knows what emotions are. Emotions are very much a part of us and we live with them all the time. On the other hand, emotions are a bit complex when we stop to think about it. Most definitions of emotion go something like this: *An emotion is a mental state that arises spontaneously and is often accompanied by physiological changes*. So, there are a few things involved in an emotional response. Something happens to trigger a response, either something in our lives or a mental event, such as a thought or a memory. There is some physical response occurring in our body. And, we are mentally conscious of the reaction. Because we are aware of these physical changes, we might label or describe this emotion, i.e. "I'm really *angry* at Sally for not inviting me to the party" or "I'm *anxious* about driving in this weather" or "that movie was so *sad*."

So, an emotion is the product of events, physiological changes happening in our bodies, and how we label or describe what's happening. Does trauma play an important role in how all of this occurs? Absolutely. As we saw in the chapter called *Childhood Harm and the Body*, a history of trauma directly affects how our bodies react to events. And, what we describe as our emotions are intimately connected to these body-based reactions.

If this feels hard to connect with, consider Reynold, a man who experienced significant physical and emotional abuse, as well as abandonment. During a session late in the day, a noisy cleaner was working in the hallway outside the consulting room. Every time there was a sound, the therapist noticed that Reynold would 'jump', sometimes looking over his shoulder at the door behind him. His therapist said, "Reynold, are you okay? You seem quite jumpy."

> **"Yeah, I'm okay. This always happens. I'm just very sensitive to noises like that."**

Reynold was actually minimising what a big problem this was for him. Reynold's body was automatically reacting to harmless noises in the hallway. Like many people who experience trauma, Reynold had a very sensitive 'startle response', meaning his body and brain react quickly to certain events. If he were to describe his emotions, he might use words like *anxious*, *scared* or *on edge*. His body and brain are generating emotional experiences today which are directly connected to a history of past abuse. Childhood trauma is an emotional problem.

As we will explore in some detail, those who experienced childhood harm got 'set up' to struggle with emotions. If you can struggle with your emotions, this chapter will hopefully support insight, encourage self-compassion and offer some ideas for coping.

Childhood harm and emotional difficulties

Everyone can struggle with emotional difficulties from time to time. It's very human. But, as we will explore, emotional difficulties can be more common and intense for many who experienced childhood harm. The way that people who experienced childhood harm relate to 'negative' emotions is often quite different from people who did not get abused or neglected. Some can feel frightened by their own emotional lives. This was true of Pete, who was physically and sexually abused.

> **"I'm scared my anger will get out of control. I don't want to hurt people or smash up my apartment. And I don't want to go back to prison either."**

Others can be fearful of being afraid. The experience of threat was genuine and significant in the past. As an adult, perhaps they have had panic attacks or suffered from distressing episodes of anxiety. As a result, anxiety is not seen as a normal emotion we experience when doing something new or challenging. Anxiety is viewed as a scary emotion – an emotion which is to be avoided. Everyone can feel low in mood at times. If you weren't abused or neglected, you'll probably see feeling low as part of life's 'ups and downs', and you'll be confident that things will pick up. But even normal low moods can worry individuals who have experienced bouts of depression. They are scared of going through *that* again.

Also, it's not just 'negative' emotions that can be challenging. This may seem counterintuitive, but many people who experienced abuse or neglect don't trust positive feelings. One individual we worked with captured this issue well:

> **"When I got into art school I was so happy... for about 10 minutes. And then... I just felt depressed. Actually, I felt empty. It was weird. Something good was happening, so why was I feeling so bad?"**

As we will explore, many people who experienced childhood harm are (yet again) at a disadvantage in terms of feeling confident that they can cope with their emotional lives. Understanding and managing distressing emotions is a skill we are not born with. Skills for understanding and dealing with emotions must be learned, just like any other skill.

You will note that we don't mention the emotion of shame in this chapter. This is because shame is such a significant and complex emotion that it deserves a separate chapter.

What is emotion regulation?

Put simply, *emotion regulation* is the process of understanding and responding to our emotions. It's sometimes referred to as *emotion self-regulation.* Emotion regulation can involve accessing emotions (often an automatic process), labelling or describing emotions, or modifying emotions. Emotion regulation is a part of everyday life. It's as common as breathing, walking or thinking. However, it's worth looking closely at this area because there is evidence that, through no fault of their own, people who experienced childhood harm can have a genuinely difficult time with their emotions.[1]

The language used to describe emotional difficulties sounds technical, but hang in there because there are some useful ideas here. Sometimes an individual may feel overwhelmed or 'flooded' by strong emotions like anger or fear. If this is happening, we can say that the emotions are *under-regulated.* This just means we haven't got sufficient control over our emotions. States of under-regulation can be frightening, distressing and confusing. The individual might feel out of control, and sometimes other people can experience the person this way. Natalie spent much of her childhood between a care home and a series of foster placements which never worked out. As an adult, she can get flooded by powerful emotions, especially if she imagines she is being neglected or abandoned.

"Jerrod was talking to the waitress about his stupid motorcycle. I went to the toilet because I just wanted to kill him. On the way back to the table I walked through an empty pool room. I felt like I wanted to scream and I picked up a glass and walked outside and threw it at a wall and it smashed. A car alarm went off and I sat down and started crying and I hated that I felt like that."

At the other end of the spectrum, some individuals may *over-regulate*, constrict or inhibit emotions. This might not happen by design, but these individuals are often cut off from their emotions, and they might feel flat or depressed. Some depressive states can be less an emotion itself, but rather a lack of access to emotions. As a therapy group member, Glen was often very quiet and appeared lost in a fog. During one session, he described what it feels like to have lost access to emotions, i.e. over-regulation.

"I'm not angry, but I don't feel happy either. I used to care about things like work. I'm just sort of... numb."

The term *emotional dysregulation* is used to describe states in which emotions are either under-regulated or over-regulated. While over and under-regulation of emotion can seem quite different, they are really 'two sides to the same coin'. They are different ways of experiencing emotional problems, which often have roots in past experiences of threat, fear or loss. And, while individuals who experienced childhood harm can have a tendency towards being under-regulated (overwhelmed by strong emotions) or over-regulated (emotionally numb), it's not this clear-cut. It is possible to experience either state at different times. And, by discussing emotional dysregulation, we are not talking about the normal emotional 'ups and downs' many people experience. We're talking about confusing emotional states which are genuinely unhelpful and prevent you from getting your needs met. Also, we are not suggesting that everyone is supposed to have some perfect emotional balance – everyone can have bad days and difficult emotional states. States of emotional dysregulation are more extreme and can relate to problematic anger, immobilising fear, depression, self-harming, dangerous behaviour, substance abuse and disturbed sleep.

Emotion regulation skills are simply the skills we use to understand and manage our emotional experience and all that goes with it, e.g. physical sensations, thoughts, impulses or behaviour.

Why people who experienced childhood harm may struggle with emotional dysregulation

We are not born with the skills necessary for understanding and managing our emotions. We have to learn how to do this. Infants and children are highly dependent on caregivers and their family environments to learn about their emotions and the way their emotional lives connect to their self-concept and relationships. People who experienced childhood harm were often at a disadvantage in learning how to cope with emotions and get their needs met. Below are five reasons why this can be the case. See what you can identify with.

Lack of a 'secure attachment' or emotional attunement

It's normal for children to feel emotions strongly. We have all been in a shopping mall or supermarket and witnessed a young child 'losing it' while a parent struggles to remedy the situation. Young children are often very emotionally sensitive, whether fearful of being separated from a parent, angry at a perceived injustice, or guilty of a misdeed. But a child's mind is underdeveloped and they have little experience of the world, so they are *highly dependent* on adults to help them understand and soothe distressing emotions.

As mentioned earlier, a child requires at least one relationship which is affectionate, close, enduring and safe.[2] In other words, when infants and children experience powerful emotions such as fear, anger, or guilt, they need a 'secure attachment' with a carer who can soothe and help them. A parent can calm and reassure their child through physical affection, comforting words, and an explanation of events. Through many such experiences, a child begins to 'internalise' the ability to soothe and calm themselves. Along the way, they learn about distressing emotions and how to cope with them. They are also learning to trust others to help them with painful emotions.

Related to the need for a 'secure attachment' is the notion of empathic or emotional attunement. It was the Austrian-American psychoanalyst Hans Kohut, writing in the 1970-80s, who emphasised the need for empathic attunement.[3] When a parent is empathically attuned to a child's emotional world, they understand the child's feelings and how those feelings are connected to the child's growing self-concept. Empathic attunement allows the parent to validate the child's feelings. Through repeated experiences of empathic attunement by caring adults, the child develops a *stable sense of self* through which they can understand and trust the feelings they encounter. As an adult, they may experience criticism, rejection, or insults, but they have acquired a sense of self which can often 'ride it out'.

Many people who experienced child abuse or neglect did not have a 'secure attachment' to a parent figure who consistently soothed painful emotional states or helped them understand how to cope. And, they did not have a parent figure who was emotionally attuned to their experiences. As a result, the capacity to understand emotions, 'self-soothe' painful emotional states, and trust others to help can be less developed. As adults, they may be less prepared to cope with distressing circumstances and the powerful emotions that come with them.

Problems with emotion regulation may have started out as way to get safety

For some children, having or expressing emotions wasn't safe. This was true of Molly, who we met earlier. She was emotionally abused and neglected by her mother.

> **"I learned pretty quickly that it wasn't a good idea to be sad or to cry. You'd get told *stop your whining, I'll give you something to cry about*, or you'd get a whack. And getting angry with my mom? No way – you didn't even think of that!"**

As an adult, Molly tended to over-regulate (over-control) her emotions. She often appears like she wants to say or do something, but she looks stuck and cut off from emotions which should help with self-expression. However, Molly had spent her entire childhood constricting or hiding her emotions. It just wasn't safe for sadness or anger to spill out. Over the years, emotional constriction (over-regulation) had been a means of survival, and today it was an automatic habit for Molly.

We met John earlier, a man who had been physically and emotionally abused by an alcoholic father. He'd done a few stints in prison as a younger man for theft and assault.

> **"I was so angry when I was a kid – always getting into fights in the neighbourhood or blowing up at school. I'd kick my desk over sometimes. I got suspended a lot and I know the teachers hated me. But I was scared most of the time. That's what people didn't see."**

John was scared and got hurt at home. He continued to feel afraid at school and in the neighbourhood, and his out-of-control anger was meant to protect him. This caused all sorts of problems. As an adult, fear and anger were always close to the surface and could get triggered easily. Fear and anger were under-regulated (under-controlled) for John, and this caused all sorts of social and legal problems. What had started as a way to get safety in childhood had led to serious problems with emotion regulation.

A bad emotional education

Many people who experienced childhood harm were simply never taught how to understand and cope with emotions and related needs; in fact, many were given bad advice.

Exercise 1: Emotional education

Some unhelpful instructions children can receive are below. You may have been directly or indirectly taught some of these instructions. Tick any which apply.

___ Don't trust others
___ Don't show weakness
___ Don't cry
___ Don't ask for help
___ Don't express anger
___ Don't expect anything from anyone
___ Don't show your emotions
___ Act impulsively on your emotions
___ Get them before they get you
___ Don't have any needs
___ Don't assert yourself
___ Conflict is terrible – avoid it
___ Fight anyone you need to

Learning through observation

Back in the 1960s, psychologists came to understand that we often learn from watching others and how they get rewarded or punished.[4] They called this form of learning 'modelling', and it applies to young children as well as adults. If we observe someone's behaviour and notice that they are rewarded in some manner, there is a tendency for us to copy the behaviour. If they are punished, we are likely to conclude that we shouldn't try to get our needs met like that. If a child grows up in a family where a parent is aggressive and appears to get what they want, they might identify with the aggressive parent and imagine they should get their emotional needs met in a similar fashion. Or, perhaps a child notices that other family members are submissive to avoid abuse; they may copy this behaviour to stay safe. Terry is a good example.

> **"My mother was an emotional nutcase. She was always the centre of attention and if she wasn't getting what she wanted she'd**

scream at everyone in the house. We were all terrified of her as kids, and my dad just wanted a quiet life. He never stood up to her, and he'd disappear a lot. I copied my dad. The problem is that I'm still doing it, and people don't respect me."

Possibly due to Terry's temperament, he watched and identified with his submissive father. If he was a different sort of person, he might have identified with his mother, who got (or tried to get) her emotional needs for importance and safety met through aggression.

Exercise 2: What were you taught through observation?
Did you learn how to cope emotionally and get your needs met by watching significant others? If so, how did this happen?

What did you learn about conflict?
Your childhood experiences may have led you to conclusions about emotions that made sense back then, but are less helpful today.

Exercise 3: What did you learn about conflict?
Tick the statement below which makes emotional sense to you. Don't tick the statement which you think is the correct answer, but the statement which *feels* true.

___ Conflict is bad because people get hurt, dominated and scared and nothing really gets resolved.
___ It's good to be able to have conflict because it's how people understand each other's views and needs – it's how things get resolved and people can feel closer later on.

Many people who experienced childhood harm tick the first statement because that is genuinely how they have experienced conflict. People got hurt or dominated, and the only resolution was that somebody 'won' and somebody 'lost'. Many simply believe that conflict must involve destructive expressions of anger, fear and guilt. Such individuals might conclude that conflict should be avoided, or, if there is conflict, they sure as hell have to win or limit the damage.

However, conflict is a normal part of all important human relationships, and differences in opinions or needs will occur. For some people, a feature of recovery is discovering that it's possible to have conflict in ways which support understanding, resolution, compromise and closeness. Choosing relationships with people who can manage conflict with sensitivity can be a feature of this.

Exercise 4: Why might you struggle with emotion regulation?
We described five reasons you may have been at a disadvantage. Tick any explanations below that are relevant for you.

___ I lacked a *secure attachment* with an adult who was *emotionally attuned* to what I was experiencing.
___ Problems with emotion regulation started out as a way to get safety
___ I had an unhelpful education about how to cope with emotions
___ Adults around me 'modelled' or showed me ways of managing emotions which were not helpful
___ I was taught or shown that conflict is dangerous and should be avoided

Two myths about emotions

You are welcome to agree or disagree with what follows. There are a couple of myths about emotions. The first myth is that *you should always trust your emotions*. Some people firmly believe this. They will say things like, how can your emotions possibly be wrong? It's not so much that emotions can be wrong. Sometimes we should trust our emotions and allow them to act like a good guide. However, other times emotions can be misleading or unhelpful. Saying you should always trust your emotions is like saying you should always trust people. Some people you should trust – other people you shouldn't. If emotions like fear or anger are based on a realistic appraisal of events, they can provide us with essential information and should be trusted. However, emotions like anger or fear can also be driven by past experiences of trauma and may not be realistic in our present circumstances (more about this in a moment).

The second myth is that *distressing emotions like fear, anger, guilt and sadness are necessarily bad or destructive*. It's understandable that people who experience childhood harm will believe that certain emotions are simply bad or harmful. Their experience of these emotions during childhood probably *was* bad. But emotions that *feel bad* can also be important and necessary, which we explore below.

The value of all emotions

Humans evolved as biological and social beings, and our emotions evolved right along with us. All emotions, whether they are positive or distressing, are designed to help us in some way. Being able to experience all emotions is essential for two reasons. Emotions (1) help us understand or 'read a situation' and (2) put us in touch with our needs and motivate us. All emotions were designed to be our friends. This can seem like an unusual idea for some people who, through traumatic circumstances, may believe that certain emotions such as anger or fear are simply harmful or bad.

Ginette grew up in a home where domestic violence was common. Her parents got into frightening arguments which could turn into physical abuse, and her two brothers often bullied her.

> **"I was at the recycling centre and this guy was complaining about having to pay to drop something off, and I had to get away. I went to the other end of the centre, into this shop they have there, and waited until he left. I don't like anger. If someone starts raising their voice, I just react."**

For Ginette, any expression of anger is scary, which is understandable. The problem for Ginette is that she is cut off from her own feelings of anger as well. In instances where Ginette is not being treated fairly or with respect, she can't access anger, and so she doesn't realise when she is meant to assert herself or express her needs. Anger is being over-regulated (over-controlled).

The chart below explores the helpful expression of certain distressing as well as positive emotions.

Chart 1

Emotion	Biological and Social Importance
Fear	Allows me to appreciate threat or danger. Motivates me to keep myself or others safe.
Anger	Allows me to appreciate injustice or unfairness. Motivates me to get needs met for fairness or to express my needs to others.
Guilt	Allows me to appreciate that I have harmed or let someone down. Motivates me to make amends or sort relationship problems.

Sadness	Allows me to understand that something has been lost or is missing. Motivates me to slow down, to care for myself or seek out solace from others.
Love/attraction	Allows me to know that I want to be close and connected to someone. Motivates me to seek or maintain a bond which can serve the purpose of connection, safety, care, or personal development.
Happiness/joy	Allows me to appreciate that I am having my needs met in some way. Motivates me to continue to seek experiences or relationship bonds connected to happiness.

So it's important to have access to all emotions because they contain important information. However, emotions such as fear, anger or guilt can be problematic for many people who experienced childhood harm. Fear can be so out of proportion to any actual threat (under-regulated) that an individual will withdraw from others or avoid interesting opportunities. Anger can get misdirected, stuck, chronic, or out of proportion to events. Guilt can be inappropriate, excessive, or stuck, i.e. an individual may feel guilty about events they weren't responsible for.

Emotion regulation skills

There are many different emotion regulation skills and entire books written on this topic[5,6]. What follows is just one perspective on emotion regulation skills, so if you think this area is important for your recovery, there are plenty of additional resources (see the recommended reading section at the end of the book).

States of consciousness characterised by positive feelings such as joy, pride, contentment, enthusiasm, or love don't usually require interference. Positive emotions often serve as feedback that we are on the right path and getting our needs met. The only exception to this rule might be instances where positive emotions are driven by substance abuse or behaviours which are in some manner self-defeating.

Emotion regulation skills are normally required when an individual finds themselves in a distressed or painful state (i.e. emotional dysregulation). In such a state, emotions can be overwhelming or out of control (under-regulated) or related to numbness, depression or alienation (over-regulated).

The emotion regulation skill below is 'trauma-informed', meaning that it was designed with people in mind who experienced past abuse, neglect or abandonment. It involves three progressive questions to help you reflect and respond to a difficult emotional state.

1. *Can you label the emotion?*
Many people who experienced childhood harm lacked a close and safe 'attachment' with an adult who helped them to understand and express emotions. As a result, it may not even occur to some people to consider what emotion they are feeling, and perhaps they were never encouraged to do this – maybe no one cared about what you were feeling. If you cannot confidently name the emotions you are experiencing, it's difficult to know how to think about your situation, what you need, or what to do.

Question one is this: Can you label the emotion you are experiencing? Can you give it a name? There are a few things that may help. A. What is the situation you are encountering? B. What's happening in your body? And C, are thoughts and impulses pushing you to act in some way? By labelling the emotion, you are slowing down and getting into your reflective or learning brain. Considering an 'emotion pallet' can be helpful. There are many examples of emotion pallets on the internet, and we have provided ours below.

- *Anger*: annoyed, rage, resentment, bitterness, outrage, hostile, exasperation, frustration, vengeful
- *Fear*: anxiety, dread, nervousness, terror, panic, edginess, apprehension
- *Sadness*: grief, loss, disappointment, sorrow
- *Depression*: alienation, despair, hurt, hopeless, loneliness, gloom
- *Guilt*: remorse, regret
- *Jealousy*: relationship insecurity
- *Envy*: desire, covet, sense of lacking
- *Dislike*: contempt, hate, resentment, loathing, aversion, repugnance, disdain
- *Disgust*: revulsion, repulsion
- *Numb*: shut-down, disconnected, detached, dissociated
- *Happiness*: joy, bliss, pleasure
- *Love*: affection, warmth, fondness, care
- *Contentment*: ease, comfort, relaxation

Sometimes labelling an emotion is straightforward. *Bob borrowed my car without asking, and I need to drive to the shop. I'm tense all over and have thoughts and impulses to yell at Bob.* Of course that's anger, an emotion we feel in response to perceived injustice – no mystery there. However, psychologists like Leslie Greenberg have taught us that labelling an emotion can sometimes be more complex.[7] Sometimes, what we feel on the surface is **not** the deepest and most relevant emotion. Can you recall the example of Natalie described above? Her partner had been talking with a waitress, and she'd smashed a pint glass against a wall outside a pub. She had clearly been feeling very *angry* at her partner, but anger had been more of a superficial emotion she was experiencing. By slowing down and reflecting on her body and thoughts, she realised that another emotion was hiding underneath the anger. Because her partner was talking to a waitress, she was *afraid* that he would leave her, something which had happened many times before.

Psychologists call the immediate and superficial emotions we feel *secondary emotions* and the deeper feelings lying underneath *primary emotions*. Sometimes the immediate emotion we are experiencing is all there is to the situation. We can identify and label that emotion, which is a good start to dealing with a state of emotional dysregulation. Other times, we need to ask ourselves: is what I'm feeling on the surface the most relevant emotion, or is there a deeper emotion I need to pay attention to? So, in labelling an emotion, using an emotional pallet can be useful. And, perhaps don't always take the emotion closest to the surface at 'face value'. Ask yourself – is this the truest or deepest emotion I need to consider?

2. Is my emotional state reality-based or is it trauma-based?

If a person experiences childhood trauma, it doesn't mean that every distressing emotion they experience is 'trauma-based'. If someone insults you or steals your phone and you experience anger, that's not necessarily because of your childhood trauma. Feeling anger or violation may well be realistic. That feeling of anger can help you understand that these situations are unfair and may motivate you to assert yourself. If you step into the road and become aware of a car coming at you quickly, experiencing fear is reality-based. If your child is very sick, it makes sense to feel anxious or worried. If your dog or cat dies and you feel sadness for a while, this makes sense.

However, there can be times when an emotional reaction is trauma-based. If an emotion is being driven by past trauma, it may be misleading or just really out of proportion to events. Once you have labelled the emotion you are experiencing, there are a couple of questions you can ask yourself. Is this the correct emotion for this experience? And, is the intensity of emotion I'm feeling proportionate to the situation?

Nancy never had a safe or close attachment with her mother and was abandoned by her father when she was five. She had a safe and healthy relationship with her partner Sally, but periods of separation could be difficult.

> **"Sally went out to her book club and I spent the whole evening feeling really upset. I was angry with her for going out and leaving me alone. I know it doesn't make sense, but I had these angry fantasies of ending our relationship. I was quiet when she came home and then I was so upset I couldn't sleep."**

Nancy had every reason to feel reasonably secure in her relationship with Sally, but childhood experiences of abuse and abandonment were driving the emotion of anger.

We met Brandon earlier, a man who was emotionally and physically abused by his mother and bullied at school.

> **"This work colleague of mine had set up a home cinema and he invited me and a few people over to have dinner and then watch a film. I'd never been to his place. When I'm anxious I get locked up – like I can't talk. I had a panic attack when I was waiting for the bus and I texted him and said I had a migraine."**

Brandon was pretty upset with himself that he didn't make the get-together. The emotion he was struggling with was clearly fear and panic. It's a new situation and an opportunity to develop friendships, something Brandon sorely needed. It's a situation many people might feel some mild anxiety about. However, Brandon's fear is really out of proportion to any threats. The intensity of emotional response was the clearest clue that past experiences of abuse and rejection are in play.

So, once you have labelled the emotion, the challenge is to explore whether the emotion is reality-based or trauma-based. Trauma is very good at convincing you that whatever emotion you are experiencing is 'the truth'. As Nancy sits at home while Sally is out at her book club, the idea that Sally will meet someone and leave her seems 'true.' As Brandon waits at the bus stop, the idea that he will have nothing to say and get rejected or humiliated seems 'true.' Assuming you are basically safe today, here is a truth that trauma doesn't want you to see: danger was real in the past but it's over now. In many ways, recovery is about your body and mind realising that the danger is over.

3. How do I want to respond to this emotional state?

How you respond to this question is very specific to your situation, so it requires reflection and creative thinking. At this point, hopefully you have been able to label the emotion or emotions – to give your emotional state a name. The emotional pallet can help if you are struggling. And, you've considered whether this emotional state is reality-based or driven by past trauma.

Only you can know what to do now. If the emotional state is reality-based, the emotion can be like a good friend, providing you with guidance. Remember, evolution designed us to have emotions for very good reasons, illustrated by chart 1. If you're scared and there is a genuine threat, find safety as quickly as possible. If you have been mistreated or are experiencing genuine injustice and feel angry, that anger is encouraging you to assert yourself. If you are sad in response to a loss, sadness is asking you to slow down, find support, or attend to yourself.

What do you do if you realise your emotion is trauma-based – if your emotional response doesn't make sense or is out of proportion to events? This is complicated, and no simple answer can be provided here. In fact, much of the recovery section of the Guidebook comes at this question in one manner or another. However, we will mention a couple of ideas as 'food for thought'. The way you respond to any situation involves how you decide to *think* and what you *are going to do*. Our tools for responding include our minds and our behaviour. As mentioned, what this means is specific to your situation. However, there is a general point that is true for almost every emotion which is being driven by past trauma. If an emotional reaction to a situation is trauma-based, what you are searching for can be described in one word – *reassurance*. If the trauma-based emotion is fear, you want reassurance that you are reasonably safe. If the trauma-based reaction is jealousy, you need reassurance that you have value too. If the trauma-based reaction is rage, you want reassurance that it will be okay. If the reaction is trauma-based guilt, you need reassurance that you are not responsible. If trauma drives numbness and you feel dead inside, you need reassurance that it's safe to feel again and start moving.

So if the emotional reaction is trauma-based, the question you are often exploring is *how do I find reassurance?* How you find safety or reassurance in any situation is a big question, and we would be doing you an injustice by providing a simplistic answer here. It's a question which will get explored as we go along and from several different perspectives. However, the skill below allows you to begin bringing your creative thinking to this question.

Exercise 5: Three questions in your wallet, purse or pocket

The emotion regulation skill we have described asks you to reflect on three questions in relation to a particular situation. These are:

1. Can you label the emotion?
2. Is my emotional state reality-based or is it trauma-based?
3. How do I want to respond to this emotional state?

You can do this exercise in a couple of ways, and it might help to use both methods. Right now, you can think about a time when you were experiencing a difficult emotional state. If you can manage it, allow some images to come to mind of what happened and its effect on you. You can then progressively consider the three questions above with respect to this memory. Because you are working with a memory, you may need to rephrase the third question to: how should I have responded to the emotional state? Then, you can do some journaling with these three questions (see below).

The other way to do this exercise is *in real time*, right in the context of your life as it's happening to you. You can write or print out the three questions above and keep them handy in your wallet, purse or pocket. If something occurs and you experience a distressing emotional state, you can pull out the questions and try to work with them, doing some writing if possible. This encourages you to slow down and reflect, and can help you get out of the reactive survival brain and into your learning brain.

If you find this exercise straightforward and helpful, we are pleased. However, it's not unusual for those who experienced childhood harm to find it challenging or confusing. If this happens, we recommend that you are patient with yourself. Keep bringing the three questions to new situations. You will likely begin to see patterns, and these patterns can eventually encourage insight. Talk to others you trust if you can. It's a process which requires experimentation, time and creativity.

1. Can you label the emotion?

2. Is my emotional state reality-based or is it trauma-based?

3. How do I want to respond to this emotional state?

References

1. Ehring, T. & Quack, D. (2010). Emotion regulation difficulties in trauma survivors: The role of trauma type and PTSD severity. *Behavior Therapy*, 41(4),587-598.
2. Brown, D. (2009). Assessment of attachment and abuse history, and adult attachment style. In C. A. Cortious & J. D. Ford (Eds.), *Treating complex traumatic stress disorders* (pp. 124-144). New York: Guilford.
3. Kohut, H. (2009). *The analysis of the self: A systematic approach to the psychoanalytic treatment of narcissistic personality disorders.* Chicago: University of Chicago Press.
4. Bandura, A. (1963). *Social learning and personality development*. New York: Holt, Reinhart, and Winston.
5. McKay, M. and Wood, J. C. (2019). *The Dialectical Behavior Therapy Skills Workbook: Practical DBT Exercises for Learning Mindfulness, Interpersonal Effectiveness, Emotion Regulation, and Distress Tolerance*. Oakland: New Harbinger.
6. Spradlin, S. E. (2003). *Don't Let Your Emotions Run Your Life: How Dialectical Behavior Therapy Can Put You in Control Paperback*. Oakland: New Harbinger.
7. Elliott, R., Watson, J. C., Goldman, R. N. & Greenburg, L. S. (2004). *Learning Emotion-Focused Therapy: The Process-Experiential Approach to Change*. Washington, DC: American Psychological Association.

Chapter 15

Healing Shame

Charlie: "I'm a bad person."
Therapist: "What makes you say that?"
(long reflective pause)
Charlie: "I don't know – I just feel that way."

You may be looking forward to this chapter, but it's possible you're not. Certain people who experienced childhood harm can feel uncomfortable even thinking about the role of shame in their lives. It can seem like quite a dark, unpleasant or complicated subject. If you don't have very positive feelings about this subject, we'd encourage you to take your time and stay with it for a couple of reasons. First, shame is a subject which deserves its own chapter. It's *that* important. Second, shame probably *is* a dark, unpleasant and complicated subject, but getting to grips with this feeling is usually an important and necessary step for recovery. While the first part of this chapter focuses on understanding how shame may operate in your life, the second part will actively support you in taking some steps in healing shame.

What is shame?

Shame is a negative emotion which occurs in relation to my sense of self. Shame is the felt sense of badness, defectiveness, or not okayness. However, to really understand this emotion for our purposes, we need to make a distinction between *normal shame* and *trauma-based shame*. And, it's useful to look at the difference between shame and guilt. If this all feels complicated, please stay with it. Understanding and dealing with this complex emotion can be a powerful tool for overcoming the negative impacts of childhood harm.

Let's look at what we will call *normal shame*. Like other negative emotions, normal shame developed as humans evolved over millions of years. Our capacity to experience normal shame has a survival function. Humans are a communal species, and our survival has always depended on being a member of social groups. Rejection and social isolation are a threat to our very survival. Our capacity to experience normal shame encourages us not to behave in ways which put us at risk of rejection from a group. We can even imagine the shame we might feel in certain situations, and this shapes our behaviour. I may have an impulse to have an affair with my assistant, but I imagine the shame I will feel if it all comes to light. I may have an impulse to steal a laptop from work, but I can imagine the shame I will feel if I am caught and get fired. If I feel an impulse to get really drunk, I may recall how ashamed I felt about my behaviour the last time I did that. The experience of shame, or even imagining shame, encourages me to engage in behaviours that protect me from rejection by groups. This is normal shame.

Like normal shame, *trauma-based shame* involves a sense that I am bad, defective, unworthy or not okay. However, normal and trauma-based shame are very different for two reasons. First, normal shame is simply a product of how our emotions evolved and is designed to help us stay connected to groups. Trauma-based shame is a product of abuse, and we will look at how this works in more detail in a moment. Second, normal shame is usually attached to a particular situation, like feeling ashamed because you stole that laptop from work and got fired. Trauma-based shame can appear to be attached to situations, but it's fundamentally an emotion an individual 'carries around' with them. Trauma-based shame is not really a sense that I was bad or defective with respect to a situation. It's the sense that my whole self is bad or defective. With trauma-based shame, it's not really about doing something specifically wrong – it's the sense that my whole self is wrong. Trauma-based shame will quite willingly attach itself to a lot of situations.

People who experienced childhood abuse can take shame with them everywhere they go, like you might carry around a suitcase. Some can feel a strange impulse to look for evidence in their lives that confirms that they are bad or inadequate. While this experience of 'badness' or inadequacy can express itself through our thoughts, some will say they can feel a sense of shame in their bodies. This is sometimes described as a 'bodily-felt sense of shame'. Physically and emotionally abused by his mother, Brandon described this sense of carrying shame around with him.

> **"I always have this feeling like I did something wrong, or someone is mad at me. Sometimes I look at people's faces and I wonder – can they see it? It's really not rational."**

Let's look at the emotion of guilt. Like normal shame, the emotion of guilt can be helpful. If I have upset or inconvenienced someone, I may feel appropriately guilty, and this can help me understand that I need to make a repair with someone or set something right. Here is what is important to understand. Unlike normal shame or appropriate guilt, trauma-based shame is **not** helpful. Trauma-based shame, resulting from childhood abuse, damages self-esteem, induces bad feelings, and undermines personal development.

Looked at psychologically and in the context of childhood abuse, trauma-based shame is a useless emotion.

In fact, it's worse than useless – it's destructive. A body of research connects trauma-based shame to a host of problems. When trauma-based shame becomes a part of one's sense of self, alcohol and drug abuse is more likely.[1] Trauma-based shame is also connected to eating disorders, domestic violence, and physical assaults.[2] Sadly, trauma-based shame is more common in people who contemplate suicide or engage in deliberate self-harm.[3] So, trauma-based shame needs to be seen as something which is getting in the way of your recovery. When we use the word shame during the rest of this chapter, we will be referring to trauma-based shame.

As we listen to people who experienced childhood trauma, we often hear 'the voice of shame' in their descriptions. It sounds like Barry, a man in his 30s who was emotionally abused and neglected by his parents before being placed into the care system, where things did not improve much.

> **"When I walk into a room I imagine other people look at me and think, *what's wrong with that guy*? It doesn't make sense that I should think that, but I do."**

It sounds like Marjorie, who experienced childhood sexual abuse.

> **"I have this male friend who is very huggy. He's a really nice guy and he hugs lots of people. But when he hugs me it just makes me feel... dirty. I want to go and take a shower straight away."**

Notice how Barry's feeling of defectiveness and Marjorie's feeling of dirtiness seem to be about events. Barry walked into a room of people – Marjorie was hugged by a male friend. But these reactions are not really about the events – Barry and Marjorie's shame-laden feelings are deeply connected to a sense of self that was shaped by childhood abuse.

Another feature of shame is that *shame wants to hide*. When people experience shame, they want to disappear, shrink away, or fade into the background. Many people we work with have managed to have relationships and feel a part of a community. But, many are disconnected from others and spend a lot of time alone. When shame has become entrenched in an individual's personality, this can help explain the relative isolation or lack of intimacy in the relationships they do have. It's understandable. If shame is felt as a sense of 'badness' or defectiveness, a person may worry that others will see these traits – that they will be 'found out'. If you recognise this shame-based impulse to hide from others, please don't despair. Shame is a problem you can work on.

Below is a summary of the three ideas we used to describe shame psychologically.

1. Normal shame and appropriate guilt are about a mistake or something you specifically *did wrong*. Trauma-based shame is a consequence of childhood harm. It may attach itself to certain situations, but you carry it with you, and it's a sense that your whole self *is wrong*.

2. Many 'negative emotions' can contain useful information. Trauma-based shame, as a consequence of childhood abuse, is fundamentally unhelpful and limits our development.

3. Trauma-based shame wants you to hide from others, making it difficult to feel a sense of connection or intimacy.

Signs of shame

While shame is a problem for many people who experienced childhood harm, the extent of shame a person *carries* can vary. How big an issue shame is can relate to the type and severity of abuse and neglect and how robust your biological temperament is. And, some individuals have had relationships in adulthood which have helped to heal shame to some extent, which can help. However, others have had further damaging experiences as adults, which only reinforces a sense of shame.

As mentioned, shame is a sense of 'badness', defectiveness, or not 'being enough'. However, on a day-to-day basis, shame can express itself in various ways, encompassing how you think about yourself and others and how you respond to situations. The questionnaire below presents a list of common shame-based experiences or reactions. It may give you a clearer idea of how significant a problem shame is for you.

Shame Questionnaire

Answer each of the questions below with a 1, 2 or a 3
Answer 1 if the issue is not a problem
Answer 2 if the issue is a moderate problem
Answer 3 if the issue is a significant problem

1. I don't feel comfortable when someone compliments or is positive with me ___
2. I feel responsible when things go wrong, even when it doesn't make sense ___

3. When I make a mistake, I can feel bad for hours or days ___
4. I spend a lot of time punishing myself with my own thoughts ___
5. I find myself imagining that I have upset someone or caused trouble, even when it probably doesn't make sense ___
6. I find myself apologising a lot, even when it's not really necessary ___
7. It's odd, but when someone is nice to me or helps me, I feel bad about it ___
8. I don't feel comfortable with eye contact or with people looking directly at me ___
9. I focus a lot more on my failures than my successes ___
10. I have negative feelings about my body or appearance which are painful ___
11. I often imagine that others are having negative thoughts or feelings about me ___
12. It can seem easier to trust substance misuse or other compulsive behaviours than it is to trust people (either past or present) ___
13. I can ruminate or obsess over past things I did which I think are bad ___
14. Whatever I do doesn't seem good enough to me ___
15. I can feel this need to avoid or hide away from others ___
16. I have this odd feeling like I'm an imposter and people will find out ___
17. As an adult I have a history of being in relationships with people who treat me badly ___
18. I don't like to ask others for what I need___

Add up the scores for all questions and place the total here ___

If the total is 18-25 this is an indication that shame is less of a problem for you.

If the total is 26-35, shame is likely somewhat of a problem and needs some work.

If the total was 36-54, shame is likely a significant problem and healing shame may well be an essential part of your recovery.

Exercise 1: Can you identify with the problem of shame?

Shame is a sense of 'badness', defectiveness, or not being okay, which can seem related to events, but it's more a general sense of how you feel about yourself. You have also been able to fill in the shame questionnaire above. Please reflect on the description and the questionnaire and consider the following question: how big a problem does shame seem in your life?

How does shame get generated?

If someone carries a lot of shame, they very likely were on the receiving end of shaming behaviours. Children are not born with shame. Shame is the product of experiences where children feel humiliation, powerlessness or worthlessness. In other words, shame is generated by verbal, sexual or physical abuse, and exacerbated by neglect or abandonment. The problem of shame in adults has been strongly connected to childhood sexual abuse and verbal humiliation,[4] as well as physical abuse.[5]

If abuse merely produced shame *during* childhood, that would be bad enough. However, the sense of shame elicited during childhood becomes a part of the individual's self-concept, and it tends to endure into adulthood. This is why shame today is less about some current situation and more a feeling about who you are.

We mentioned George previously, a man who experienced childhood sexual abuse and substantial bullying at school from peers and teachers. He told us about a deeply engrained traumatic memory which serves as a striking illustration of how shame gets generated.

> **"I can't remember what I had done, but my teacher told me to come up to the front of the classroom. He had actually made this paddle out of a piece of pallet wood. He beat me in front of the class with the paddle. It was... humiliating."**

Any form of abuse *normally* generates shame, and this is certainly true of sexual abuse. Due to the subtle grooming process used in many instances of sexual abuse, shame can seem especially confusing. Martine, mentioned previously, was sexually abused by a stepfather between the ages of 5 and 11.

> **"I didn't know that what was happening was wrong or that it didn't happen to other kids. He paid a lot of attention to me and it was nice to feel like I had a father like other girls I knew. But when I got older I began to know how wrong it was and then I felt disgusting because of what happened."**

The experiences of George and Martine illustrate powerfully why children are especially vulnerable to shaming experiences. If abuse occurs to adults who did not experience childhood harm, they may have a robust sense of self which can resist any inclination to feel shame. The adult may think, 'this is wrong – I shouldn't be treated this way'. A healthy sense of self is like a shield that protects us from abusive or shaming experiences. But a robust sense of self takes many years of development and much support from a nurturing carer. Children who lack a safe and supportive 'attachment' are unlikely to develop a robust sense of self which can resist shaming experiences. The shame just 'goes right in'.

Making sense of responsibility for shame

Many people who experience childhood harm struggle with the sense of 'badness' or defectiveness which are features of shame, but they can also feel responsible for these feelings. Not only do individuals think 'I'm bad or inadequate', but they can also think 'it's my fault I'm this way'. In other words, they imagine they feel a sense of 'badness' because *they are bad*, rather than seeing that they feel a sense of 'badness' because what happened to them *was bad*. One explanation for why they are 'stuck' with shame is because they are taking responsibility for the shame they feel, rather than being able to locate responsibility with the people who harmed them. Experiences of shame occurring in the present moment have become *disconnected* from the original abuse that underlies it. A feature of recovery is to see that shame *is* connected to the harm which occurred, and that you should not have been harmed.

There is a compelling metaphor which can help illustrate the role of responsibility as related to shame.[6] Suppose you have an attractive and good-quality record player, but the only records you have ever been given are badly scratched and warped. The music is going to sound awful. A child is like the record player. There is nothing wrong with the child. All the shaming messages which result from abuse are like the damaged records. The music is very painful to hear, but it's *not* the responsibility of the record player (the child); the problem is the horrid records (abusive messages/shame). But it's practically impossible for children to see the situation as it is. Children don't have the developmental capacity to understand that they are not 'bad' – that the 'badness' is in what is happening to them. Even as adults, people often still believe *they are* the scratched and warped records. And, it can then be difficult to imagine that other records even exist – that there are much better records which can play some really good music.

Jerry experienced physical abuse throughout childhood, and he really managed to see shame for what it was.

> **"Shame is just a way I got taught to see myself. It's only real when I allow it to be real."**

If you struggle with shame, it's essential to see that you did not originally generate the feeling of shame. The experience of shame requires *social circumstances* where you were shamed by others (most likely occurring through abuse). Here's a 'thought experiment' to illustrate this point. Suppose it were possible for you to grow up on a desert island where you had no contact with other human beings. You will certainly experience some distressing emotions like fear and loneliness. But how are you going to experience shame? No one has ever treated you in an abusive manner which induced shame.

Have you ever felt especially shameful in the presence of a pet? Unless you have a very strange dog or cat, the answer is normally 'no'. Why is this? Because pets do not treat us with behaviours which are shaming. The point of the desert island scenario and example of our pets isn't to suggest that we should have no relationships or only relationships with our pets. The point is that it's far better to have safe and caring relationships rather than shaming ones.

You are responsible for working to heal the shame you carry, but it's important to locate responsibility for shame with those who shamed you. Having the problem of shame is bad enough. Feeling responsible for the problem amounts to 'adding insult to injury'. The shaming experiences you encountered should never have happened. The record player was fine. It still is. You were just given some really bad records.

Exercise 2: Connecting shame to an abusive childhood experience

We are going to focus on verbal or emotional abuse as it is the simplest way to do this. Take a few minutes and recall an event from childhood where someone was verbally abusive to you in a way that induced bad feelings about yourself (e.g. feelings of defectiveness or worthlessness). Choose a memory which feels manageable. Imagine yourself as a child, during and just after the event, and get a good sense of how you felt about yourself *as a child*. When you've got a sense of those bad feelings, reflect on this question: can you still have similar bad feelings about yourself today?

If you can see that childhood feelings produced by abuse are the sort of feelings you can still have about yourself today, you are getting a sense of how shame became a part of yourself and how it still endures. Journal any thoughts below which seem relevant concerning this exercise.

Shame-based anger or aggression

At the outset of this chapter, we mentioned shame is a complicated emotion. Part of the reason for this is the relationship between shame and anger. We will describe this relationship here in a way we hope will provide clarity for you.

As mentioned, trauma-based shame is a sense of 'badness', inadequacy or 'not okayness' that a person carries around. In this respect, shame can be seen as anger directed at oneself. *I'm bad, worthless, pathetic, a loser*. It's not unusual to even hear an individual say things like *I hate myself*. So, shame can be seen as self-directed anger. For individuals with more of a submissive style of coping, it's possible that this is where all the shame-based anger gets directed - at themselves.

However, some people who experienced childhood harm may be more demonstrative characters. The childhood abuse they experienced means they struggle with shame as well, but they may cope differently. If they imagine they might be criticised or humiliated in a way which would trigger shame, they defend themselves through outward expressions of anger or aggression. This is why simplistic 'anger management training' often doesn't work for people who experienced childhood harm; such training rarely addresses the underlying trauma and associated shame.

John is a good example of how anger can be directed outward to defend against feelings of shame. We mentioned John previously, a man who had been emotionally and physically abused by an alcoholic father. On countless occasions, he had been humiliated by his father, and as a result, he carried a lot of shame (a sense of defectiveness and insecurity). John had planned to cook dinner for his family. He told us:

> **"Janet [wife] asked when we were having dinner. I said I don't know and then I'm getting angry at her about all the work I have to do to keep the house from falling down and I'm shouting and she's really upset and the kids can hear. I go upstairs and stand in the hallway and I'm shaking and thinking... what am I doing?"**

When we explored John's anger, things made more sense. John explained that he was going to make a chicken-based dinner, but he needed paprika and barbecue sauce, and he'd realised it was Sunday and the stores were now closed. He hadn't explained his oversite to Janet and he was afraid she'd be disappointed or annoyed and maybe the kids would be as well. Anger or aggression was a way that John sometimes defended against any criticism which might elicit the shame he had carried since childhood.

As mentioned in the chapter entitled *Emotions*, anger is an important emotion which can be useful as a self-protective response when you have been mistreated. But, shame-based anger, when directed inwardly or outwardly, can be confusing and unhelpful. Shame-based anger is like a coin with two sides. The coin itself represents childhood harm and associated shame. Just like a coin has two sides, the angry expression of shame can be directed at the self or the world. But, where ever it's directed, it comes from the same place. It comes from the historical harm you experienced.

There are three ways to identify when anger is based in shame and past abuse. 1. The anger feels out of proportion to events, 2. the anger seems to be about more than the current situation, and 3. the anger doesn't seem helpful. In the final section, we look at some ideas for beginning to heal shame. However, healing shame can also be thought of as healing shame-based anger.

Exercise 3: Your thoughts on shame-based anger

Can you identify with shame-based anger? In other words, can you feel anger which is out of proportion to events, seems to be about more than the current situation and doesn't seem helpful?

Healing shame

It's definitely possible to make progress at healing shame, but it's also important to be realistic. As mentioned, shame is less an emotion connected to particular events and more like a part of an individual's identity. So, shame can have some fairly deep roots. You can think of shame as 'the terminator' of trauma-based feelings. You can deal with it some days or in certain situations, but *it'll be back*. This should not be a cause for cynicism, but it's useful when dealing with shame to take the 'long-view'. Because shame is a part of your self-concept, you'll probably have to respond to it many times; but every time you do, shame may lose a little bit of its hold on you.

Shame-busting in three steps

In the same way people can take their phone, wallet or purse with them, many individuals take shame with them every day. This sense of shame likes to pop up and attach itself to many experiences. It's possible to deal with an experience of shame in three steps: detect shame, challenge shame/reassure yourself, and let shame go.

Step one of healing shame is developing your *shame detector*. This just means spotting shame when you are experiencing it. Whenever you suddenly feel some sense of inadequacy, defectiveness, unworthiness, etc… see it for what it is and 'call it out': "Aha - this is shame I'm feeling. I'm feeling this because people harmed me in the past." Keep in mind that you might experience shame directly, or shame might be hiding behind anger you are feeling towards others.

You can personalise and use your *shame detector* in whatever way works best for you. Adele experienced childhood sexual abuse, and we like how she went about it.

> **"I never thought of what I experienced as shame. I just thought that I was a useless waste of space. But now, when it happens, I just say *shut up stupid shame.* I have to say that a lot."**

Adele did have to say that a lot, and that's one of the challenges of developing and remembering to use your shame detector. Shame is not going to go willingly. Shame is like a bad tenant who makes a lot of noise, breaks things, doesn't pay their rent, and doesn't want to leave. To have any chance of getting rid of it, you have to see it happening in your daily life… again and again and again.

Shame is subtle and crafty, and there is a common problem that can 'throw off' your shame detector. Once you detect that you are feeling shame, it can seem very 'natural' to *rationalise it*. In other words, you may find reasons why you're supposed to feel inadequate or defective! You may think, 'I'm supposed to feel bad about me because… (fill in the blank with your favourite way of rationalising shame).

Ryan's words below represent a good example of how many individuals rationalise shame. Ryan was physically and emotionally abused by both parents and had isolated himself for much of his adult life. Following some months of therapy, he joined a poker group he had been avoiding for years.

"I didn't have much to say, so I just played poker. Everyone else was laughing and telling stories. They were all having a lot of fun. I felt so useless."

Can you see how Ryan rationalised the need to feel shame? He decided he was useless because he said less than the others. Unless you think undermining your confidence and impeding your personal development is a good idea, there really is no good rationale for trauma-based shame. Shame… is not your friend.

A healthy shame detector will also be able to distinguish shame from guilt. Recall that if you feel bad because you have genuinely upset or inconvenienced someone, that's guilt. You can often make some repair to deal with your feelings of guilt. Like guilt, shame involves having bad feelings about yourself, but in the absence of having inconvenienced, upset or hurt anyone. With shame, you didn't *do* anything wrong; you just feel you *are* wrong. Unless you think feeling defective or worthless is important, trauma-based shame is pointless.

Once you have detected shame ('aha, this is shame I'm feeling'), you can then *challenge shame/reassure yourself* (**step 2**) and *let it go* (**step 3).** How you stand up to shame depends on the circumstances and the particular expression of shame. Julie, an individual who experienced childhood neglect and multiple forms of abuse, was ten minutes late for her GP appointment.

"The receptionist told me to have a seat. When I was waiting I just felt so awful. I was so angry with myself and I felt sure my GP was upset with me. How could I have made such a mess of things?"

You can get a sense of the 'badness' or defectiveness Julie was feeling, and how it's less about the situation and more about the sense of shame she brought to the situation. However, once Julie detected that she was experiencing shame, she told herself, "I'm just ten minutes late to an appointment. I haven't done anything terrible and I was late because there was traffic works that I didn't know about. My GP is a kind person and she knows that I'm always on time so I'm sure she'll understand [**challenging shame/reassuring yourself**]. Now, stop beating yourself up about it and check your emails" [**letting go of shame**].

And that… is standing up to shame/reassuring yourself, and letting it go. But it's also Julie's way of dealing with that particular shame reaction which occurred in that particular situation. Responding to shame will involve some creative thinking on your part.

Some individuals have found it useful to write shame-challenging statements down on a card and then carry the card in a purse or wallet. If the idea of carrying statements seems silly, consider this: if you're going to carry shame with you, why not also carry some statements that can be used to stand up to shame? Why not level the playing field?

Avoid shame-inducing relationships – seek relationships which help heal shame

If you were shamed by people when you were a child, you may be vulnerable to getting into relationships with people who continue to induce or reinforce the feeling of shame (recall the chapter on re-traumatisation and relationship patterns). You might not even recognise that you are in a relationship with someone who is reinforcing shame because this type of relationship may seem 'normal' or what you deserve. And, if shaming relationships are familiar to you, you might feel uncomfortable or mistrustful in relationships which could help heal shame.

There is a fairly straightforward way to know whether you have a relationship with someone who reinforces the feeling of shame or who helps to heal shame. You just need to consider some questions: how do you feel while with them and just after seeing them? Do you feel better about yourself and life, or do you feel worse about yourself and life? Do you feel safe with them? This question works for all relationships, whether a friend, partner, colleague or family member.

The information in chart 1 can help you consider whether your current relationships reinforce or heal shame in more detail.

Chart 1

Reinforcing shame	Helping to heal shame
Speaking down to you	Speaking to you as an equal
Demeaning comments	Comments respectful of your feelings
Comments attacking personal attributes	Comments supporting personal attributes
Taking advantage of you	Respecting you
'Putting down' your views or personal projects or interests	Respecting your views or personal projects or interests
Not listening to you	Paying attention to you
Disregarding/discounting your views	Attending to your views
Not feeling safe with them	Feeling safe

Exercise 4: Considering your relationships in respect to shame

Reflect on the people you are spending the most time with and consider whether these people reinforce or help to heal shame. When thinking about these relationships, consider the main question we mentioned: when you spend time with them, how do you feel while with them and just after seeing them? Do you feel better about yourself and life, or do you feel worse about yourself and life? You can also refer to chart 1 to consider these relationships and use the space below for any journaling.

Reducing shame-reinforcing behaviours

We mentioned that shame often expresses itself as a self-perception of inadequacy, 'badness', or lacking worth. People who experience childhood harm seem especially vulnerable to behaving in ways that reinforce these self-perceptions. In other words, an individual's behaviour can help shame to stay stuck. The fact that this can happen needs to be seen with self-compassion and insight. After all, the emotional difficulties such individuals experience seem to require more extreme coping. Shame is part of an individual's sense of self, and anything deeply rooted in our self-concept wants us to keep going in the same direction.

We mentioned Jerry previously, a man who was physically and emotionally abused by his father, and you can see the way shame gets stuck for him.

> **"After work I often tell myself to stop at two or three pints, but then I just don't. When I look at my face in the morning I look like crap, and I feel like crap. I hate that I keep doing this."**

Marjorie's relationship to deliberate self-harm is also a good illustration of how shame can stay stuck.

> **"It's not like I want to self-harm, but there are times when I feel so awful and stressed that it can seem like I have to do it to feel some relief. But after I've self-harmed, I hate myself for having to rely on it. It makes me feel weak and pathetic."**

Substance abuse or deliberate self-harm are just two examples. It may work differently for you, but we are talking about any behaviour you feel compelled to do that leaves you feeling worse (more shameful). Compulsive eating, spending, gambling or sexuality can all represent shame-reinforcing behaviours.

We will mention one final example because it not only illustrates a shame-reinforcing behaviour, but it's just one of those discussions you never forget. Karen was emotionally abused throughout childhood. During one group session, she said, "I fall down the stairs a lot. Like maybe once or twice a month I just trip and go down the stairs."

Another member said, "that's awful. Do you get hurt?"

"Sure," said Karen. "Sometimes. It depends on how far I fall."

"Karen," said a therapist, "do you know why you keep falling down the stairs? Have you seen a doctor?"

Karen smiled. "Oh no, there's nothing medically wrong with me. I wear slippers and I just don't seem to pay attention to where I'm going."

This was a humorous moment in the session, but something serious was also going on. During further exploration, it was clear that Karen's lack of attention and self-care was not only causing her real harm but reinforcing shameful feelings about herself.

Exercise 5: Shame reinforcing behaviours

Can you identify any behaviours which serve to keep shame stuck? Are there ways you may wish to drop or reduce such behaviours?

References

1. Dearing, R.L., Stuewig, J. & Tangney, J.P. (2005). On the importance of distinguishing shame from guilt: Relations to problematic alcohol and drug use. *Addictive Behaviors*. 30 (7), 1392-1404.
2. Mills, R.S. (2005). Taking stock of the developmental literature on shame. *Developmental Review*. 25 (1), p. 26-63.
3. Brown, M.Z., Linehan, M.M., Comtois, K.A., Murray, A., & Chapman, A.L. (2009). Shame as a prospective predictor of self-inflicted injury in borderline personality disorder: A multi-modal analysis. *Behavior Research and Therapy*. 47 (10), 815-822.
4. Negrao, C., Bonanno, G.A., Noll, J.G., Putnam, F.W. & Trickett , P. K. (2005). Shame, humiliation, and childhood sexual abuse: Distinct contributions and emotional coherence. *Child Maltreatment*. 10 (4), November, 350-363.
5. Sekowski, M, Gambin, M., Cudo, A., Wozniak-Prus, M, Penner, F, Fonagy, P, & Sharp, C. (2020). The relations between childhood maltreatment, shame, guilt, depression and suicidal ideation in inpatient adolescents. *Journal of Affective Disorders*. 276 (1), November, 667-677.
6. The record player metaphor was described by Counselling Psychologist and Psychotherapist Agnieszka Dixon during an HTP group therapy session in May, 2021.

Chapter 16

Traumatic Core Beliefs: Getting to Know Them

"There are a few mirrors in my house, but I never look into them. Well, maybe for a second, just to be sure I'm not too much of a mess. I hate mirrors."
Tim

Understanding and managing traumatic core beliefs can be a powerful way for many to create a more positive and compassionate view of themselves. Getting to grips with traumatic core beliefs can also help with developing healthier relationships, feeling more confident in getting needs met and expressing one's unique abilities. This chapter will support you in developing an understanding of traumatic core beliefs. The chapter that follows will support you in developing ways of overcoming the negative impact of traumatic core beliefs.

Introducing traumatic core beliefs

The HTP draws on ideas and skills from several therapeutic traditions. The concept of traumatic core beliefs is most closely associated with what is known as cognitive behavioural therapy (CBT). The development of CBT got off the ground in the 1960s and 1970s. The two most significant figures are Aaron Beck, who created what became known as *Cognitive Therapy*,[1] and Albert Ellis, who developed *Rational Emotive Behavior Therapy*.[2] Cognitive Behaviour Therapy (CBT) is today an umbrella term which comprises the ideas of these original thinkers, plus many later developments.

What made CBT different from other approaches to mental health problems was its emphasis on the way an individual *interprets* events through their thoughts. Put simply, if something occurs, we have to give meaning to the event. We have to interpret the event, and we do this through how we think about it. But, the way an individual thinks about an event is subjective and may be very different from how somebody else will think about the same event. For example, if Bob and Janet do the same job and work for the same company and they are both made redundant, they might have very different ways of thinking about what occurred. Perhaps Bob thinks it's a disaster and Janet thinks it's probably for the best. And, how Bob and Janet think about redundancy will impact them in different ways, e.g. Bob gets depressed, withdrawn and drinks more alcohol, and Janet starts looking for other jobs and buys new clothes with her redundancy pay. The way we think about events affects how we experience ourselves, others and life. It's a simple idea, but one with powerful or even life-changing implications. As we will explore, the experience of trauma can have a significant impact on how we interpret our experience.

In the early days of CBT, there was a lot of emphasis on depression and anxiety disorders and the immediate conscious thoughts people seem to have (sometimes known as 'automatic negative thoughts'). This early version helped people with milder problems. However, it was less helpful for people who experienced childhood trauma and whose style of thinking occurred across many areas of their lives. CBT had to advance in a way which could help these individuals. Aaron Beck and his colleagues re-developed Cognitive Therapy to do just this.[3] And, a psychologist named Jeffrey E. Young and his colleagues developed Schema Therapy, a model which is well-suited to individuals who experienced childhood trauma.[4,5] Beck and Young realised that many people who experienced childhood trauma had a *style* or *pattern* of reacting to many events that went deeper than simple automatic negative thoughts. This deeper or more pervasive *style of thinking* was described as *traumatic core beliefs* or just *core beliefs*. The similar term *schema* is used by Young, Beck, and others.

So, what is a traumatic core belief? A traumatic core belief is a concept or an idea meant to help us understand certain psychological experiences. There are three features of a traumatic core belief. 1. A core belief is a deep theme which drives how a person typically experiences themselves, relationships or life; 2. A core belief was created through an interplay of experiences of childhood harm and biological temperament; and 3. A core belief can get triggered by many events and tends to drive how a person typically thinks, feels and copes. If any of this is sounding overly academic or hard to follow, please stay with us. Understanding how core beliefs developed and continue to operate in your life is one of the most powerful tools available for recovery.

In a previous chapter we mentioned *the adapted self*. The adapted self is who a traumatised child becomes to try and stay safe and get some needs met. There is a connection between the adapted self and core beliefs. We could say that the adapted self is made up of traumatic core beliefs. Or, it's core beliefs that keep the adapted self going. So, if you want to pull apart and dispose of the adapted self, understanding and dealing with core beliefs is important. We could also put it this way: if you want to get a better sense of who you really are when trauma is not in control, you will likely need to deal with core beliefs.

We will describe core beliefs in more detail in a moment. However, ideas are most meaningful when they are personal, so below you have an opportunity to fill in a questionnaire which can help explain how core beliefs operate for you.

Traumatic Core Belief Questionnaire

Rate each statement below with a number which describes how true or untrue that statement is for you. You're not rating each question specific to a given situation, but rather how true that statement seems across many different situations and over your life. Try not to agonise over the questionnaire – just go for your 'gut' response.

5 definitely true of me
4 mostly true of me
3 not especially true or untrue of me
2 mostly untrue of me
1 definitely untrue of me

1. People are likely to take advantage of or manipulate me ___
2. I am quick to imagine that someone might harm me emotionally or physically ___
3. I don't tend to feel safe in crowded places or with people I don't know ___
4. In general, I can't trust most people ___

5. I haven't really felt like people have understood or cared about me ___
6. Partners or friends seem more interested in their needs than my own ___
7. I haven't really felt important to others ___
8. I seem to imagine that relationships won't last or I will get left ___

9. I tend to think others will eventually see my flaws and reject me ___
10. I don't understand why people would like me or want to spend time with me ___
11. I have this sense that there is something basically defective about me ___
12. I talk to myself in quite punitive ways ___

13. I've often believed that I won't be able to cope with life's problems ___
14. I have a pattern of not trying at something because I imagine I'll fail ___
15. I tend to imagine I'm less capable than other people ___
16. I don't trust myself to make decisions. I seem to want others to do that ___

17. I don't know why other people seem to be so positive about life ___
18. I seem to latch onto all the bad news and pain in the world. Existence is pretty bleak ___
19. There just doesn't seem to be much point to life ___
20. I tend to imagine things will remain the same or get worse, rather than get better ___

21. I often imagine something bad is going to happen to me or people I care about ___
22. Life seems filled with danger like sickness, financial threats, etc… ___
23. I tend to worry about a disaster occurring ___
24. I have to do things in a certain way or keep things in order or something awful could happen ___

Scoring your questionnaire

How many core beliefs there are is a matter of judgement. For the purposes of this chapter, we have highlighted six that are quite common. For those who want to work in more detail with core beliefs (schemas), see the end note to this chapter.*

Add the scores for questions 1-4 and place the total below next to *people will harm me*
Add the scores for questions 5-8 and place total below next to *people will neglect or abandon me*
Add the scores for questions 9-12 and place total below next to *I'm inadequate or unacceptable*
Add the scores for questions 13-16 and place total next to *I can't cope; I will fail*
Add the scores for questions 17-20 and place total next to *life is pointless*
Add the scores for questions 21-24 and place total next to *life is unsafe and something bad will happen*

People will harm me	___
People will neglect or abandon me	___
I'm inadequate or unacceptable	___
I can't cope/I will fail	___
Life is pointless	___
Life is unsafe and something bad will happen	___

Scores below 11 represent little or no problem with this core belief
Scores of 11-13 may represent milder difficulties with this core belief
Scores of 14-16 may represent moderate difficulties with this core belief
Scores of 17-20 may represent significant difficulties with this core belief

Core beliefs in more detail

If your questionnaire suggests that you struggle with moderate or significant difficulties with core beliefs, this is not something to get depressed about, and it's definitely not something to feel bad about. There is evidence that people who experience childhood harm are more likely to develop painful core beliefs.[6,7] Also, it's possible to make progress in healing core beliefs (which is what much of the next chapter focuses on).

But, let's look in more detail at these core beliefs. Scoring core beliefs mathematically is just one way of seeing how relevant they are. The extent to which you can identify with the descriptions below is at least as important as what the math suggests.

People will harm me

People who 'carry around' the core belief that people will harm them are likely to have difficulty trusting others. They may be quick to imagine that others will deceive, manipulate or hurt them physically or emotionally. They can be hyper-vigilant for 'hidden agendas' or ulterior motives. They can be anxious with people they don't know and may avoid social situations. Being mistrustful of others in a biased way is often a natural result of having been abused or deceived in childhood. If people hurt you in the past, you are likely to imagine this will happen again.

People will neglect or abandon me

People with this core belief tend to imagine that other people will not truly care about them or meet their needs for love or affection. Because they expect that others will not really care about them, they may accept being neglected in their relationships because 'that's just how it is'. Abandonment is the ultimate expression of emotional neglect, so individuals may also expect that people will leave them or the relationship will end. In childhood, such people often experience emotional neglect or abandonment.

I'm inadequate or unacceptable

People who carry around this core belief have poor self-esteem and self-worth. They tend to see themselves as less desirable, unworthy, flawed or unlovable. They are quick to imagine that others have negative thoughts or feelings about them. They have a tendency towards self-blame when something goes wrong. They tend to talk to themselves in quite negative or punitive ways. They may carry around with them a sense of shame. Individuals with this core belief were often abused physically, emotionally or sexually. Children who are abused often feel to blame for the abuse, which forms the basis of a core belief of inadequacy in later life.

I can't cope/I will fail

Individuals who carry around this core belief lack confidence that they can cope with life's challenges, whether those challenges are educational, financial, occupational or just everyday problems. They are quick to imagine that they will fail if they try something and are rather avoidant of new challenges. They might be dependent on others they see as stronger as a means of coping. These people often had the confidence 'knocked out of them' during childhood through emotional or other forms of abuse. Abusive experiences and neglect convey a message to the child that they are *incapable and will fail.*

Life is pointless

Individuals who carry around this core belief tend to see existence as monotonous, meaningless, futile or dreary. If they come across an opportunity, they have a genius for spotting how it will lead to nothing of value. They are often pessimistic, critical and depressed. Beneath the view that existence is pointless is a perception that they have little control over improving their lives. We might have called this core belief "same shit-different day," except that's not very professional. Individuals who struggle with this core belief often did not have nurturing and enlivening experiences in childhood. They may have had to grow up quickly, or they grew up in situations which encouraged a pessimistic or cynical view of existence.

Life is unsafe and something bad will happen

This core belief is a counterpart to *other people will harm you*. Rather than feeling easily threatened by other people, this core belief relates to seeing life itself as dangerous. These individuals may worry incessantly that something bad will happen, and their worry can attach itself to any number of possible calamities – financial disaster or homelessness, illness, accidents and so on. They may have phobias (irrational fears), and some are inclined to obsessive-compulsive coping. Some can worry that they will be in 'big trouble', though they might not know how exactly. Such individuals were often abused or had chaotic childhoods where disasters really did happen. Life was not safe when they were young, so they are quick to imagine that the world continues to be a threatening place.

Exercise 1: Your thoughts on core beliefs

You've had an opportunity to complete a questionnaire and read descriptions of six core beliefs. You may have found that many or even all core beliefs are difficult for you. Or, you may see that there are particular core beliefs which seem especially challenging, while others are less of a problem. Please reflect on the questionnaire and descriptions and describe below your thoughts about how core beliefs seem to operate for you, i.e. are there some core beliefs which seem especially difficult? If so, why might this be the case?

Core beliefs and 'automatic negative thoughts'

It's useful to understand how CBT distinguishes core beliefs from 'automatic negative thoughts'. Automatic negative thoughts are the moment-to-moment thoughts going through an individual's mind. Core beliefs are the 'deeper' and more pervasive aspects of an individual's personality which act as the driving force behind many automatic negative thoughts. The word *automatic* is used because that is often how thoughts occur when we experience a threat. When a core belief gets triggered, people don't decide to think the way they do – the thoughts seem to come pretty much automatically to mind. When a core belief gets triggered, it typically causes you to experience the present as if it were the traumatic past.

If this sounds complicated, here is a straightforward way to think of it. One of the core beliefs your questionnaire explored is *people will harm me*. If an individual carries around a core belief that other people are likely to harm them, that core belief can get triggered by many different events. Sally was abused by her parents, sexually abused by a neighbour and then retraumatised in adulthood by three partners. *People will harm me* is an understandable core belief which has become a part of her. When this core belief is triggered, she will experience negative automatic thoughts specific to the current situation. If a friend texts her and asks if she can babysit, Sally may think, "she's just using me" (automatic negative thought). If a cashier gives her the wrong change and she has to correct him, Sally might think, "he tried to rip me off" (automatic negative thought). If Sally is at her book club meeting and notices two women speaking quietly to one another, Sally may think, "they're talking shit about me" (automatic negative thought). Even though the content of these automatic negative thoughts differs in each situation, the driving force underlying these thoughts is the same core belief (people will harm me).

However, it's important to point out that not all automatic negative thoughts are driven by core beliefs. For example, if you are approached by an aggressive man in a dark alley, and you think, "he might hurt me", this sounds like a healthy and reality-based thought. Automatic negative thoughts driven by core beliefs are *biased* by past trauma, and as a result, they tend to be unrealistic and out of proportion.

How do core beliefs develop?

The general view is that there are two interacting reasons why core beliefs develop. These reasons relate to the idea that we are all products of nature (our inborn biology) *and* nurture (our experiences, especially the quality of our childhood relationships).

Core beliefs develop due to mistreatment, neglect or abandonment (nurture). In a previous chapter you explored the 'messages' you received in childhood, either directly through what was said to you or indirectly through how you got treated. If the message 'you are useless' is conveyed to you through others' words or actions often enough, you absorb the message. This message is the basis of core beliefs such as *I am inadequate or unacceptable* or *I can't cope/ I will fail*. Childhood abuse originally caused the core beliefs to develop, and then the core beliefs took on a life of their own when the abuser was no longer there to send the messages.

There is also growing evidence that biological temperament (nature) plays a significant role in personality development.[8] In other words, some people are born with a biological temperament which makes them more vulnerable to abuse and neglect, if it occurs. This can help to explain why siblings exposed to similar experiences can be affected to different degrees. For certain people who experienced childhood harm, this is useful to know. Some people can feel like a failure because they seem to have been badly affected by childhood harm, whereas the impact on others they grew up with seems less significant. Biological sensitivity to trauma can help explain this.

Triggers

For those who experienced childhood harm, triggers can be anywhere. Triggers can be at the post office, some news item on the radio, the phone ringing, the mail arriving, a sudden noise, something your partner said, or the expression on a stranger's face. However, core beliefs are not constantly being triggered. Core beliefs can 'lie dormant'. They exist and are part of you because of the many traumatic events you experienced, but they are often waiting to be triggered. So, core beliefs can at any one time lie dormant, or they can be activated by a trigger. This is often why you sometimes feel better and more confident, and other times can feel awful, frightened, angry, ashamed, lonely, and so on. What will trigger a particular core belief will vary from person to person because it will depend on past experiences.

Pulling these ideas together

People who experienced childhood harm are more likely to find themselves encountering powerful and painful emotions, tortious thoughts and disturbing impulses. These difficult states of consciousness can seem both bewildering and overwhelming. One of the values of the CBT approach is that it encourages individuals to *stand back* and observe their experiences. In getting some distance, you can break down what is happening into meaningful parts. This can then allow you to feel a better sense of control. Feeling less bullied by the damaging effects of past trauma and more confident that you can handle your emotions and direct your life is important.

The chart below illustrates how experiences can be pulled apart in meaningful ways. This chart is general rather than relating to any individual's particular experience. Later in this chapter, you will have an opportunity to begin breaking down your specific experiences in ways which will hopefully be meaningful. Please look through this chart and see what you can identify with.

Chart 1

Core Belief	**Typical trauma history**	**Examples of triggers**	**Examples of automatic negative thoughts**	**Common painful emotions**
People will harm me	Physical, emotional and sexual abuse	Receiving criticism; unfamiliar social setting; being teased.	"they are talking behind my back,"; "I'll get ripped off"	Fear, anger, panic
People will neglect or abandon me	Abandonment, emotional or physical neglect	Friend does not reply to text; partner seems distracted or distant.	"I'll end up alone again"; "they don't care about me"	Sadness, fear, anger
I'm inadequate or unacceptable	Emotional abuse, neglect	Making a mistake, 'falling short', not being invited to an event.	"I'm useless, stupid, a failure"; "people don't like me"; I'm unacceptable."	Depression, sadness, shame
I can't cope/I will fail	Emotional or physical neglect, abuse	New situations or challenges; pressure; stressors; criticism.	"I'll mess things up"; "I'm not capable of dealing with this"; "best to quit".	Anxiety/fear, depression, shame
Life is pointless	Emotional and physical neglect; all forms of abuse	Getting out of bed in the morning; setbacks concerning projects.	"This won't work out"; "I won't be appreciated or recognised"	Depression, despair, anger
Life is unsafe and something bad will happen	All forms of abuse and neglect; abandonment; poverty; crisis and loses	Any small potential threat; changes to routine.	"I'll get ill"; "I'm in trouble with the authorities"; "I'll be poverty-stricken or homeless"	Fear, panic

Three reasons not to despair

If you appreciate that core beliefs are derailing your sense of self, relationships and personal development, this is a dilemma we believe can be viewed with some optimism.

1. Traumatic core beliefs and related automatic negative thoughts are not 'the truth'

Is the light on or off in the room you are currently sitting in? Putting aside some potential heavy philosophical arguments, you probably can feel fairly certain you know what's true about the light being on or off. However, much of everyday human communication is much more complicated. To understand what is 'true', we often have to make guesses or inferences about other people's behaviour, thoughts or feelings. Childhood trauma and the resulting core beliefs can encourage individuals to make guesses that are heavily biased.

Marta grew up in a family where abuse and neglect were frequent. She was invited to a work party. A part of her wanted to go, but another part didn't want to. We asked her why.

> **"Because they all hate me. They all joke around with each other and I'm always left out. The only reason they invited me to the party is because they have to. They don't really want me there and if I go I'll just end up on my own."**

When we explored Marta's relationships with her workmates, we could see evidence that some people liked and accepted her. But Marta's childhood experience of abuse and abandonment had created a powerful core belief that she was somehow inadequate and would get neglected or abandoned. Her description above is 'the voice' of at least two core beliefs: *I'm inadequate or unacceptable* and *people will neglect or abandon me*. These core beliefs were so strong that Marta experienced her automatic negative thoughts (e.g. "they all hate me") as 'the truth', rather than merely guesses she was making. And, with some exploration, it's clear these guesses were unfair and biased. Core beliefs can be so powerful and deeply rooted that many simply see related thoughts as 'the truth'.

Reason number one not to despair is this: appreciating that core beliefs and the automatic negative thoughts they generate are not necessarily 'the truth' offers individuals some 'room for manoeuvre'. If you can recognise when you are in the grip of a core belief, you then have some control over how you want to respond to it (more about this in the next chapter).

2. The pain is often in your thoughts

Not *all* pain is generated by my thoughts. If I accidentally hit my hand with a hammer or someone is threatening me, the source of physical or emotional pain is real. However, core beliefs and the automatic negative thoughts they generate exist in my head. And, these are *my* thoughts. They may have deep roots in many historical experiences of abuse, neglect or abandonment, and they might be triggered by something happening now, but the thoughts I'm having are *in my head*. This might sound like an obvious or even pointless thing to say. However, for many people who experienced childhood harm, the psychological pain they are feeling can seem to be caused by *events* outside of their control.

Many people we work with know the experience of ruminating for hours over some perceived threat or insult and the intense fear or anger it generates. In such states, an individual can imagine they are helpless because the cause of the pain seems to be 'out there' in another person or some event. In such a state, it's hard to appreciate how much pain is generated by one's mental thoughts and images.

Marion was abandoned by her mother at six and did not feel emotionally attached to any carer throughout childhood. When she discovered that her ex-husband had a new partner, she spent days in a state of anger and depression and ruminated constantly. It was hard work, but eventually she saw that so much of her psychological pain was being generated inside her head. We really liked her use of the word *liberating* in the quote below.

> **"I'd been so angry and distraught that I'd hardly slept in days. It was all I could think about. I kept imagining him with his new girlfriend. And then it hit me. I'm hurting myself with all of the thoughts and pictures in my head. I don't *have* to keep thinking about it. It was sort of liberating. It didn't just make the thoughts go away, but it made me feel like I had some control over how miserable I was going to be."**

Reason number two not to despair is this: you are the owner and proprietor of all that goes on inside your head. You can have *some* control over core beliefs and associated automatic negative thoughts because they exist in your head. We highlight the word *some* because we appreciate how very deep and powerful core beliefs are. The extent to which individuals can control core beliefs and related automatic negative thoughts does vary. Some individuals can develop substantial control, but it may be a much more difficult task for others. What's important is that people can move in a positive direction, and even gaining 10-15% more control represents progress.

3. The existence of core beliefs is not your fault

Our view is that individuals should take responsibility for managing core beliefs that generate misery, but the existence of such core beliefs is not the person's fault. If you glance over the descriptions of the six core beliefs above, you will note that at the end of each description we highlight the typical childhood experiences which generate each core belief. And, for some individuals, biological temperament may play a role. Harmful experiences (and sometimes biology) *are* significant causal factors of core beliefs. The existence of core beliefs is not an indication of some personal flaw or defect. Reason number three not to despair is this: the fact that you struggle with painful core beliefs is not your fault, so go easy on yourself.

Observing and recording trauma-based core beliefs

Thus far, you have been reading about core beliefs in a theoretical way. This can be a good start for many, but *your* core beliefs are not theoretical. They get triggered within your daily life and have a very real impact on your emotions, physiology, relationships and personal development. To get intimately acquainted with your core beliefs and all that goes with them, you have to *observe* them in action. In a previous chapter you worked on developing your 'observing self', and this capacity is just what you are accessing to notice core beliefs when they occur. The exercise that follows represents a structured way to use your observing self to track core beliefs.

We want to highlight an issue based on our experience of working with many people who experienced childhood harm. You may feel some resistance to journaling core beliefs. The resistance may express itself in 'forgetting' about doing it, deciding you're too busy, telling yourself that you already know all about it or worrying that you won't do it correctly (this last one applies especially to those with core beliefs such as *I'm inadequate or unacceptable* or *I can't cope; I will fail*). If you feel resistance to journaling, the reason might be as follows: core beliefs do not want to change. They are so much a part of an individual that successfully challenging them might seem about as likely as deciding you will be three inches taller. We can sometimes be more comfortable with what is causing us pain than with what might be otherwise, so changing might not seem possible or even a good idea.

Below is some journaling a person we worked with named Barbara did concerning three situations. Barbara was never able to bond with an alcoholic mother and was physically and emotionally abused by an older brother. How you journal situations in your life will be very specific to those situations and your core beliefs, but Barbara's journal serves as an example.

Barbara's Journal

Trigger (what happened?)	Automatic negative thoughts (immediate conscious thoughts)	Emotions, physical sensations, impulses	What is the core belief(s) driving this?
I'm sitting in the café and Martin is 15 minutes late. He hasn't replied to my text.	"He's not coming. He doesn't care about me and can't even be bothered to reply to my text. He's just another friend that doesn't give a shit."	Really tense and stressed. Anger. Frustration. Dejected. Sad. I want to leave the café.	People will neglect or abandon me
A letter from the job centre arrived.	"It will be something I can't cope with. They'll want me to do something I can't handle. I'll have panic attacks again."	Scared. Heart pounding. Want to run from this. I don't want to open the letter.	I can't cope/I will fail I'm inadequate or unacceptable
A teacher asked to meet with me after our class	"She's disappointed in me. I'm in trouble for something. They'll kick me off the course. This isn't fair."	Frightened, suspicious, angry. I want to ignore the meeting and just leave at the end of class.	People will harm me

Exercise 2: Journaling core beliefs

As mentioned, trauma-based core beliefs drive *biased and unrealistic* ways of thinking about yourself, others and life. Sometimes an interpretation (thought) about an event is realistic, and your feelings are in proportion to some disappointment or threat. In this case, you haven't unearthed a traumatic core belief. You're just doing some clear-headed thinking which probably contains some useful information. *Part of the challenge is to see the difference between reactions driven by core beliefs and reactions which are in proportion to real threats or disappointments.*

Here are three tips for using the journal below. First, the triggers do not need to be massive or represent some crisis – even small events can trigger core beliefs. The more times you can journal situations and reactions, the more practice you get at spotting historical trauma's biggest adversary.

Second, most triggers are events occurring in your life. But, a trigger can also be thoughts, images or memories in your head. This is sort of an 'internal event'. You can journal triggers whether they are external events happening in your life, or internal events happening in your head. You can find core beliefs either way.

Third, it's helpful to have a copy of the journal that you can take with you in a purse, wallet or pocket. You'll want to fill it in as soon as you think a core belief is being triggered. If a core belief is triggered, you're likely to be most aware of strong negative feelings, physical sensations and automatic negative thoughts. You can fill in the journal from left to right or in any order. You can start with emotions and automatic thoughts if you like, then work backwards to the trigger, and then the core belief. The next chapter will focus on healing core beliefs. All you need to focus on now is noticing and describing them.

Trigger (what happened?)	Automatic negative thoughts (immediate conscious thoughts)	Emotions, physical sensations, impulses	What is the core belief(s) driving this?

* Jeffrey Young's model of Schema Therapy (and Beck's cognitive therapy) use the term 'schema' to describe the pattern by which people react to stressful events. A schema includes not only core beliefs, but the typical pattern of emotional, physical, and behavioural responses as well. In this chapter, we have used the term core beliefs for simplification. Schema Therapy originally suggested there are eleven schemas,[5] and more recent versions of this approach have highlighted eighteen.[4] If you have found this chapter and the next helpful and want to work on core beliefs/schemas in more detail, we strongly recommend reading Young and Klosco's *Reinventing Your Life* (see reference below). While written in the early 1990s, it's still the best personal development guide we are aware of on this topic.

References

1. Beck, A.T. (1975). *Cognitive therapy and the emotional disorders*. Madison, CT: International Universities Press.
2. Ellis, A. & Greiger, R. (1977). *Handbook of rational-emotive therapy*. New York: Springer Publishing Company.
3. Beck, A .T., Freeman & Davis, D. D. (2015). *Cognitive therapy of personality disorders (3rd ed.)*. New York: Guilford Press.
4. Young, J. E., Klosko, J. S. & Weishaar, M. E. (2003). *Schema therapy: A practitioner's guide*. New York: Guilford Press.
5. Young, J. E. & Klosko, J. S. (1993, republished 2019). *Reinventing your life*. New York: Plume.
6. Messman-Moore, T. M. & Coates, A. A. (2007). The impact of childhood psychological abuse on adult interpersonal conflict: The role of early maladaptive schemas and patterns of interpersonal behavior. *Journal of Emotional Abuse*, 7, 75-92.
7. Crawford, E. & O'Dougherty Wright, M. (2007). The impact of childhood psychological maltreatment on interpersonal schemas and subsequent experiences of relationship aggression. *Journal of Emotional Abuse*, 7(2), 93-116.
8. Canli, T. (2006). *Biology of personality and individual differences*. New York: Guilford Press.

Chapter 17

Traumatic Core Beliefs: Taking Control

"I had this moment where it occurred to me, *I don't have to think like this. I can decide how I want to react*. It might not seem like a big deal, but it was for me."
Tom

The previous chapter offered an opportunity for you to develop an understanding of how you are affected by traumatic core beliefs, automatic negative thoughts and the painful emotions that come along for the ride. But learning about how core beliefs affect you does not in itself help you respond to them. This chapter explores skills for managing or even healing core beliefs.

Before going further, we need to offer a note of realism. Perhaps you recall our discussion of *neuroception* in the chapter called Childhood Harm and the Body. Neuroception explains how, at a subconscious level, our bodies continuously scan the environment, searching for signs of threat or safety. This helps us appreciate why a physical and emotional reaction is almost immediate when you get triggered. Learning about your core beliefs and developing skills to deal with them will unlikely prevent them from being triggered. So, what is critical is *how you respond* once a core belief and related emotions get triggered. We don't believe this should come across as pessimistic, for a couple of reasons. First, over the past sixty years, talented clinicians such as Albert Ellis, Aaron Beck, Jeffry Young and many others have developed skilful ways of coping with core beliefs. Second, with time and dedicated practice, the triggering of core beliefs can begin to lose its hold over you.

Problematic ways of coping with trauma-based core beliefs

Before exploring healthy skills for responding to core beliefs, we want to share some coping styles it's possible to fall into when core beliefs get triggered. Not only is it necessary to feel confident that you can respond skilfully when core beliefs get triggered, but it's useful to be aware of what can get in the way of your progress. There are three coping styles that can encourage core beliefs to remain stuck and powerful. In the 1920s, a psychologist named Alfred Adler identified coping styles referred to as *avoidance* and *compensating*,[1] ideas that Aaron Beck and Jeffrey Young developed. The third means of coping, *submitting*, was developed most significantly by Jeffrey Young.

Avoidance

Jason had been emotionally abused by his father and stepmother and then bullied in school. These experiences formed the basis for two powerful core beliefs: *People will harm me* and *I am inadequate or unacceptable*. At 22, Jason's main means of coping when these core beliefs get triggered is to *avoid* social situations. He doesn't work or attend school, only has a couple of online friends and spends his days playing video games. Avoidance keeps his anxiety in check, but he isn't meeting his needs for belonging, self-esteem, self-expression, or meaning. Unmet needs on this level are the source of the chronic depression he experiences.

But sometimes, it's not just other people that are avoided. It's possible to feel a need to avoid painful feelings such as anger, depression, loneliness and anxiety. Some individuals may avoid or numb such feelings with alcohol and drug abuse, self-harming, dangerous behaviours, unhealthy eating, other addictive behaviours, etc…

Another expression of avoidance is to never ask for what you need, confront a person or express yourself. Some individuals pay little attention to their needs and will not assert themselves. It's often a way of avoiding conflict or preventing others from leaving them.

Submitting

Jeffrey Young discusses another means of coping when a core belief (or schema) gets triggered, which he calls submitting.[2] Rather than avoiding, the individual just accepts the core belief. They see the core belief as 'true' and accept all the automatic negative thoughts and painful emotions that go with it.

Robert serves as a good example. He experienced all manner of abuse, neglect and abandonment. Robert had been playing cards with the same four male friends for years. One evening he was telling a story, and before he could finish it, a friend said, "Hey, Robert, does this story have a punch line or at least an ending." The other guys laughed, Robert made a face and went quiet, and they started playing cards. Had Robert not been badly abused and abandoned, he might have shrugged it off or found a way to assert himself. Instead, what happened was that core beliefs such as *I'm inadequate or unacceptable* and *people will neglect or abandon me* were triggered. All that evening and for days following, Robert kept thinking, "I'm boring and have nothing interesting to say" or "They aren't really my friends and probably don't want me as part of the card group" (automatic negative thoughts). He got quite depressed about it and felt rather lonely. Robert wasn't coping by avoiding people, places or his feelings. Robert simply believed that his core beliefs and automatic negative thoughts were true, and his feelings made sense to him. He couldn't look at it in any other way. He was *submitting* to the core beliefs.

Compensating

In a sense, compensating is the opposite of submitting. If I submit, I accept the core belief and related thoughts and feelings as true. I get rather immobilised by the core belief and thoughts. With compensating, I defend against the core belief by thinking or acting the opposite of what I really feel. Or, I might push the issues or feelings onto someone else. If this seems confusing, here are some examples. If the core belief *I'm inadequate or unacceptable* is triggered, I might project these feelings onto someone or something else ("It's not me that's bad or inadequate – it's you or the situation."). Or, perhaps I will compensate for feeling inadequate by bragging or embellishing accomplishments. If a core belief of *someone will harm me* is triggered, rather than just feeling scared and immobilised (submitting), I might act tough, become threatening, or try to scare someone else. Imagine how a peacock or a blowfish compensates when they feel threatened. If a core belief of *life is unsafe and something bad will happen* is triggered, I might compensate by checking for threats obsessively or throwing myself into compulsive rituals. If a *people will neglect or abandon me* core belief is triggered, I might act distant, decide I don't care about this person, or even dump them before they do it to me. With compensating, an individual often wants (unconsciously) for someone else to feel what they are feeling ("I'm not crap -your crap"; "I'm not failing – you're failing"; "I'm not unloved – you're unloved").

Compensating, as a means of coping, brings to mind the words of Queen Gertrude in Shakespeare's Hamlet: "The lady doth protest too much, methinks." Some individuals can cope through what Lublin and Johnson refer to as dumping.[3] Compensating, especially when we blame or frighten others, can sometimes take the form of dumping, i.e. 'dumping your stuff' on others.

Compensating, avoidance and submitting are probably rooted in human evolution. All animals will fight, take flight or freeze when feeling threatened. Fighting is related to compensating, flight (running away) is related to avoidance, and freezing is related to submission. These can all be good defences when we are genuinely threatened, but unhelpful when the reaction is trauma-based. Bessel Van Der Kolk uses different language, but he too is describing these three ways of coping.[4] He uses the terms *disengaged shutdown* (avoidance), *subservient compliance* (submitting), and *angry defiance* (compensation). These three coping responses seemed hard-wired into us, but you can use whatever language works best.

Exercise 1: Your reflections on avoiding, submitting and compensating

It's possible you cope through avoiding, submitting *or* compensating at different times. But perhaps you can identify with one of these styles more than the others. What are your thoughts about how these styles operate in your life?

What's the point of dealing with traumatic core beliefs?

What's the point of managing your core beliefs? For us, the point relates to something we've explored in different ways and at different times during this programme. Historical trauma and neglect mean that, as a child, you did not get your needs met sufficiently for safety, love and belonging, self-esteem, self-expression and meaning. Child abuse and neglect produce traumatic core beliefs, and these core beliefs can prevent an individual from getting these important needs met as an adult. Core beliefs, when triggered today, can sap an individual's confidence, induce unhelpful levels of anxiety and mistrust, and instigate feelings of being unwanted or unloved. Core beliefs can also be the driving force behind experiences that retraumatise individuals today. The point of dealing with core beliefs skilfully is this: managing (or even healing) core beliefs gives you a better chance of getting your needs met for safety, love and belonging, self-esteem, self-expression and meaning.

A core belief triggered: Mapping out the experience

Below is a map which describes what usually happens when a core belief gets triggered. Having the map below with you or in your head can be a good resource in case a core belief gets triggered… and you feel 'lost' in terms of knowing how you want to deal with the situation.

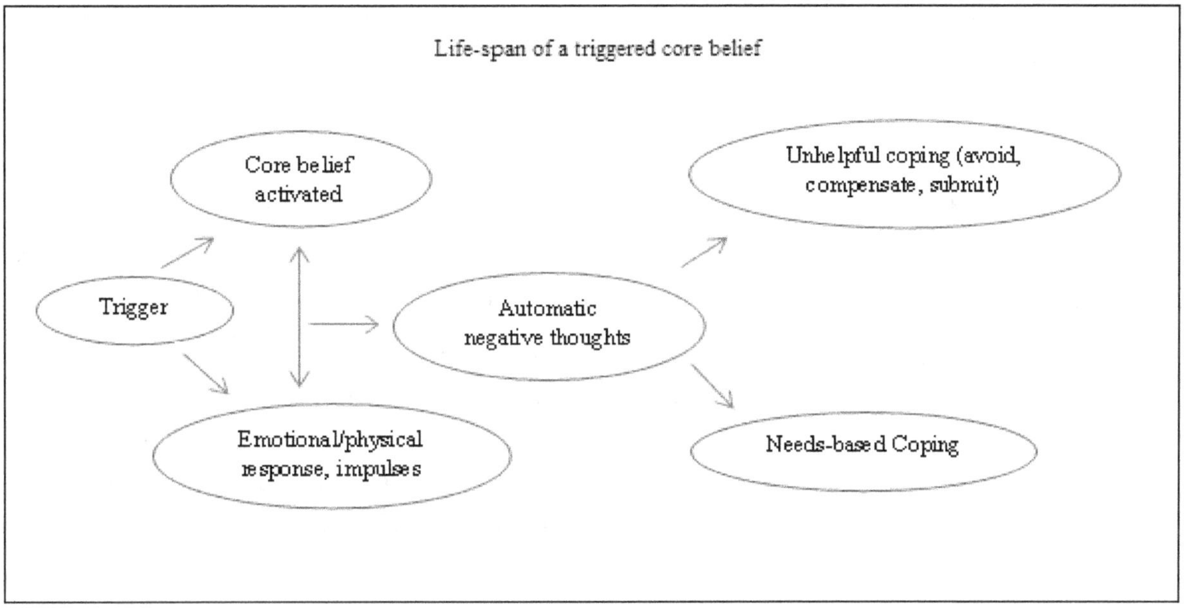

Let's walk through the map above, allowing the experience of Margaret to act as a guide. Margaret is a singer and guitarist. She was asked to audition for a band which consisted of four other musicians – all of whom were men she didn't know. Margaret had experienced multiple forms of abuse as well as emotional neglect throughout childhood. She also experienced retraumatisation as an adult, which included physical abuse from previous partners, one of whom was a musician. Today she is in a relationship with a man who does not harm her, but she still finds it hard to tell him how frightened she can get in certain situations or ask him for help.

Considering the map above, Margaret had an opportunity to audition with the band (**trigger**). A powerful **core belief** (*people will harm me*) was activated. Simultaneously, Margaret experienced fear and strong physical responses such as a pounding heart, shallow breathing and feeling shaky (**emotional/physical response**). Whenever she imagined auditioning with the four male band members, she'd think, "they are going to hurt me," and she had images of getting emotionally abused, humiliated and even physically or sexually assaulted (**automatic negative thoughts**). She cancelled one audition date, explaining that she had a throat infection (**unhelpful coping in the form of avoidance**). She felt awful about herself for cancelling, which likely triggered another core belief (*I'm inadequate or unacceptable*).

Margaret's experience clearly illustrates how past trauma creates a core belief that, when triggered, can generate all sorts of problems and make it difficult to meet needs. The one bit of the map we have not illustrated through Margaret's story relates to **needs-based coping**. The rest of this chapter focuses on those skills which support needs-based coping. And, before we finish, we will return to Margaret and see what needs-based coping looked like for her.

Needs-based coping

Unhelpful coping (often in the form of avoiding, compensating or submitting) tends to keep core beliefs powerful and results in unmet needs. *Needs-based coping*, as we are defining it, are ways in which an individual thinks or behaves which leads to needs getting met. And, needs-based coping will also weaken traumatic core beliefs. What represents needs-based coping will depend greatly on the situation (trigger) and the individual's present needs. There are several skills we can discuss that can support needs-based coping, but you will need to do some creative thinking regarding how you apply any skills to a particular situation.

Here is a simple way to know whether your response to any core belief represents *unhelpful coping* or skilled *needs-based coping*. If the way you think and act in response to a core belief means that you (and others) don't get important needs met, that's unhelpful coping. If the way you respond when a core belief gets triggered results in you (and others) getting important needs met, that's needs-based coping. It sounds simple on paper but only makes real sense when observing your core beliefs and coping through real-life circumstances.

Observing your reactions: The 'primary' skill

As a prelude to discussing skills for needs-based coping, it's useful to consider what we have control over. To be fair, there is much we have little or no direct control over. For example, whether our partner or friend will be in a good mood, the traffic, whether the bus will show up on time, the government, the weather, the genetics we were handed at birth, the economy, and so on. And, we often don't have much control over when or how our trauma-based core beliefs will get triggered. However, we all have some direct control over three areas of ourselves:

- The choices we make and our behaviour
- Our thoughts
- Our body

Observing your reactions to events is the most primary skill. This was the focus of the last chapter, and you looked at this in depth when we discussed 'the observing self' in a previous chapter. When core beliefs get triggered, it's not theoretical – it's personal! The automatic negative thoughts, emotions and impulses which follow can be powerful. In such a state, individuals can be *so close* to their experience that it's difficult to imagine they can direct their thoughts or actions.

The key is to get some distance from what you are experiencing – to observe it. The previous chapter covering mindfulness can be useful in this respect. If, for a moment, you can look at what you are experiencing as 'interesting news' rather than 'the truth' or a crisis, you have created some distance from the reaction. Recall our earlier suggestion that being driven by your emotional reaction is like being inside a washing machine. Observing your reaction is like being outside the washing machine and watching what's going on through the glass window.[5] It's not easy because when your core beliefs get triggered, you are likely to get whacked by powerful emotions and impulses, making it difficult to step back from your experience. You have to be able to slow down. Slowing down, stepping back, and observing your experience is the basis for all other skills.

So what is it you are observing? You can observe and identify what is triggering the reaction. You can also observe automatic negative thoughts and painful emotional/physical reactions; you can identify the core belief(s) you imagine are driving everything. These aspects of your experience will sound familiar because they were what you observed in the exercise from the previous chapter. In addition, you can observe impulses to cope in ways that are unlikely to help you meet your real needs (avoiding, submitting, and compensating).

The other thing you can get in touch with when you get triggered is your needs. We are not talking about what you need *in general*, but what you need *right now*, in any situation where a core belief is getting triggered.

Those who experienced childhood harm often struggle to know what they really need in any particular situation. What you need in any situation is something only you can understand, but Abraham Maslow (discussed earlier in the programme) gave us a good guide to universal human needs. What you need when a core belief is triggered is very likely a particular expression of the core human needs Maslow identified. The list of universal needs below is a slight modification of what Maslow said, but is true to his intentions.

- Safety (emotional, physical or material)
- Belonging (love, connection, intimacy, affection, friendship, community)
- Self-esteem (self-worth, self-respect, confidence)
- Meaning (self-expression, creativity, personal development, industry)

You can't know how you want to think about a situation or how you want to respond to a situation unless you know what you need. And what you *really* need might be different than the apparent needs which are driven by a traumatic core belief and powerful emotions kicked off by the survival brain.

John, a person who experienced multiple episodes of abandonment in childhood, can help us distinguish apparent needs from real/deeper needs. He had checked Facebook and discovered that there had been a party that he'd not known about. He felt really angry, and his immediate impulse was to defriend several people he knew on Facebook. He even felt a wish to smear the guy he imagined was mainly at fault on social media. On the face of it, he needed revenge and was likely to cope by trying to get it (compensating). But, when he could slow down and think it through (with help from his sister), he could see that his needs for belonging and self-esteem had been badly dented. Being in touch with these 'deeper' needs puts him in a position to respond that makes it more likely these needs would get met. This was fortunate because when he talked to a friend, he discovered he'd been invited to the party through an email that had ended up in a spam folder.

To summarise: when you are in the grip of a core belief and the resulting painful feelings and impulses, stepping back from the reaction is essential. It's the basis for gaining control, and feeling a sense of control is vital. Control is what you didn't feel when you were a child and probably later in life. So, what is important to observe is:

- The trigger (what happened to set this reaction off?)
- My reaction (emotions, physical sensations, impulses, automatic negative thoughts)
- Traumatic core belief(s) driving this reaction
- My real need(s) in this situation

If this seems like a lot of information to keep in mind, don't worry. At the end of this chapter, we offer another journal that pulls many of these ideas together and helps you apply them to real-life circumstances.

Skills for needs-based coping

Below we describe some of the needs-based coping skills we have seen work well for many individuals, but it's important to note that this is not a comprehensive list. The situations people find themselves in are so unique and varied that we couldn't possibly list every skill that may be helpful. So, we encourage you to be creative in discovering other healthy ways of responding to triggers.

So, you've been triggered, your experiencing painful emotions, you have some idea of the unhelpful coping you might fall into (avoiding, submitting, compensating), and you have accessed what you need. What can you do?

Challenging or reframing automatic negative thoughts

Core beliefs and the negative automatic thoughts they spawn often represent highly biased ways of looking at yourself, others and the world. Have you ever found yourself with someone who is *bullying you* - someone who is saying things that are hurtful, untrue and unhelpful? It's important to stand up to this person and set them straight, or get away from them. Core beliefs and the negative automatic thoughts they engender are like *bullies* that need challenging because they are frightening or discouraging you.

Sharon was a young woman who experienced childhood physical and emotional abuse. She gave us a memorable example of challenging negative thoughts that resulted from a core belief. Sharon had left a new and expensive mobile phone on a bus, and when she called the bus company, the phone could not be found. She raged against herself and her 'stupidity' for hours that evening, calling herself every name she could think of. She was in so much emotional pain that she started drinking vodka and then had impulses to self-harm. While literally holding a knife in her hand, she recalled the therapy she was doing. Losing her mobile phone (trigger) had elicited an *I'm inadequate or unacceptable* core belief, and she was directing a whole range of horrible automatic negative thoughts at herself ("I'm useless and stupid"). At that moment, she accessed what she needed: the lost phone and her reaction had seriously dented her self-esteem. She needed to get things into perspective to repair the damage to her self-esteem. She put the knife down and challenged automatic negative thoughts resulting from the core belief.

> **"Leaving my mobile phone on the bus was a silly thing to do and I should be more careful. But it doesn't mean I'm useless and a waste**

of space. It's just one mistake and a phone can get replaced. I'm doing better now in a lot of ways. I've stopped using drugs and I'm doing well on my course."

Sharon caught herself before falling into unhelpful coping (getting drunker and self-harming – a means of *avoiding* feelings). She was able to challenge and reframe the negative thoughts, and she felt better about herself, which she needed in this situation. Challenging thoughts means directly standing up to them. Reframing means looking at things differently. She did both.

Challenging and reframing is something many people have to force themselves to do for a while because it's so natural to experience automatic negative thoughts as 'the truth'. Challenging and reframing can work well as a means of responding to negative thoughts elicited by any of the core beliefs.

Ask for help

Many people who experienced childhood harm find this extremely difficult to do. The reason is that in order to ask for help, you have to show somebody that you *need* help. Being abused or neglected taught a lot of people that they should *never* show vulnerability or rely on anyone, because that would be dangerous. The problem is that everyone has to rely on others at various times for practical and emotional reasons, which means being able to show your needs (even vulnerability) and ask for help. Challenging core beliefs or thoughts is something you do for yourself. But sometimes we cannot get our needs met on our own, and we have to ask for help.

Jonathan came from a chaotic family and spent time in the care system. Whenever his wife left for her night shift, he felt agitation and an unreasonable anger. He felt as though he was being abandoned again, and he'd convince himself that his wife didn't care about him (core belief = *people will neglect or abandon me*). Sometimes skills such as challenging core beliefs or self-soothing could work for Jonathan, but sometimes there was just no way he could get his needs met on his own. What did he need at such times? He needed emotional safety, belonging and connection. Sometimes he coped with his fears by getting angry with his wife (compensating), but this would push her away. With encouragement from his therapist, Jonathan began explaining his background and vulnerabilities to his wife, which allowed him to occasionally ask for reassurance from his wife in ways which didn't interfere with her work.

Graded exposure

Graded exposure is one of those terms that sound perfectly normal to clinicians but ridiculous (or even rude) to the general public. However, graded exposure can be a powerful skill for responding to triggered core beliefs and difficult emotions, especially anxiety.

Anxiety or fear is a common problem for many people who experienced childhood harm. These individuals had genuine reasons to be afraid when they were young, and many had reasons to feel afraid later in life, especially if they were retraumatised. Graded exposure simply means breaking down a feared situation into steps that can be taken, one at a time. In other words, you are *exposing* yourself to what is feared, but doing it in a *graded* (step-by-step) fashion.

Kevin was physically and emotionally abused by his father, sexually abused by a neighbour and bullied at school. Now in his mid-thirties, he has a wife and two children and works as a painter-decorator. All things considered, he seemed to be doing well until two events conspired to throw him into an anxious depression. His father died, and shortly after, by chance, he saw the man who had sexually abused him. He had a couple of panic attacks, lost confidence, took sickness absence from work and didn't leave the house for two weeks. For Keven, recent events had activated core beliefs such as *people will harm you* and *life is unsafe and something bad will happen*, and he had fallen into avoidance as a way of trying to stay safe. He needed to feel safe again, reconnect with people and get back to doing what felt meaningful to him.

With help from a therapist, Kevin created a list of places and people, starting with more manageable ones and working up to those that were really frightening. Visiting his mother – going to the library – going out bicycling – seeing a friend – shopping at Tescos – high street shopping – going to the mall, and finally – returning to work. He felt anxious at every step, but being able to manage each situation gave him the confidence to deal with the next one.

That was how graded exposure worked for Keven, but it needs to be applied differently for each person who may benefit from it. It can be a good strategy, especially for core beliefs such as *people will harm you, life is unsafe and something bad will happen, I can't cope/I will fail* and *life is pointless.*

*The power of the word '**stop**'*

The automatic thoughts which are driven by a core belief can be really persistent. Even when you can identify them as unrealistic, trauma-based, or out of proportion to any real threats, these distressing thoughts can keep popping into your head. If it's hard to think about anything else, we can probably say you are obsessing. You want to get on with your life, but the disturbing thoughts won't leave you alone. What can you do if you recognise that the thoughts are trauma-based, over the top, and getting in the way of your happiness? You can face the thoughts and say STOP. Say it out loud or in your head. If you wish, you can also visualise a stop sign. Does this technique sound too simplistic to be useful? Not for a lot of traumatised people we've known.

You met Marsha before, a woman who had been physically and emotionally abused by her father. She'd sent a WhatsApp message to four friends the day before suggesting a social get-together, and no one had yet replied.

> **"I'm trying to do the simplest things – clean the house, pick my son up from school, sort the bills.... I just keep thinking what a bunch of assholes my friends are. And, I'm having fantasies of getting a bunch of new friends, and then I tripped on the rug and banged my knee. I was on the floor crying and that's when I remembered about just saying *stop*. The thoughts kept coming, but I'd say *stop* each time and try to focus. It didn't stop the thoughts from coming, but having a way of responding made me feel I had a little more control."**

The core belief mainly being triggered was *people will neglect or abandoned me* and her coping style was to *surrender* to the core belief. The stop technique gave Marsha enough space to access her learning brain. We felt she responded in quite a skilled way. She sent another message to her friends, one which was humorous but made a point. *'Hey gals – did you get my message from yesterday or have you all been kidnapped? What's up.'* Her friends started responding, and most of them had just been busy at the time she sent the message.

Past trauma often works like this. Our body and brain experience the present as if it were the past. It often does this by spitting out a stream of automatic negative thoughts which are driven by a core belief. Saying *stop* is a way of helping your brain and body understand that the danger is over.

Breathe and relax

If an event triggers emotions such as fear or anger, your body will react by pumping more oxygen and constricting muscles. Your neurology is preparing you to fight (compensating), run (avoidance) or freeze (submit). This is fine if you or someone else is genuinely in immediate danger. However, it's possible that a pounding heart, muscle tension and rapid/shallow breathing are responses to a core belief having been triggered. If this is the case, what you need now is reassurance and the feeling of safety. As discussed previously, you can directly get control by slowing and deepening your breathing.

"Don't let them win"

This isn't a skill, exactly. It's more of a perspective, but it's one we think must have validity because it has been suggested by several people we have worked with. Martine voiced this perspective while talking about her stepfather, a man who sexually and emotionally abused her between the ages of seven and thirteen.

> **"Sometimes I get so angry thinking about what he did and what a mess my life has been. I can get crazy with it and then I don't sleep and I can be horrible with Steve [partner] and my friends. But then I think – he [expletive] ruined my childhood – he's not going to ruin the rest of my life. I'm not going to let him win."**

Anger can be destructive, whether it's a storm inside an individual's head or expressed outward at others or the world. Martine seemed to be channelling her anger at her stepfather constructively. It was coming out as a stubborn refusal to allow the effects of her stepfather's abuse to ruin her life.

If all else fails...

Sometimes, the anger, frustration or despondency might seem so powerful that many of the skills mentioned previously will seem wholly inadequate. More likely, in the grip of a really powerful core belief, many people will lose contact entirely with skills that can help at other times. If you're getting overwhelmed, perhaps all we can suggest is to *stay in the moment and do the next thing*. States of consciousness are just that – they are states. They change. If your anger is driving homicidal fantasies or your despair is driving suicidal impulses, perhaps remind yourself that this state of consciousness will change. A horrible state of consciousness is immobilising and separates you from life and other people. So, see if you can reassure yourself that this can't last, stay in the moment and do the next thing… And, until it passes, try not to make it worse. Most people have enough experience of making things worse to know what we are talking about. Drugs/alcohol, picking a fight, self-harming, and so on. See if you can avoid making it worse until this crapstorm of a state of consciousness blows itself out.

And, if you do fall into ways of coping which make it worse, see if you can learn from it rather than punishing yourself. What's important is making progress – not pursuing perfection. Making progress usually involves a lot of missteps. You're not a failure – you just got side-swiped by a very powerful trigger and a persistent core belief.

Exercise 2: Skills for needs-based coping

The skills suggested here include challenging or reframing automatic thoughts, asking for help, graded exposure, breathe and relax, interrupting trauma-based obsessions with the word *stop*, 'don't let them win' and stay in the moment and do the next thing. Which of these skills seem potentially helpful for you to develop? Are there other skills not mentioned here you think can be helpful?

Responding to core beliefs through journaling

The journal you used in the last chapter was designed to help you identify triggers, reactions, and core beliefs. There is a blank journal for you to use at the end of this chapter which does this, but also encourages you to discover and apply needs-based skills. As an illustration, below is a version of this journal that was completed by Margarett, who we mentioned earlier in this chapter. If you recall, Margaret experienced multiple forms of childhood abuse and was frightened to audition for a promising band. She'd experienced retraumatisation as an adult from men that was compounding experiences of childhood abuse. Margaret's use of the journal was very specific to her situation, core beliefs and patterns of coping. Your journaling will be unique. Please examine Margaret's journal entry below to support your understanding of how to use the journal.

Margaret's Journal

What is the event which is triggering the reaction? This can be an actual event or an internal event, i.e. thoughts.	What's occurring inside? What are the distressing feelings, automatic negative thoughts, physical sensations or impulses?	What is the core belief(s) you think are being triggered?	What might be the unhelpful coping response in terms of thoughts or behaviours?	What do you need in this situation?	Use of needs-based coping. How do you want to think and act in order to get your (and others) real needs met?
I want to audition with this band. It's a really good opportunity.	*I'm scared and my heart keeps pounding. I keep thinking, "they are men and they are musicians - they are going to hurt or humiliate me. I'm useless not being able to deal with this"*	*It's mainly* ***people will harm me.*** *There is some* ***I'm inadequate or unacceptable***	*Avoidance. I cancelled on them once and told them I had a throat infection. I don't want to face this.*	*I want to feel* ***safe*** *(emotionally and physically).* ***Self-esteem*** *(I feel like an idiot that I can't face this).* ***Meaning and self-expression*** *(this is important to me).*	*I need to challenge the core belief and thoughts. "I'm safe. This is now – not what happened then". Use breathing. I asked my partner to drive me, but I went in on my own and he waited in the car.*

When a core belief is triggered, individuals often have thoughts and feelings that are heavily biased. Margaret was very sure these musicians were going to harm her, and her fear was really out of proportion to any actual threat. She used *a combination* of needs-based skills to help her manage the emotional reaction to resist falling into further avoidance as a way of coping. She challenged the core belief and automatic thoughts, focused on her breathing to reduce the anxiety response, told her partner what she was experiencing and asked for his help. The way in which her partner supported her was also a form of graded exposure (it was a step on the way to being able to audition with no support). She still felt fear, but her skilled response to core beliefs helped her face the situation. She wasn't chosen as band singer, but was asked to sing backup vocals for recording sessions. In this situation, standing up to core beliefs helped her get needs met for safety, self-esteem and meaning/self-expression.

The way Margaret coped and her use of the journal is useful as an illustration, but it's a fairly ideal illustration. In practice, it can be messier and more confusing, especially when someone is new to journaling. Journaling can be a powerful way to develop insight, but it can take some experience to feel confident about it.

Exercise 3: Journaling your experiences

The best way to develop your skills for dealing with core beliefs and getting your needs met is to practice in relation to the natural events arising in your life. You probably won't have to wait long for a core belief to get triggered. The journal below allows you to track everything discussed in this and the previous chapter. Here are a few suggestions:

- Keep in mind that the clearest indication that a core belief has been triggered is the experience of strong feelings, physical sensations or impulses. Fill in the journal as soon as possible. Making copies of the journal you can keep with you is often helpful. Also, it may make sense to fill in the journal from left to right, but you can do it in whatever order is most helpful.
- The page following the journal offers additional information that has helped many people reflect on their experiences and fill in the various parts of the journal.
- Keep in mind that the needs-based skills discussed in this chapter may or may not be what is going to help you in any situation. You may have to do some creative thinking or talk it through with others. If you feel you need help with any particular column, try and speak with anyone you trust.
- The more situations you journal, the more experience you will gain. When individuals have journaled several experiences, they inevitably see patterns developing. Reoccurring themes can include triggers, certain core beliefs, unhelpful coping impulses and particular needs. Seeing these patterns offers opportunities for increasing insight. And, the purpose of using the journal is to help you 'internalise' your capacity for observing and coping with core beliefs and other reactions. With enough practice, individuals don't need to actually use the journal.

Journal for responding to trauma-based core beliefs: When you feel strong and distressing emotions/impulses, a trauma-based core belief could be getting triggered. As soon as possible, sit down and fill in the journal below. Please use the information on the following page to help you fill in the journal in the most helpful way.

What is the event which is triggering the reaction? This can be an actual event or an internal event, i.e. thoughts.	What are the distressing feelings, automatic negative thoughts, physical sensations or impulses?	What is the trauma-based core belief(s) you think are being triggered? **See next page for list of possible core beliefs.**	What might be the unhelpful coping response in terms of thoughts or behaviours **(see next page eg. submit, avoid, compensation)**	What do you need in this situation? **See next page for core human needs.**	Use of needs-based coping. How do you want to think and act in order to get your (and others) real needs met? **See next page for some needs-based strategies.**

Trauma-based core beliefs and related thoughts	**Coping Styles**
People will harm me: "Somebody is going to humiliate or hurt me emotionally or physically. Someone will manipulate or take advantage." People will neglect or abandon me: "They don't really care about me. Or, I think I'm going to get left and end up alone. I'll be rejected." I'm inadequate or unacceptable: "I am bad, incompetent, useless, etc…I'm not as smart, attractive, lovable, etc… as others." I can't cope/I will fail: "I can't do this on my own. I'm going to mess things up. I can't trust myself to get this right." Life is pointless: "There is little reason to do anything. There is nothing but pain and drudgery. Existence is futile." Life is unsafe and something bad will happen: "Something awful is going to happen. I must stop a calamity from occurring, e.g. sickness, financial, legal,	Surrender: Giving into and accepting the core belief as "true". Being stuck or immobilised by the awful thoughts and feelings. Avoid: 'cutting off' from or avoiding the situation or feelings, e.g. avoiding people, places, challenges, using drugs/alcohol, self-harming, etc.… Compensating: 'Hitting back' or dumping your pain on somebody. Acting or feeling the opposite of the core belief. NEEDS-BASED COPING: Seeing the core belief and related issues for what it is. Thinking and acting in ways which will lead to you (and others) getting their needs met.
Some Needs-based coping strategies	**Core Needs**
❖ Challenging or reframing core beliefs or automatic negative thoughts ❖ Use self-compassion, self-soothing, reassurance ❖ Ask for help or assert yourself – avoid isolation ❖ Graded exposure to what is feared. Take gradual steps to beat avoidance ❖ Breathe, relax your muscles… ❖ "Don't let them win". ❖ If it's really bad - stay in the moment and 'do the next thing'. Let it pass Be creative. Use any strategies which work for you	Safety (physical, emotional, material) Belonging (love, affection, connection, community Self-esteem (self-worth, self-respect, confidence) Meaning (self-expression, creativity, personal development)

References

1. Adler, A. (1964). *Social interest: A challenge to mankind* (J. Linton & R. Vaughan, trans.). New York: Capricorn Books. (original publication 1924).
2. Young, J. E. & Klosko, J. S. (1993). *Reinventing your life*. New York: Plume.
3. Lublin, H. & Johnson, D. R. (2008). *Trauma-centred group psychotherapy for woman: A clinician's manual*. New York: The Hayworth Press.

Chapter 18

Relationships and Community

"My relationship… or as I like to refer to it… my *relationshit.*"
Dane Cook, stand-up comedian

We mentioned Sally previously, an individual who experienced childhood physical and sexual abuse. We were struck by something she said during a session.

> **"All I saw around me [as a child] were people that ignored each other, shouted at each other, hit each other or threw things around the house. There was no affection and no one really listened to anybody. Then I was married to that idiot for ten years. How would I know what a healthy relationship is?"**

The 'idiot' Sally was married to was a man who physically and emotionally abused her, which is a good example of retraumatisation. Sally's words serve to illustrate an important point. If much of what you experienced while growing up or during adulthood represents dysfunction or painful relationships, how would you know what a healthy relationship is? It's difficult to recognise something you have little experience of. What if someone asks you, *do you like the taste of poutine?* Unless you are Canadian, you are likely to say, *I have no idea – I've never had it.**

If a child experiences safety, affection, love and genuine care, they come to know what this is. As an adult, it's then easier to recognise if someone is providing them with the sort of good experiences they had in childhood. And, if they meet someone likely to neglect or harm them, it's easier to realise that this is *not* healthy because they have a basis for comparison.

Childhood trauma occurs within relationships, and recovery from childhood trauma also occurs within relationships. This is not the sort of news many people who were traumatised want to hear. Many people who experienced childhood harm would prefer to do their recovery work in silence and relative isolation. On the face of it, this can appear to make sense.

* Poutine is French fries (chips) smothered in cheese curds and brown gravy.

If you got hurt within relationships, why would you want to rely on relationships to help you recover? However, there is a problem with this approach which is captured by Bessel Van Der Kolk: "Managing your terror all by yourself gives rise to another set of problems: dissociation, despair, addictions, a chronic sense of panic, and relationships that are marked by alienation, disconnection, and explosions."[1]

Before proceeding, we want to mention the following: if you have experienced a pattern of unhealthy or 'toxic' relationships (past or present), this chapter may feel challenging. You may feel a range of emotions doing this work, such as anger, sadness, shame or just a sense of feeling upset. We encourage you to look after yourself, be careful not to go down any sinkhole of self-blame, and use any support available.

Why do relationships have to be so difficult?

It needs to be said that everyone who experienced childhood harm is unique, and we have known people who have managed to create safe and intimate friendships or partnerships. We have also worked with people who have very good relationship skills. However, many who experienced childhood trauma will find relationships complex or difficult, either currently or in the past. And, it's worth noting that one of the six diagnostic criteria for C-PTSD is *difficulties with relationships*. Such difficulties can take the form of unstable and painful relationships, feeling alienated within relationships, or periods of relative social isolation. Self-blame for painful relationships or the experience of social isolation is common. Being able to connect childhood harm to relationship problems in adulthood can help ease self-blame and encourage self-compassion. Below are three explanations for why you may have struggled with relationships as an adult. See what you can identify with.

1. People evoke anxiety and avoidance

The experience of childhood abuse, neglect or abandonment occurs within relationships – you were harmed by other people. So, it makes sense that being in public spaces, meeting new people, or intimacy may evoke anxiety. Something as harmless as being looked at by someone can trigger a sympathetic nervous system response. Normal social experiences which offer fun and opportunities to develop friendships or partnerships can be experienced with a sense of dread or fear. Those with a history of childhood harm don't plan it that way – it just happens. A person's body, brain and emotions signal danger in safe social situations. When prospects for closeness present themselves, rather than enthusiasm, the reaction can be an impulse for distance and protection. The consequence is that opportunities for intimacy or a sense of community can get missed.

2. The role of shame

As we explored in a previous chapter, shame is a common consequence of childhood harm. Trauma-based shame is experienced as a personal sense of inadequacy, defectiveness or brokenness. However, shame is *relational* – it was created with relationships and then is reactivated within later relationships. When people who struggle with shame meet someone new or intimacy begins to occur, they may think, *this person will discover how awful, repulsive or broken I am.* There are many ways people will then try to protect themselves from 'being found out'. They may create distance or end relationships, construct fake personas, or 'act out' their inner sense of defectiveness to test the relationship. None of this tends to happen by conscious design, but the problem of shame often results in feelings of alienation and social disconnection.

3. Relationship skills have to be learned

If someone wants to be a computer technician, nurse or artist, we assume they will need to learn a set of skills. For some reason, many people don't see relationships as requiring skills which have to be learned. But relationships require many complex skills, and no one is born with these skills. As children, we need to be taught or shown relationship skills by the people who are meant to be caring for us. If you did not have a caring adult who took the time to teach and show you relationship skills, you were at a disadvantage. It's also possible that the people you grew up with were unskilled within their relationships. So, just watching what was happening around you amounted to a bad education in relationship skills.

Exercise 1: Were you disadvantaged concerning relationship development?

We suggest there are three reasons why those who experience childhood harm may be disadvantaged in terms of developing safe and rewarding relationships. Appreciating these explanations can help you look at a history of relationship problems with insight and self-compassion rather than self-blame. Tick what you feel applies to your childhood experience.

___ I may avoid social situations or intimacy due to anxiety which is related to childhood abuse, neglect or abandonment.

___ I struggle with trauma-based shame. This means I imagine that other people have negative thoughts or feeling about me, and this undermines my social confidence.

___ I didn't get taught or shown important relationship skills when I was growing up.

Are there any additional thoughts you have on this subject?

Identifying 'toxic' patterns in others

There is probably no such thing as an individual with a perfectly healthy personality or who always relates to others with wonderfully healthy behaviour. We all have blind spots, can have bad days, and may not always relate in a 'perfectly' healthy manner. However, certain people spend much of their time relating to others with behaviour which can be considered 'toxic'. By toxic, we mean insensitive or ego-centric behaviour, or behaviours which are harmful or draining for others.

Some people who experienced childhood harm can have a difficult time identifying those who exhibit toxic behaviours. This is understandable. If the caregivers you grew up with related to you with toxic styles of behaviour, this may seem 'normal', or simply 'the way people are'. Later in life, you may accept similar toxic behaviours in others because (without a good basis of comparison) it's harder to recognise how 'abnormal' these behaviours actually are. Recovery requires being able to spot people who tend to exhibit toxic behaviours as well as people you can have safe and nurturing relationships with. When we refer to *relationships* in this chapter, this can mean any type of relationship, e.g. partner, friend, work or schoolmate, family member, etc.

Below are descriptions of what we identify as seven 'toxic' styles of relating. Before exploring this area, we need to make a couple of points. First, notice that we refer to 'toxic behaviours' rather than using the descriptor 'toxic people'. This is because we don't see people who relate in toxic ways as fundamentally bad people or necessarily incapable of change. Some people who relate through toxic behaviours may have been abused or neglected, may have been taught to get needs met in toxic ways, and may not be fully conscious of how their behaviour impacts others.

Second, it's not a simple matter of saying that some people have toxic styles of relating and other people don't. People are more complex than this, and toxic styles of relating can exist along a spectrum. All of us can at times relate to others with behaviours which are occasionally or to some extent toxic. And, people may exhibit toxic behaviours in certain relationships and not in others. For example, some people may express toxic behaviours within their intimate personal relationships but not at work or in other social contexts.

The main point of exploring the seven styles of toxic relating is to recognise if you have been or are currently in relationships with people who relate in toxic ways. The point is also to protect yourself and work on your development. But it's normally impossible for individuals to do this work without also considering whether they too can sometimes act with toxic patterns of behaviour. If you discover this to be the case, please don't beat up on yourself. There will be reasons why you fell into such styles, and it's something that can be worked on. You'll have an opportunity to explore your own behaviour at the end of this chapter.

As you read the descriptions below, consider whether you have been in relationships with people expressing toxic behaviours, either in the past or currently.

The controlling bully style

This individual can have intimidating, critical, and controlling behaviour; they generally have to have their way, and others must accept how they see things. They may put people down, make others feel defective, and act to control others' lives and relationships. In more extreme expressions, this style leads to direct physical or emotional abuse.

How do you know? The feeling state around this individual is one of *fear*. If you're in a relationship with someone who relates as a controlling bully, you are often 'on edge' or 'walking on egg shells'. You don't feel confident expressing your views or needs, and you may feel small or inadequate around this person.

The ego-centric neglecter style

This individual's style tends to see their needs, ideas, and wishes as simply far more important than yours. They don't really listen to you, are poor at genuine empathy or concern, and the focus of attention needs to mainly be about them, not you.

How do you know? The feeling state around this person is one of *neglect* or being unvalued. Your needs, views, wishes, etc... don't seem to matter much. Spending time with this person can leave you feeling unimportant or uncared for.

The manipulative exploiter style

This person may express concern, care or interest in you, but there is a hidden agenda. Rather than being fundamentally interested in you, they focus on what they can get from you. They may lie or present themselves or their intentions in ways which are deceptive.

How do you know? This style can present more covertly than other styles, so you may not know for a while. But the feeling state with this style eventually is one of *mistrust, frustration or anger*. You can eventually see that you are being treated as a 'resource' rather than a person.

The emotionally unstable style

If you're in a relationship with someone with this style of behaviour, it isn't easy to know how they will be from one day to the next, or even one hour to the next. They can flip between emotional states quite dramatically, going from happy to critical or angry, enthusiastic to despondent, and so on. The web of relationships they are a part of can seem like some daytime TV drama, and you can get dragged into these dramas.

How do you know? The feeling state around this person is often one of *anxiety* because you just don't know what's coming next. Their volatile emotional states tend to infect others around them, so you can end up absorbing their feeling states, and you may be expected to play a role in the relationship dramas they often seem caught up in.

The dependant style

With this individual, there always seems to be something wrong or an overwhelming dilemma they need help with. The problem is that if you manage to help them in one respect, more problems or needs suddenly arise. They may seem to appreciate your help, but their appreciation of you as a person depends on *you* helping *them*, which is largely a one-sided affair. Inevitably, you end up being the giver/carer, and they don't reciprocate in an equitable way.

How do you know? The feeling state you experience (sooner or later) tends to be one of *frustration* or *resentment*. There is a growing sense that your needs will just not get met.

The passive-submissive style

This individual has a very difficult time knowing and expressing their needs or asserting themselves. They tend to have poor self-esteem, and they feel guilty if they express their needs or views.

How do you know? It can seem nice to spend time with the passive-submissive style. After all, they are very attentive to your needs. But after a while, it can feel a bit unreal because you aren't quite sure you know who this person is, how they see things, and what they want. They almost seem to invite exploitation, and that can feel unsettling.

The nihilist style

Life can be rubbish and human beings can commit atrocious acts, but most of us can see the other side of the equation as well. The nihilist style, however, sees human beings as fundamentally bad and life as quite pointless. They seem to have a genius for pointing out the negatives of a situation, seeing the bad side of people or dismissing opportunities as a waste of time. *Nihilism can be an interesting place to visit, but you wouldn't want to live there.*

How do you know? The feeling state you experience if you spend enough time with this individual is *despair*, and the confidence you feel in yourself and life may begin to ebb away.

Exercise 2: Identifying 'toxic' styles

Scan back over the descriptions of the seven 'toxic' styles of relating, and ask yourself the following questions.

1. Am I *currently* in a relationship with someone exhibiting toxic behaviours?

2. *Thinking back over your life*, can you recognise any pattern of being in relationships with people exhibiting toxic behaviours? Is there any particular style of toxic relating that you have encountered more than others?

A strange question

On occasion we spontaneously ask clients with trauma histories an apparently straightforward question that can turn out to be anything but straightforward. The question is below. Have a look at it and see what spontaneously comes up for you.

Exercise 3:

Set aside any work relationships in respect to this question as we are only interested in non-work relationships. What is the point of relationships? Go with your 'gut answer'. Jot down whatever comes up for you, trying not to look ahead in the book.

Do not feel badly if this question seemed weird or difficult. A number of people with trauma histories find this question perplexing. Some may reply in a pessimistic manner, e.g. "There is no point to relationships." Some focus exclusively on their role in caring for others, e.g. "It's about looking after others." Some are just 'stuck' or lack confidence in answering, e.g. "I'm not sure"; "I don't know." Some feel defensive, e.g. "that's a pretty stupid question."

An explanation may relate to the fact that children (just like most mammals) are naturally 'wired' for spontaneous play. From the moment they get up to the moment they go to bed, the point of life is playing and having fun. However, in order to play a child needs to feel safe and have opportunities to play. Play can be solitary, but much of the time play involves relationships – other children and adults you play with. If you feel safe and cared for and have other children and adults you can enjoy playing with, you learn to see relationships in this respect.

So, later in life if someone asks you the question *what is the point of relationships?* your answer might be something like: The point of relationships is that they are fun or interesting. You see that essentially relationships involve 'playing', although the manner of playing may resemble something other than Lego or Barbies. Relationships are also for caring and being cared for, but they are fundamentally supposed to be fun and interesting.

A child exposed to abuse and neglect comes to see relationships as something you have to protect yourself from or survive, rather than opportunities for fun. It's understandable that as an adult, some will continue to see relationships the same way. Dinner parties or other social gatherings are not seen as opportunities for 'playing', but something to survive or at least get through.

Children who grow up with safety and love do not need to learn how to play – it comes naturally. For some adults who didn't have safety and love as a child it can feel like playing is something they need to learn or get used to. There is no simple or single way forward in this respect. Some people have told us that they learned how to play when they themselves had children who they needed to play with. Others have told us how they found playing with their dogs, cats or other animals to have helped in this respect. Some managed to develop a safe relationship with someone who was very playful. If you struggle to feel safe enough to 'play', perhaps just being aware of the issue is a good start in encouraging you to reflect on the challenge.

Identifying features of healthy relationships

The challenge for those who experienced childhood harm is not just realising when you are in a relationship with someone with toxic behaviours. It's also about identifying people who can offer opportunities for safe and nurturing experiences, and finding the confidence to develop relationships with them. This can be less straightforward than it may appear because people who experience childhood harm can feel jaded concerning relationships. However, there are many people who are largely capable of healthy relationships.

Below are features which can be associated with healthy relationships. For comparison, we contrast these features with related unhealthy expressions. These are not 'facts', but ideas for you to reflect on. Also, you may have additional ideas we neglected to mention, which you can add to our list. The first seven keys for healthy relationships apply to all manner of relationships. The final factor applies only to partnerships involving sexuality.

Chart 1

Healthy Relationships	Unhealthy Relationships
1. Feeling fundamentally physically and emotionally safe.	1. Feeling physically or emotionally unsafe. 'Walking on eggshells'.
2. Trust, open communication and basic honesty.	2. Deception, lies, hidden agendas, suspicion.
3. Being able to work through conflict with mutual respect for each other's feelings and needs.	3. Conflict is painful, people get hurt and there are frequently 'winners and losers'.
4. Mutual commitment to the relationship despite times of difficulty.	4. Relationship is fundamentally insecure with abandonment a real possibility.
5. Equity in the relationship with each person shouldering a share of responsibilities.	5. Inequity in dealing with responsibilities, usually with feelings of resentment.
6. Genuinely liking each other and wanting to spend time together. Affection and intimacy.	6. Not fun to spend time together and a lack of interest in one another. Lack of affection and intimacy.
7. Interest in supporting each other emotionally and with life projects.	7. Disinterest in one another's emotional well-being or life projects.
8. Sexual experiences that are safe and mutual (for partnerships).	8. Sexual experiences which are distressing or unpleasant for at least one partner (for partnerships).
9. Add other ideas important to you	

There are a couple of points which need to be made. First, the eight factors in the left column represent an 'ideal' relationship. Ideal relationships only exist in certain films or within the lyrics of some songs. Even good relationships, in times of stress, can fall into periods of difficulty and dysfunction. However, within a healthy relationship, there will be a core of trust, safety, mutual interest, affection and respect. This is the relationship's 'default setting'. A healthy partnership or friendship may hit some hard times where things get a bit dysfunctional for a while, but it tends to find its way back to the healthy default setting. A healthy relationship is like an ocean-going yacht with a solid keel. There will be storms and the boat will get tossed around for a while, but the keel will keep it from capsizing, and there will mostly be stable periods of sailing. In an unhealthy relationship, there are frequent storms, people are often scared, and there is a good chance the boat will capsize.

Second, one of the features indicated for a healthy relationship is trust, open communication and basic honesty. A phrase you will often hear concerning recovery from complex trauma is the need to 'break the silence'. This is much more than some bland cliché. We explored in a previous chapter how very common it is for children to keep what's happening to them a secret, and we looked at the many reasons why this occurs. Not being able to acknowledge what happened and its impact on yourself creates a divide within an individual. The HTP asks you to look at what happened directly and with insight, which may help heal this inner division. However, if you have a friendship or partnership that provides sufficient trust and safety, this can be the context through which you can 'break the silence' with someone else. If you are listened to, supported, and accepted, this can help heal the separation a traumatised person feels between themselves and the rest of the human race.

Exercise 4: How healthy are your relationships?

1. Scan through the list of healthy/unhealthy features in relationships in chart 1, and consider the following – how healthy are your current relationships?

2. Is your need for healthy relationships feeling relatively sorted at the moment, or is this something you need to work on?

Believing you deserve healthy relationships

The previous chapter on retraumatisation goes some way to explain why certain individuals are more likely to end up in unhealthy relationships. As discussed, children who were abused or neglected are more likely to experience further harm through adult relationships because: 1. It's what they expect to happen, 2. It's what they feel they deserve, and 3. It's what they are 'comfortable' with (i.e. they might feel uncomfortable being loved and cared for).

The issue of self-worth gets to the heart of why many people find themselves stuck in unhealthy relationships. So many individuals struggle to feel they deserve good relationships – relationships where they are thought about, valued and treated well. Shelly is a good illustration. She was badly emotionally neglected and then placed into care at the age of twelve. From age fifteen through her late twenties, she used heroin and had numerous sexual relationships with men. Therapy helped her see what had been going on.

> **"Men wanted to have sex with me, so I let them. Sometimes they would give me drugs or money, but I also did it because of the attention I got from them. For a while I thought maybe I did it because there was something messed-up about me sexually – that maybe I was a sexual masochist. But that's not it. The only reason I had all these temporary relationships with men who wanted sex off me was because that's all I thought I could hope for."**

In other words, Shelly never felt deserving of something better than being used by men for sex. Getting off heroin allowed her to think carefully about her past and how it damaged her self-worth. She needed to develop better feelings about herself before accepting that she deserved to be treated with respect and care. It was slow work, but feeling that she deserved to be in a healthy relationship was a cornerstone of Shelly's recovery.

We are asking you to consider to what extent you feel deserving of healthy relationships because unless you get to grips with this issue, you are unlikely to ever break a chain of unhealthy relationships. Even if you recognise that you are in an unhealthy relationship with someone exhibiting toxic behaviours, unless you feel deserving of something better, this insight probably won't make any difference to your life.

Exercise 5: Do you feel deserving of healthy relationships?

This exercise might feel silly or strange, but please humour us, and do it anyway. You are going to read out the statements below and pay attention to how you are feeling and any thoughts that occur. These statements relate closely to the features of a healthy relationship you saw earlier in chart 1. If you have the necessary privacy, it's best to read the statements out loud. After reading all the statements, you will have a chance to reflect on the experience. Keep in mind that the term 'relationships' can refer to any important relationship, e.g. partner, friend, or family member.

1. In my relationships, I deserve to always feel physically and emotionally safe.
2. In my relationships, I deserve feelings of trust, open communication and basic honesty.
3. In my relationships, I deserve to work through conflict with mutual respect for each other's feelings and needs.
4. In my relationships, I deserve a sense of commitment, even in times of difficulty. I shouldn't have to fear abandonment.
5. In my relationships, I deserve equity, with each person shouldering a share of responsibilities.
6. In my relationships, I deserve affection and intimacy – a sense of genuinely liking each other and wanting to spend time together.
7. In my relationships, I deserve to be supported emotionally and with life projects.
8. In my partnership, I deserve sexual experiences that are safe and pleasant.

Please answer the questions which follow. Did the things you were saying feel comfortable, right or self-evident, or did these words feel somehow wrong or implausible? Did you notice yourself having certain thoughts as you read these statements?

If you felt comfortable doing this exercise and the statements you read felt correct or self-evident, this is a good sign. It suggests that you believe you deserve healthy relationships. But if it felt uncomfortable to read these statements or if you found it hard to believe what you were saying, this suggests you have work to do.

No simple suggestion can tell you how to feel more deserving of relationships where you are safe, cared about and feel valued. For some people, just developing insight into the problem of not feeling deserving of healthy relationships is an essential step. This insight can *raise awareness* in the context of current relationships, as illustrated by Cloe.

Cloe had been abandoned by her mother at a young age and her father had been too busy with work and a string of relationships to women to care much about her. Cloe was currently in a relationship with a man who didn't listen to her, frequently put her down, forgot birthdays and spent time largely with his drinking buddies (his behaviour struck us as a mix of the *ego-centric neglecter* and the *controlling bully* styles). When Cloe came to appreciate how little she felt she deserved a healthy relationship, she began to relate differently to her partner's behaviour.

> **"Martin was sitting on the couch and I told him about something that happened at work earlier, and he totally ignored me. I know he heard me, but he literally stared into space and didn't bother saying anything. He'd done this hundreds of times over the years, but I thought to myself, this is so wrong. He shouldn't treat me like I don't exist."**

Avoiding or protecting yourself from people with toxic behaviours

What can you do if you think you might be in relationships with people who exhibit toxic behaviours? Sometimes a good starting place is, like Cloe, just observing what happens in your relationships, reflecting on your understanding of what's healthy and toxic, and paying attention to your feelings, thoughts and needs. It may be a matter of questioning what was once seen as acceptable or tolerable.

But what if you see that you are clearly in an unhealthy relationship with someone who exhibits significant toxic behaviours? There is no simple advice which can be given because so much depends on the situation and nature of the relationship. One option, of course, is to end the relationship. This may be a good idea if it's pretty clear your needs are not being met, you are quite sure this individual isn't going to change, and it just makes sense to move on. Sometimes, however, the relationship might feel important, and you think things can change. Option two can mean asserting yourself and letting them know what you need, which may give the relationship a chance to move in a healthy direction.

What about instances where a person's behaviours are clearly toxic, there is little chance they will change, but you still don't want to end the relationship? This can sometimes be the case with family members. Option three can be about setting boundaries to protect yourself from the toxicity. When people find themselves in a relationship with someone who exhibits toxic behaviours and is unlikely to change, they sometimes try to *control* the person or their behaviour. This rarely works, and you can get into an ongoing struggle for control which feels like you have stepped into quicksand. Rather than attempting to control their behaviour, it's often better to simply set boundaries. We mentioned Kerry previously. She had been emotionally abused by her mother, a woman she described as an 'unstable drama queen'. Despite this history, Kerry did not want to end the relationship and created some healthy boundaries to protect herself.

> **"I made it clear to mom that I would visit on Sundays with my two girls, but that we would stay for an hour. And, if she becomes unpleasant, then we will leave. I had to leave a couple of times when she started being mean to one of my girls."**

Notice that Kerry wasn't trying to control or get her 70-year-old mother to change who she is – she is just being clear about boundaries and what's acceptable. Boundaries can exist in terms of limiting the time you spend with someone or ending phone calls or visits when you reach a point where behaviour is unacceptable. These are physical ways of setting boundaries, but you can also protect yourself psychologically or emotionally by setting boundaries in your own mind. The voice you may need to find might sound something like this: *you can act in toxic ways if you want to, but I am not going to be confused or hurt or distressed by your behaviour.*

Reparative relationships

The idea of a reparative relationship was mentioned during the chapter on retraumatisation. Briefly, a reparative relationship is one in which at least some of the harm from childhood gets mended. If a child is physically or sexually abused, they often come into adulthood imaging that the world and people will hurt them. Having a relationship with someone they feel safe with helps to repair some of the earlier harm and supports the belief that the world and other people will not necessarily cause harm. If a child is emotionally neglected or abandoned, they tend to arrive at adulthood imagining that others are likely to neglect or leave them. A relationship in which they feel genuinely cared for, valued and secure helps repair some of the previous harm.

Creating or accepting reparative relationships is often an important part of an individual's recovery. Alesha's childhood history had been one of physical/emotional abuse and abandonment, and her description below illustrates a reparative relationship.

> **"We have our problems like most couples, you know, stresses about money and that sort of thing. But, I know Don won't hurt me and I know he really cares about me. I've been horrible to him sometimes, and he doesn't leave me, so I don't think he will."**

Reparative relationships are not always partnerships. They can come in many forms, such as friendships, a relationship with a teacher, a relationship with an older individual who seems like a parent figure, or a relationship to a sibling. A reparative relationship can occur in adulthood, but certain individuals can identify someone from their childhood who helped cushion the trauma they were experiencing, such as a teacher or coach. A relationship with a pet can also be reparative, as was illustrated by Toby, a man who experienced childhood physical and emotional abuse.

> **"For years I wanted a dog, but I was worried that I wouldn't be able to look after it the right way. Kelly is a collie mix breed, and he was a rescue dog. People who say that a dog only cares about you because you feed them don't know what they're talking about. Kelly is very affectionate and I know that I'm important to him. He's very protective of me and goes mad whenever the postman arrives at the door."**

However, creating or accepting a reparative relationship can be difficult for many. When meeting someone who might be able to offer a relationship in which they would feel safe, cared for or valued, they might not trust it. So, they might avoid opportunities to create such relationships or find ways to push away the people they need.

Exercise 6: Three questions concerning reparative relationships

Can you identify relationships which have been reparative, either in the past or the present?

Can you identify ways you avoid or undermine opportunities to have reparative relationships, e.g. do you avoid relationships? Do you create distance in your relationships? Do you push people away or create conflict in your relationships?

If you currently are in a reparative relationship, in what way is it reparative? Or, if you need a reparative relationship, what would that relationship be like?

Relationship skills

We explored how relationship skills must be learned and that many people who experienced childhood harm were disadvantaged in this respect. If you struggle with social confidence or feel you need to develop relationship skills, this is nothing to feel badly about. However, there may be a complication that needs considering. People who have healthy and rewarding relationships tend to make relationships a priority in their lives. If a person has been hurt within childhood and adult relationships, they can lose trust in relationships. This can result in a cynical view of relationships. We mentioned Alice previously, who put things quite bluntly when she said, "I don't like people." Alice's words illustrate the dilemma. Her life is a self-fulfilling prophecy. She has a long history of being hurt by people, so she does not trust or like people. Therefore, she does not see relationships as a priority, and so there is little point in developing relationship skills. It's little wonder she does not have healthy and supportive relationships.

It's possible that, despite your experiences, you have good relationship skills and feel confident in social situations. But, if you struggle with social confidence and skills, this area is just another facet of your recovery. A detailed description of relationship skills is beyond the scope of this chapter, but there are many books and online resources you can access. Seeing relationships as a priority in your life is the motivation for this form of development. If you want to work on relationship skill development but are not sure where to begin, Alan Garner's *Conversationally Speaking* has helped untold numbers of people. Despite being written over 40 years ago, it's still one of the best resources, and a new addition came out in 2021 (co-written with Caporaletti).

Your contribution to healthy relationships

Early editions of this chapter asked readers to consider patterns of toxic behaviours in others, as you did previously. However, we did not ask people using the Guidebook to reflect on whether they may at times fall into coping through toxic behaviours. During one group therapy session many years ago in which we were discussing this chapter, an older gentleman named Julian said something that we were struck by:

> **"I get why it's important for us to consider how we've been in relationships with people who have toxic behaviours, but how come you don't ask us about our own toxic behaviours? I got lots of those." (said with a broad grin).**

Julian's remark was well-timed and got a good laugh, but it was a useful moment of learning for us clinicians. On reflection, Julian's advice makes sense for a particular reason. Two considerations are likely important: 1. Avoiding or limiting time with people who display significant toxic behaviours, and 2. Self-reflection which can allow us to recognise when we may fall into coping through toxic behaviours. Julian made us aware that the chapter was only focusing on half of the story.

Since adding a new section to the chapter, we have seen a number of people manage some very self-honest reflection with respect to how they can at times fall into certain toxic behaviours. Rob serves as a good example of this personal development work. He experienced childhood neglect and abandonment and had felt lonely and scared for much of his life. Rob came to appreciate that he was treating his wife in a highly controlling way, checking her phone and email records and getting her to call or text him several times a day concerning her whereabouts (controlling bully style). One day he happened to watch a movie featuring a very controlling man, and he identified with the character in a way that shocked and upset him.

> **"I just thought, oh my god. I'm like the guy in the movie. I'm really controlling. I'm just scared she will leave me, which is why I act this way. But... I've got to do something about this."**

There are of course a range of toxic behaviours anyone can fall into if under enough stress, and Rob illustrates just one way this can play out. The exercise below will ask you to explore any toxic behaviours you may fall into at certain times or within certain relationships. If you recognise such patterns and it feels upsetting or elicits a shame response, we advise you to try und see any past behaviours *psychologically* rather than through the lens of self-punishment or shame. If you at times cope through such behaviours, you are much more than just those behaviours. Rob managed it by recognising that he was falling into the controlling bully behaviour, but could see that he was scared of being abandoned, and this was in turn a consequence of childhood abandonment and neglect.

Exercise 7: Your contribution to healthy relationships

We would ask you to briefly review the seven toxic behaviours you explored previously. When you have gone over this information, try to address the following question with as much self-honesty as possible.

Are you vulnerable at times of falling into certain toxic behaviours? If so, which behaviours stand out? Do you have thoughts about how you may wish to work on this?

Finding community

Human beings are communal animals. Just like elephants, gorillas, penguins, honey bees and even jellyfish, millions of years of evolution designed us for communal experiences. Loneliness and associated emotions remind us that we were constructed to be a part of a group or groups of other humans. However, there is a common dilemma faced by people who experienced childhood harm. Most of these people were harmed *in the context of a group*. Many experienced danger in the first group they were part of – their family. School is often the second group we belong to and some experienced abuse or rejection there. This sets up a contradiction. Evolution designed us for group membership, but our experience has taught us that groups can be dangerous. As a result, our nervous system may signal danger when we have opportunities for group experiences.

There is no single solution to this dilemma, but we can offer three ideas and the story of Mark, a man who did find a way forward. First, isolation or social avoidance will not work in the long run because it goes against the very fibres of what makes us human. So, if that's the solution you have in mind, it's probably helpful to give up on it. Second, certain people who experience social disconnection or isolation can feel unsure about how to find a sense of group belonging, often because their confidence in themselves and others has been compromised. For some, the question can be: where do I begin? If this is the case for you, there is a principle which can help. Human beings often form groups with respect to a shared interest. Photography, cars, every expression of sport, gym groups, book clubs, art or crafts, politics, etc....Whatever your interest, there is a group of human beings who seem to find each other, and the internet has made this easier today than at any time in human history. There is (no joking) a Cloud Appreciation Society and Extreme Ironing Bureau in Britain. Third, if past trauma means that your nervous system gets badly triggered when in a new group, it may help to go gradually, be open about the difficulties you have, and ask for support if you can. Some find that online groups are an easier place to begin. Society is probably more 'trauma aware' today than ever before, and most people will understand and support you. Mark is a good example.

Mark had experienced quite serious abuse and neglect within his family home before being shipped off to boarding school, where he experienced more abuse. Aside from contact with his daughter and two grandkids, his only social connections were through volunteering as a moderator for a gaming site, which provided no real intimacy. As therapy was nearing the end, he expressed frustration that little progress had been made with the chronic feelings of anger, generalised anxiety, and poor sleep which had caused him to seek help. His therapist challenged him, pointing out that he had worked hard at developing insight, but that he hadn't yet taken risks in creating social connections.

During therapy, Mark had developed an interest in mindfulness meditation. His therapist encouraged him to attend a local mindfulness meditation group which met monthly. Just the idea of joining such a group elicited significant anxiety, and it required another two sessions of preparation and planning before Mark was able to join his first session. Email communication and then a phone call Mark had with the group leader helped. Explaining how anxious he gets in groups allowed the leader to reassure him in ways which made that first session possible. Insight had been essential, but the sense of belonging he eventually experienced produced noticeable reductions in the chronic symptoms he had brought to therapy.

References

1. Van Der kolk, B. (2015). *The body keeps the score: Mind, brain and body in the transformation of trauma*. London: Penguin Books.

Chapter 19

Self-compassion and Self-care

"I don't really like the idea of self-compassion. Just the word makes me feel uncomfortable."
Belinda

Some might imagine that the topics of self-compassion and self-care would be easier than other areas in this programme. It can be for certain individuals, but these topics can feel challenging for a surprising number of people who experienced childhood harm. If your response to this chapter is one of enthusiasm, that's fine. But if these topics feel uncomfortable, this is common. As we shall explore, there are several reasons why many can be 'slow to warm' to this material.

Also, for some people the ideas of self-compassion and self-care can seem strangely new. This experience was captured well by Robert, an individual we mentioned earlier who had experienced significant childhood neglect. His clinician had spent some time describing self-compassion and self-care and had noticed a bemused expression on his face. The clinician asked Robert what he thought about these topics. His response was interesting, if not humorous.

> **"Um... I don't know. (nervous laughter). I've never really thought about this stuff."**

To provide some orientation, we offer brief definitions of self-compassion and self-care below. The rest of the chapter represents an opportunity to explore these areas in detail, as well as develop your capacity for self-compassion and self-care.

Self-compassion includes acknowledging mistakes or lapses in judgement but also means relating to yourself with kindness, soothing and encouragement. Self-compassion is an internal experience – it involves how you *think about* or *talk to* yourself.

Self-care is the capacity to look after your physical and psychological well-being. It involves behaviours – *what you do* to care for your body and organise your life or relationships.

SELF-COMPASSION

There are countless ways in which human beings can get things wrong. Whether we are aware or unaware of our behaviour, we sometimes cause upset or inconvenience to others. Or, sometimes, when we believe we have 'fallen short', it's not something we did to someone else – it's because we feel we have not lived up to our standards. But, whether we believe we have caused harm to others or fallen short of our standards, everyone makes mistakes, gets things wrong or screws up. The British poet Alexander Pope put it more succinctly: 'to err is human'.[1]

Does the simple fact that human beings make mistakes have any special relevance concerning childhood trauma? It turns out it does. While those who experienced childhood harm share in the human experience of making mistakes, there is evidence that they are much more likely to relate to themselves negatively *when they do make mistakes*.[2] In fact, one of the key diagnostic criteria for Complex Post-traumatic Stress Disorder (C-PTSD) is 'negative self-concept'.[3] Punitive self-talk is both a cause and a consequence of having a negative self-concept. In other words, while such individuals make mistakes like everyone else, they are more likely to be self-judgemental in ways which can induce feelings such as worthlessness, guilt or shame.

So how does this work in practice? Relationships come in three different forms: our relationship with the world, others and ourselves. The practice of self-compassion relates most intimately to the *relationship you have with yourself.* For some people who experienced childhood harm, the idea that they have a relationship with themselves is something they haven't given much thought to. This can sometimes be a consequence of a history of neglect. As you go through the day, thoughts go through your head, and some of these thoughts involve how you think about or talk to yourself. This can be referred to as *self-talk*, and everyone does it. As mentioned, there is evidence that people who experience childhood abuse or neglect tend to be more punishing in how they think about or talk to themselves.

We mentioned Bertrand previously, an individual who was physically and emotionally abused by his father. Bertrand had avoided opening a letter which contained a parking citation, which resulted in a £40 penalty.

> **"I'm such a f****** idiot! How stupid can I possibly be? I am constantly doing this shit."**

If Bertrand had experienced a moment of annoyance with himself over his mistake, that would be one thing. But he had spent a lot of time punishing himself in the three days before we spoke with him. And, interestingly, Bertrand wasn't 'constantly doing this shit'. He was normally a fairly organised guy. His reaction represented some very punitive self-talk and difficulties accessing self-compassion.

Why do people struggle to be self-compassionate?

The skill of self-compassion is *not* difficult to understand, but for many who experienced childhood harm, it feels difficult to *actually do it.* To have some confidence in self-compassion, it's often necessary to understand the part of you that is likely to be resistant. Below we explore four reasons those who experienced childhood trauma can struggle to practice self-compassion.

Misunderstanding what is meant by self-compassion

Some people see self-compassion as unacceptable because they think it means:

- Being irresponsible (being able to say or do whatever you want or letting yourself 'off the hook' for your mistakes)
- Being selfish
- Being weak
- Seeing self-compassion as the same thing as self-pity

Let's return to our definition of self-compassion. *Self-compassion includes acknowledging mistakes or lapses in judgement, but also means relating to yourself with kindness, soothing and encouragement.* Notice that a feature of self-compassion includes having the **strength** and **sensitivity** to appreciate and learn from your mistakes. So, this is not about being irresponsible, selfish or weak.

Associating self-compassion with weakness was exemplified by John, who was physically abused by his father throughout childhood.

> **"This self-compassionate stuff – it just seems so wet. When I try doing it, I feel sort of... pathetic."**

Also, when people use the word self-pity, they usually are referring to someone who is feeling sorry for themselves for reasons which are not justified. That's not self-compassion. Self-compassion means relating to yourself with kindness, soothing and encouragement in circumstances where this is necessary and healthy.

The internalisation of the abuser's voice

Emotional abuse represents an attack on the child's sense of self. In an unconscious manner, people who experienced childhood harm can *internalise the voice of the abuser.*

In other words, they can talk to themselves in a similar way that the abuser used to talk to them. When you talk to yourself in a punishing way, it probably sounds like your voice, but if you pay attention, you may notice that it sounds similar to how an abuser used to speak to you.

Mark was emotionally abused for years by his father. An auto-mechanic, one day he left a toolbox out in the rain which resulted in tools collecting some rust.

"I hate making mistakes. I'm so stupid. Why am I such a loser?"

Mark's therapist replied, "so this idea that you are stupid… that you are a loser… who's voice does that sound like?" The look of recognition on Mark's face was immediate. Mark had internalised his father's voice, and now he was very adept at punishing himself severely for many mistakes.

The belief that you are supposed to be punished

Self-compassion often just doesn't 'feel right' for people who were harmed as children, an issue that can be compounded if they experience further abuse as an adult. Many such people seem to carry around with them 'a sense' that they are bad and are supposed to be punished. Barbara experienced childhood neglect as well as physical and emotional abuse.

"I swear, even if something isn't really my fault, I still feel responsible. Self-compassion feels weird because… I just sort of feel like I'm supposed to be punished."

If you experienced harm that was punishing in childhood, it doesn't mean you are supposed to be punished for the rest of your life. Other people should not continue punishing you, and you don't need to punish yourself. The past doesn't have to be the present and the future. With this in mind, self-compassion becomes possible.

You were never shown or taught how to be self-compassionate

From a developmental perspective, children are inexperienced, their brains are underdeveloped, and they are physically clumsy. All of this means that they will make thousands of mistakes and messes before they arrive at adulthood. Whether a child learns the value and skill of self-compassion depends greatly on what they see in childhood and how others respond to their mistakes.

An 8-year-old receives a 'D' on a math test at school and is upset with herself. She is speaking with her mother below.

Child: "I'm useless at math. I can't do any of it. Next, we are doing division and that's even harder."

Mother: "You really revised for that test. English comes easy for you, but math just seems trickier. But I'm sure you will learn it, and I can help. You're trying, and that's what's important. You shouldn't be so hard on yourself."

By being compassionate with her daughter, this mother is teaching the skill of self-compassion. We *learn* how to relate to ourselves through how others relate to us. If a child has adults around them who are compassionate and supportive, they learn to be compassionate and supportive with themselves. We 'internalise' the behaviours and thoughts of others and make them our behaviours and thoughts. How I relate to myself will reflect the way others related to me.

Sadly, this is also true in the case of abuse and neglect. If the mother above had responded to her daughter's test score of a 'D' with verbal abuse and shaming, the child is likely to learn that self-punishment and shame are necessary when she makes mistakes or 'falls short'.

Also, some people watched an important adult relate to themselves punitively. A child can learn from watching others that beating up on yourself psychologically or even physically seems necessary.

Exercise 1: Why might self-compassion be difficult for you?

We have explored four reasons why self-compassion may not come naturally to people who experienced childhood harm. Tic any you think help explain why self-compassion can be difficult for you.

___ You believe self-compassion means being irresponsible, selfish or weak.

___ You 'internalised an abuser's voice', i.e. you became punitive with yourself in ways reflecting the punitive voice of past abusers.

___ You acquired the idea that you are bad and therefore have this 'sense' that you are supposed to be punished.

___ Adults were not compassionate with you, and so you didn't learn to be compassionate with yourself. Or, you learned to be self-punishing by watching important adults act this way.

Below you can describe any further thoughts or feelings about the above exercise.

The skill of self-compassion

The idea that self-compassion is 'a skill' might sound odd. However, like cooking, driving a car, or repairing a computer, it requires some knowledge, and you need to do something in a clever way. The initial step in self-compassion requires that you recognise and let go of its opposite: *the self-punitive loop*. We need to say a bit about what this is. The self-punitive loop has two features.

1. Punishing yourself inwardly through self-talk for some period of time in ways which induce feelings like worthlessness, shame or guilt. These thoughts feel like 'a loop' because you are stuck in them, or they keep reoccurring.

2. If you pay close attention to the self-punitive loop, you will notice there is no practical benefit or resolution, unless making yourself feel terrible is seen as a benefit (which we would not agree with). The nature of self-punishing thoughts is that they don't help you or others.

Below is a description of the skill of self-compassion, but we need to make a few points. First, the issue requiring self-compassion may have occurred 2 minutes ago or 20 years ago. It doesn't matter. Second, sometimes you will find yourself in a self-punitive loop because of a mistake you made. Other times, it's because someone criticised you. Such criticism represents an 'invitation' for you to be self-punitive. In either event, self-compassion can be equally important. Third, as mentioned above, knowing *how* to practice self-compassion is not that complicated, and it's not what gets in the way. The blocks to being self-compassionate have more to do with the issues outlined in the previous section entitled *Why do people struggle to be self-compassionate?* It's those issues that are driving you away from self-compassion and towards the self-punitive loop. To practice self-compassion, it's necessary to accept that self-compassion is a good idea.

The skill of self-compassion involves four steps:

- *Recognise that you are experiencing a self-punitive loop.* Be aware of self-punishing thoughts. You might be experiencing punishing self-talk about something you did, something which happened between you and others, or even just thoughts or impulses you have had. If you are thinking in ways that induce guilt, shame, or worthlessness, that's a clue. If you can recognise the self-punitive loop in a few seconds – that's great. If you have been in a self-punitive loop for a while before you spotted it, that's better than not seeing it at all.
- *See the big picture and appreciate why you may have acted or thought as you did.* If you made a mistake, acted insensitively or didn't live up to your expectations, there can be mitigating reasons or circumstances. Perhaps you didn't have certain information, misunderstood something, were tired or distracted, or your history of complex trauma played a role, etc..... This is not about being irresponsible or shifting blame – it's about appreciating your human fallibility.
- *Can you learn from the situation or make something right?* You might be able to learn something from this situation about yourself and how you want to do things in the future. Or, if you recognise you have made a mistake or fallen short, sometimes you can make a repair, e.g. offering an apology or sorting something out. If there is something you can learn from the situation, you can decide to try and do things differently in the future. If you can mend something between you and others, you can make a decision to do this.
- *Apply a healthy dose of self-compassion.* You have spotted a self-punitive loop, explored why you acted or thought as you did, and tried to learn from and (if possible) repair your situation. **There is nothing else you can do**, so it's time to *be* self-compassionate. This means talking to yourself with kindness, soothing or encouragement. If this sounds unlikely, ridiculous or even impossible, the journaling below (which three individuals did) may help. The first illustrates a current situation, the second occurred many years ago, and the third relates to an 'internal event'.

Tom's son misses one of his classes

Tom normally drops his son off at secondary school on the way to work. He was about to wake up his son and checked his diary. He realised that he had an unusual meeting scheduled first thing, which meant he couldn't drop his son off and his son would have to take a bus. This results in his son missing his first lesson, which he journaled.

Journal 1

The self-punitive loop	Seeing the big picture	Learning and repairing	Self-compassion
I messed up and my son missed his class. I keep imagining my son getting reprimanded, and I keep telling myself what an idiot I am. I didn't see the self-punitive loop until late in the afternoon.	I messed up, but I was distracted by financial worries the night before, which made it more difficult to be organised in the way I normally am.	I apologised to my son a few times, but it occurred to me that I could send the school an email and explain that I was responsible for my son missing his class, which I did. I make a mental note that I need to be more careful about checking my diary before bed.	*"I made a mistake, but I'm a good dad in a lot of ways. I've done what I can about this, so I need to stop beating myself up over it. Let it go."*

One interesting point about the journaling Tom did is how counter-productive the self-punitive loop can be. When caught up in self-punishing thoughts and images, you illicit painful emotional states, like anxiety, anger or shame. In this state of mind, it's very hard to think productively, such as seeing the big picture, thinking about what can be learned or whether a repair can be made.

Karen punishes herself over an accident occurring many years ago

When Karen's son was ten years old, he was jumping on a trampoline in their garden and broke his arm. Her son is now 22, and the arm mended a long time ago, but there is an obvious bump where the bone calcified, which Karen can see when he wears short-sleeve shirts.

Journal 2

The self-punitive loop	Seeing the big picture	Learning and repairing	Self-compassion
When I see the bump on my son's arm I feel terrible about what happened. I just think I was a bad mom and that this is all my fault, and I should have protected him.	I had two other young children at the time, a very busy life, and it was impossible to watch all of my kids every minute.	I don't know if there's anything to learn. I've apologised to my son so many times that he is getting sick of me bringing it up.	*"I was a good mother in lots of ways and it was impossible to keep my children safe from everything. My son is fine now and he doesn't resent me about this. Stop thinking about it."*

Mary punishes herself for violent thoughts which come into her head

Mary experienced physical abuse throughout childhood. It's very confusing for her, but she can have vivid thoughts or images of doing something violent to others which pop into her head. She has never been violent to anyone and is confident she won't. But the violent thoughts/images are very upsetting.

Journal 3

The self-punitive loop	Seeing the big picture	Learning and repairing	Self-compassion
I was walking through the high street with my two kids and I saw these homeless men and I had violent images of attacking them with a cricket bat, and later that evening the images occurred several times. I keep thinking I'm sick and disgusting to have these thoughts.	I got abused as a child, and it's confusing, but that may be why I can have these awful thoughts.	There's probably a connection between my violent thoughts and my past but it's difficult to understand this entirely. My thoughts don't hurt anyone, so there is nothing for me to fix.	*"My own abuse is probably connected to the disturbing thoughts I can have, but these thoughts are not my fault. I'm a kind person and I don't want to hurt anyone, so just accept the thoughts and get on with life."*

Exercise 2: Journaling your use of self-compassion

Self-compassion is more than an idea – it's a skill you can use. Below is a blank journal you can fill in to help you use self-compassion. When you spot that you are getting into a self-punitive loop, that's the time to use the journal. If you like, you can make a photocopy of the journal and take it with you in a purse or pocket.

There are two important points to keep in mind. First, some individuals will say, *'I didn't journal anything because I didn't get into any serious self-punitive loops'.* On exploration, we often discover there were a number of times they needed to use self-compassion. The issue doesn't have to be 'serious' to require self-compassion.

Second, the nature of the self-punitive loop is that *it's a loop*. Even when you see it for what it is and pour a dose of healthy self-compassion on it, the self-punitive thoughts or images often reoccur. What should you do? See it for what it is and use the skill of self-compassion again. And again, and again and again. You may have to use the skill of self-compassion many times before self-punitive thoughts ease off. Remember – self-punishment is not making you more insightful, it's not helpful, and it's not necessary. You have already received more punishment than you ever deserved. It's okay to be self-compassionate. You deserve to be self-compassionate.

Journal 4

The self-punitive loop	Seeing the big picture	Learning and repairing	Self-compassion

SELF-CARE

Some individuals feel an impulse to skip this section, and occasionally this is because they have come across information on self-care that was 'off-putting'. A lot of the available information on self-care (especially on the internet) can come across as simplistic, condescending, or annoying, and often consists of lists of direct advice-giving. Our view is that self-care is an essential area for individuals to explore, but we will not be providing a 'pick 'n mix list' of self-care ideas. Instead, we will look at this topic in some depth, provide you with a questionnaire and then encourage you to explore what is needed. We trust that *you* will know if changes need to be made for better self-care, and how to make them.

What is self-care and why is it important?

Self-compassion and self-care can overlap and support one another, but they are different. Self-compassion means generating inner *thoughts* that are kind, soothing and supportive to yourself. Self-care is the capacity to look after your well-being, but it involves behaviours – it's what *you do* to care for your body and organise life and relationships.

Do issues of self-care have any special relevance for people who experienced childhood harm? As was the case with self-compassion, the answer is – yes it does. There is evidence that those who were abused or neglected are more likely to experience a broad range of medical issues resulting from inadequate self-care.[4,5] If this worries you, there are a couple of reassuring points to be made. First, while the research tells us that such individuals are *more at risk for medical problems* than the general population, this does not mean it will apply to you, as there are always many exceptions to any general research finding. Second, if you can identify that your self-care is inadequate and putting you at risk for problems, you can begin making changes *now* that will protect you or help repair certain issues that may be developing.

Why might those who experienced childhood harm be vulnerable to poor self-care?

There are at least a couple of reasons why those who experienced childhood harm may not do a good job of self-care, and you will notice some overlap with a similar section on self-compassion.

We learn self-care through being cared for

Children require care when they get sick or scrap their knees; they need to be supported in brushing their teeth and having regular bedtimes; they need to be provided with nutritious food, opportunities for play and rest, etc... . All of this and more should be supported consistently by caring adults. When it is, children are shown what caring for their bodies and minds looks like, and they learn that they deserve good care. Because their bodies and minds got cared for as children, they 'internalise' a model of what good care looks and feels like. As adults, this internal model of good care expresses itself in the capacity to care for themselves (self-care). Put simply – through being cared for as a child, you acquire the skills of self-care and the sense that you deserve good care. If your body and mind didn't get cared for by adults around you, you are *less likely to have a clear grasp of what good self-care looks and feels like.*

Painful states of emotional dysregulation can result in poor self-care

In a previous chapter on emotions, we saw that people who experience childhood harm are more likely to encounter painful emotional states (emotional dysregulation), and that more extreme emotional states seem to require more extreme ways of coping. These ways of coping can include, for example, alcohol and drug abuse, junk-food binging or food restriction, over-exercise, overwork, self-harming, etc... If developed into a pattern of coping, these sorts of behaviours can represent poor self-care.

Kelly experienced childhood sexual abuse and neglect, and struggled with a mix of anxiety and depression.

> **"I know drinking 15 cans of coke a day is bad for me and I worry about my teeth, but it's this habit I've got into. When I feel bad I just pop open a can without even thinking about it."**

Whether an individual reaches for alcohol, drugs, junk food, or behaves in self-harmful ways, they are often just trying to get control over painful emotional states which have roots in childhood experiences.

Exercise 3: Why might you struggle with self-care

If you don't care for yourself as you should, we suggest two reasons this might be the case. Tic either you think may apply to you.

___ Because you were not cared for properly, you didn't learn self-care or that you deserve to care for yourself.

___ When you have painful emotional states, you might do things that represent poor self-care.

Any further thoughts about this exercise?

Exercise 4: Questionnaire for self-care

The questionnaire below asks what may feel like quite personal questions, and there is a risk that some may feel patronised by the nature of this exercise. This occurs occasionally and if it feels somewhat patronising, we are sorry. However, we have kept this exercise in the programme because of the significant number of people we work with who can really struggle with self-care. Write a number next to each question which rates your experience for each area.

1. Yes, definitely
2. Doing okay
3. Improvement needed
4. No, this is a real problem

Environment

___ Does your home environment provide a comfortable space you feel good to be in?
___ Is your living environment clean, organised and free from clutter?
___ Do you wear clothing which is comfortable and which you feel comfortable in?

Physical Well-being

___ Are you eating a nutritious and balanced diet?
___ Are you drinking enough hydrating fluids?
___ Is your use of alcohol or other drugs relatively healthy?
___ Is your bed and sleeping area comfortable?
___ Do you have routines which set you up for a good night's sleep?
___ If you get sick or unwell, do you slow down and care for yourself properly?
___ If you are sick or unwell, do you access medical help like your GP when you should?
___ Do you care for your teeth well on a daily basis?
___ Do you see the dentist when necessary? (Yes, we appreciate this can be difficult in the UK).
___ Do you engage in regular aerobic physical exercise, i.e. gets your heart and lungs pumping?
___ Hair, skin and nails: are you looking after them?

Relationships

___ Are you spending time with people who you enjoy and leave you feeling good?
___ Do you create 'boundaries' concerning people who would otherwise drain or exhaust you?

Time and finance

___ Is your time organised so you are not rushing, late or missing appointments?
___ Do you pay attention to finances in order that you don't develop any worrying problems?
___ Do you have time and space for 'recharging' when you are run down?

Personal

___ Do you make time for things you enjoy doing?
___ Are there personal or creative projects you do which are nurturing or interesting?

Other?

Indicate any other areas of self-care not mentioned which are important to you.

The space below offers an opportunity to do some personal journaling on the following question: do you need to make improvements concerning self-care? One way to reflect on this question is to look over the questionnaire you just completed. For areas you answered with a 1 or 2, you're doing okay or well. But if you answered with a 3, this may be an area you want to consider working on. If you answered with a 4, this is perhaps an area you really need to give some attention to. So, below, reflect on changes you may need to make to improve your self-care.

Final thought

People can have very different experiences concerning this chapter. Some may discover they are not doing too badly concerning self-compassion and self-care. But, it's not unusual for us to work with people who discover that these areas represent significant problems. Some clients can even feel rather shocked by how difficult self-compassion and self-care are for them. If you have discovered that you really struggle with these areas, we encourage you not to beat up on yourself or get despondent about it. There will be genuine reasons why these areas are difficult, and working at change will take time, reflection and practice.

References

1. Pope, A. (1963). The poems of Alexander Pope: a one-volume edition of the Twickenham text with selected annotations. New Haven: Yale University Press.
2. Cloitre, M., Garvert, D.W., Weiss, B., Carlson, E.B. and Bryant, R.A. (2014). Distinguishing PTSD, Complex PTSD, and Borderline Personality Disorder: A latent class analysis. *European Journal of Psychotraumatology* (5).
3. Rosenfield, P.J., Stratyner, A., Tufekcioglu, S., Karabell S, McKelvey, J. and Litt, L. (2018). Complex PTSD in ICD-11: A Case Report on a New Diagnosis. *Journal of Psychiatric Practice*. Sept; 24 (5). 364-370.
4. Gilbert, L.K., Breiding, M.J., Merrick M.T., et al. (2010). Childhood adversity and adult chronic disease: an update from ten states and the District of Columbia. *American Journal of Preventative Medicine*.48(3): 345-9.
5. The Adverse Childhood Experiences Study, go to: https://acestoohigh.com/got-your-ace-score/

Chapter 20

Meaning and Self-Expression

"I didn't have a childhood, and maybe that's why there are times I worry I won't have a life. But other times I can think, no way, that's not gonna happen."
- Juliet

"There is only one thing that I dread: not to be worthy of my sufferings."
- Fyodor Dostoyevsky[1]

Some models of therapy or personal development do not give much attention to the question of meaning. Our view is that meaning (and the related issue of self-expression) is of great importance in overcoming the effects of childhood trauma. We do not see this discussion as a diversion or philosophical indulgence.

However, we wish to acknowledge that our discussion of meaning does not represent facts or the product of scientific research. There are no 'techniques' or 'strategies' here, but there are ideas you may be able to identify with, the voices of others who experienced childhood harm and opportunities for self-reflection.

What is meant by 'meaning'?

In this chapter, we use the word *meaning* to signify what has *importance* or *value* to us. The experience of meaning relates to why I want to get out of bed in the morning, why I feel desire, and why people, projects or life matters. Meaning is often associated with the experience of interest, enthusiasm, pleasure, concentration or energy. The experience of meaning relates to feeling engaged with life in a manner which offers a sense of value or purpose.

We can also understand the experience of meaning by appreciating its opposite – an absence of meaning. There are perhaps a number of feelings associated with the absence of meaning, such as despair, despondency, anguish or hopelessness. An absence of meaning can also be experienced as a feeling of alienation (or being 'cut off') from others, existence or even oneself. The experience of depression is certainly quite troubling for many people who experienced childhood harm, and we should not discount how disturbing depression can be. But it's possible to overlook how depression coincides with the absence of meaning. Depression is about more than problematic brain chemistry. Depression can also be seen as the psychological expression of a lack of meaning.

There is another point concerning meaning which is important to mention. Western philosophy renewed its interest in meaning between and following the two world wars. This was existential philosophy, and it was mainly French and German philosophers such as Jean-Paul Sartre, Simone DeBoviour, Albert Camus, Martin Heidegger, Hannah Arendt and Karl Jaspers who got very interested in human meaning. They had intense and often confusing relationships with one another. Sartre slept with DeBoviour, Heidegger slept with Arendt, and DeBoviour asked Camus to sleep with her (he said no). Arendt and Jaspers did manage to avoid trouble and remained good friends throughout their lives. They all disagreed about many things (they were French and German, after all), but they agreed on a fascinating way of thinking about human meaning. They said that the challenge for human beings wasn't about discovering 'the meaning of life'. They believed that there was no single or universal 'meaning' to life. Instead, the experience of meaning (or value) is something every individual must *create* within the context of their lives.

And, meaning doesn't simply relate to ideas we have or a perspective we hold – we experience meaning through our actions and daily interactions. Victor Frankl, a psychiatrist and Auschwitz survivor, put it like this: "The meaning of life is to give life meaning."[2] This is both a hopeful and challenging view. Hopeful because it suggests we have at least some control in directing the creation of meaning. Challenging because we are also responsible for the creation of meaning.

The experience of meaning can provide at least a partial remedy to suffering. The oft-quoted words of Friedrich Nietzsche capture this view in a powerful and succinct manner. "He who has a *why* to live for can bear almost any *how*."[3] [Please excuse the dated use of language in this chapter with respect to certain quotes]. In other words, having something you want to live for can make suffering more tolerable. If trauma is a wound, meaning can act as a balm to soothe the pain of that wound.

Can the creation of meaning be especially difficult for those who experienced child harm?

This chapter will offer a forward-looking and encouraging opportunity for you to focus on meaning creation. However, we begin with a realistic appraisal of how meaning creation can be more challenging for people who experienced childhood abuse or neglect. If this sounds depressing, please hang in there. Some people we work with who struggle to experience meaning can blame themselves. Appreciating why meaning creation can be more difficult can provide relief from self-blame.

It's not just the physical or emotional pain of childhood abuse or neglect that matters; it's how senseless or meaningless these experiences can seem. To repeat the words of

Victor Frankl mentioned much earlier: "At such a moment, it is not the physical pain which hurts the most… it is the mental agony caused by the injustice, the unreasonableness of it all."[4]

Individuals need to make sense of the harm done to them by others, but this can be agonisingly difficult. Stan experienced multiple forms of abuse, and his words illustrate an idea we have heard from many others.

> **"Why would they do it? Why would anybody treat a child like that? They didn't want children, so why did they have me?"**

A question can be: how might I create a life of meaning as an adult when my childhood experiences of harm seem so senseless? For many people who experienced childhood harm, we believe creating a meaningful life is more challenging. There are at least a couple of reasons why this can be the case, which we explore below.

Learning brain, survival brain and meaning

In a sense, we have two brains. In a previous chapter, we talked about how the fight or flight pathway (Sympathetic Nervous System) is responsible for responding to threats through activating defences. The shut-down pathway (Dorsal Vagal system) responds to threats by collapsing. Together, we can refer to these two systems as 'the survival brain'. The present and connected pathway (Ventral Vagal system) is what we can access when we are safe, can learn and be social. We can call this our 'learning brain'. Many people we work with spent much of their childhood in their survival brain as they sought to stay safe or avoid harm. The functions of the survival brain grew strong with repeated use and, in adulthood, tend to get activated quickly and more frequently. As a result, many can be distracted by focusing disproportionately on survival, anxiety and potential harm.

Creating a life with meaning relies on feeling safe and social. If you are frightened, either by events in your life or by your internal emotional world, how can you focus on creating meaning? In a state of fear or anger, how can you focus on personal projects, personal learning, developing rewarding relationships, educational/occupational development, or any of the almost unlimited ways people create meaning? The purpose of the survival brain is to avoid harm *right now*. To create meaning, we need access to the calm, reflective and *future-orientated* learning brain. This can be more challenging for those who experienced childhood abuse and neglect. Appreciating the impact of childhood harm can allow some to be more self-compassionate with respect to how meaning creation may have been more challenging.

Self-agency and meaning

A sense of self-agency refers to the confidence a person has that they can sort problems, engage socially, and make a contribution to society. In this respect, self-agency supports the experience of meaning. Self-agency develops through caring, safe and supportive relationships the child has with carers. Parents or carers will set the child up for safe and successful experiences. We saw in a previous chapter that when a child has a 'secure attachment' to caring adults, they will play and explore the world with a sense of curiosity. If a child feels loved and important in the eyes of caring adults, they come to see themselves as having value and being capable, which is the basis of self-agency.

If a child lives with fear, they will find it difficult to approach the world with curiosity and playfulness. They spend energy searching for safety rather than exploring and learning. They are more likely to experience social and academic problems at school. Without feeling truly loved and valued at home, developing a sense of self-agency is very difficult. Feeling loved, important, and successful is the antidote to exploitation as the child grows older. Without self-agency, we know that those (especially boys) who experienced childhood trauma are more likely to 'act out' and get drawn into groups with radicalised ideologies[5] or gangs involved with criminal behaviour.[6] They give up what sense of agency they might have to leaders willing to tell them what to do. Lacking self-agency, young women may be more likely to 'act in' through self-harm, eating disorders, etc…

With a sense of self-agency, we are confident in solving problems, creating relationships, and being productive, all of which are the wellspring of meaning. Without the childhood experience of safety and love, self-agency, and therefore meaning, become much harder to get hold of.

Can there be meaning in suffering?

It can be difficult to imagine that experiences of childhood harm have any point beyond confusion, fear or loneliness. Suffering, at the time it is occurring, often seems to have no meaning. However, over time some people have been able to create meaning in ways which seem related to past trauma. They may see, for example, that there are certain positive aspects of who they became which are in some way connected to the harmful experiences they encountered. They may be creative or express themselves as a way of responding to or working with trauma. While it can be important for certain people to honour or value something which was a product of awful experiences, it's also essential to be careful with our use of language. Just because certain positives may have eventually come from past harm, this is *not* suggesting that the trauma was 'ok' or 'justified'. It in no way exonerates anyone who caused harm or gives these people power. It does not excuse or rationalise abusive behaviour.

It is also important to say that while we have worked with people who have eventually been able to see positive aspects of personality or self-expression which relate to past trauma, there are also people for whom this is not the case. Their experience can be that past traumatic experience was simply hurtful, compromised their development, and caused problems. If this was your experience, this needs recognising and respecting too.

However, below are examples from a small selection of people we have worked with who have been able to connect certain valued aspects of personality or self-expression with past harm. Mary Ann was physically and emotionally abused by her parents.

> **"If things could be different, I would never want to go through it again. I was scared a lot of the time and there was never anyone I could talk to. But what happened has made me very aware of right and wrong. I've got this moral compass that I trust, and people will often come to me for advice because I can be really clear about the right way to handle things."**

Michelle had been abandoned by her mother and was abused and neglected by her stepmother.

> **"Because of what happened to me I know that I am very sensitive to other people's pain. I can sense it, even in people I meet for the first time. I feel a lot of empathy for anyone who has been hurt, and I end up being like a counsellor to a lot of my friends and family because of that."**

Tom grew up in a family where violence was the norm, and he was on the receiving end of it as much as anybody. As an adult, he took up canvas painting, and he could make a connection between past trauma and creativity.

> **"I guess my paintings are pretty 'dark', but it's been a way of exploring what happened to me and channelling my anger. There are people who can definitely relate to them, and maybe my paintings help others in some way. It's also the best way I know to pay the bills."**

Sally experienced multiple forms of abuse which occurred throughout childhood. Her experiences eventually led her to a career which is important to her.

> **"When I was an office receptionist, staff and clients would come to me with their problems. I think that because of what happened to me I can relate to the problems people have. One day I just thought, I'm good at this – I need to get qualified. So that's how I became a social worker."**

Whether people can create meaning out of past trauma varies greatly, but it does seem possible for some. Victor Frankl even suggests that suffering may be a requirement for some forms of self-expression or creativity: "What is to give light must endure burning."[7]

Exercise 1: Think about the person you have become today. Think about what you see as strengths or positive qualities. Is there anything positive about you today related to the past harm you experienced? Are you, in some manner, a more capable or more complete person because of what you went through?

Reconnecting to meaning in early childhood

Most young children are 'wired' to find almost everything about life meaningful, interesting or stimulating. What many adults will view as mundane, children find fascinating. And, most young children start out with a natural need for self-expression.

Robert Fulghum tells an amusing story which vividly illustrates the above points.[8] He had been teaching art at different schools in Tuba, Utah (yes, that's the city's actual name). In the morning, he was working with a group of five-year-olds and asked, "who can draw?" Every child immediately raised their hand. Later that day, he worked with a group of teenagers at a secondary school. Again, he asked, "who can draw?" Only one student raised their hand. Later he reflected: *how is it that all those kids forgot how to draw?*

So it is probably normal for most adults to lose some of the confident self-expression of childhood. But many people who experienced childhood harm had these qualities squashed early on through abusive and neglectful experiences. So when individuals say things like "I didn't have a childhood" or "my childhood got taken from me," they are referring indirectly to the loss of meaningful exploration, creative play and self-expression.

However, childhood exploration and self-expression are so strong that most people can recall experiences of excitement and enthusiasm they nevertheless experienced during childhood. For some, accessing what was interesting or meaningful in childhood can be a gateway to reflecting on your need for meaning today.

Exercise 2: Can you recall a period in your childhood when you felt fascination, interest or enthusiasm for something? Imagine yourself as a child involved in this thing, and describe it below.

A tool for reflecting on meaning creation

The creation and experience throughout one's life of some sense of meaning is neither simple or easy. However, Victor Frankl put a realistic and yet positive spin on this idea when he wrote, "What man actually needs is not a tensionless state but rather the striving and struggling for some goal worthy of him."[9]

The final section of this chapter allows you to reflect on meaning creation. We are sure that this is something you have spent time working on long before you came to this programme, and we hope this does not come across as patronising. What follows is an opportunity to *build on* your previous work.

There is no single method for reflecting on how meaning can be experienced, but we offer a model below that suggests three ways to consider the experience of meaning. You may wish to keep in mind the way we described meaning previously: the experience of meaning relates to feeling engaged with life in a manner which offers a sense of value, purpose or richness.

There are at least three ways meaning can be experienced: 1. Through helping or caring roles; 2. Through self-expression or self-development; and 3. Through strong personal interests or aesthetic experiences.

Helping or caring roles

Built into most of us seems to be a need for altruism. We take pleasure in helping, caring for or assisting others. There is no end to the ways altruism can express itself within relationships—the role of parent, friend, coach, carer, teacher, etc.... Almost every work or volunteer role has an element of helping.

Sarah experienced severe childhood neglect. She was a single parent but took pride in being a good mom to her two children. Her role as mom gave her a clear sense of meaning.

> **"I know I'm not a perfect mom, but I love my kids in a way that didn't happen for me. I won't let anything happen to them."**

But experiencing meaning through helping others doesn't need to come through what we conventionally think of as a 'caring role'. We mentioned Mark earlier, a socially anxious young man. He was an auto mechanic who got meaning from his job in ways that went beyond simply fixing cars. He genuinely took pleasure in helping his customers.

> **"People come into the garage and they are worried that it will cost a fortune. But I know engines and I have a reputation for keeping**

older cars going. I love the part where I explain what's wrong and how I'm going to repair it. You see the relief on their faces."

Self-expression or self-development

The experience of meaning is intimately connected to what we can do or become. The word *existence* comes from the Latin word exsistere, which means to appear, to arise, to become, or to be, but literally, it means to stand out.[10] Existing means to stand out in some manner. To be something. To express yourself.

Everyone has particular abilities or skills. There is pleasure or meaning to be found through developing and expressing such skills. Such skills do not have to be grandiose. Any skill developed at any level counts – athletics, baking, playing chess, dressmaking, etc..... Meaning can be found in any form of creative expression—gardening, woodworking, painting, writing, and so on. The range of ways people work to develop or express themselves seems endless. We have worked with individuals who are keen to build dollhouses and who enjoy soap carving. One individual bred and raced ferrets!

Suzanne experienced serious childhood emotional abuse and neglect, and she struggled with depression, poor self-esteem, and sometimes didn't want to live. Though difficult to sometimes admit, she was good at creating hand-made cards. Getting back into her craft room at home and reconnecting to the meaning she found in making cards became an important part of her recovery.

A clinician named David Viscott captured the above ideas in the following words: The purpose of life is to discover your gift. The work of life is to develop it. The meaning of life is to give your gift away.[11]

Personal interests or aesthetic experiences

Meaning can also be found through anything we find interesting or within aesthetic experiences. The enjoyment of film, music, art, reading, the natural world, or any field of ideas. The pleasure of being with others. The pleasure we can take in eating, walking, or a hot bath. The fascination with simply existing or the riddles of the universe.

Exercise 3: Creating meaning as a feature of your recovery

Below you have an opportunity to reflect on your experience of meaning and whether there are ways to enhance this. We'd encourage you to think expansively – not to feel limited. What matters less is *how* a person experiences meaning; what matters more is that they *do* experience meaning.

We have suggested three ways in which people can experience meaning.

1. Helping or caring for others
2. Developing or expressing yourself in some way
3. Personal interests or aesthetic experiences

Consider how you currently experience meaning in relation to the above areas in the space below. And, is there something you want to develop within yourself, life or relationships which you imagine may help you experience more meaning?

Julian's notepad

There was something a man named Julian told us during a therapy group which had quite an effect on clinicians and clients alike. The comment fits quite nicely with the topics of meaning and self-expression, and the story has a humorous twist. Julian was in his later years, had spent time in the care system, and had experienced childhood physical and emotional abuse, as well as neglect. Everyone noticed that Julian always carried a small notepad and pen in his front pocket, and in one group therapy session, another client asked him what he did with the notepad. Julian said that many years ago he had developed a habit of reflecting on two questions every morning:

1. What is it that's important for me to do today?
2. How can I look after my well-being while I'm doing it?

He would then make a list of what he wanted or needed to do that day, and a note about how he will look after his state of mind. At first glance, Julian's approach might seem rather simple, even trite. After a hundred years of psychology and a few thousand years of philosophy, surely there's more to it than this, right? Well, probably. And yet, the two questions Julian asked himself and the way they helped him organise his day... well, they seemed to capture something quite essential.

During subsequent sessions, a younger man began turning up with a notebook and pen in his shirt pocket. No one felt the need to point this out. However, as we were just about to take a break during a particular session, a woman sitting next to the young man reached down into her purse and pulled out a small notepad and said to him, "I got one too." While we are certainly not suggesting that everyone start carrying notepads around with them, we thought Julian's insight was worth sharing.

Trauma, society and you

If there is something that 140 years of psychology has taught us about trauma, it's the importance of being able to remember and talk to others about what happened. Freud got this right in the 1890s, and it's no less true today. Finding safe relationships and spaces to talk about what happened can encourage self-expression and meaning. Being *unable* to remember and talk about the past not only makes recovery more difficult, but acts to separate you from the rest of society.

However, as Bessel van Der Kolk[12] and others have pointed out, historically, societal forces have been opposed to traumatised people remembering and speaking out. The trauma experienced by war veterans was ignored or minimised for decades. Abuse cover-ups occurring in a wide range of institutions, both religious and secular, serve as another example. Historically, policing did not always investigate when necessary. Many traumatised individuals can also feel inappropriately ashamed, which makes silence likely. Therefore, when society encourages silence, this is a 'double whammy'.

However, in the past couple of decades we have seen changes to the status quo which are huge and positive. The development of movements such as #MeToo, #MeTooMilitary, and #ChurchToo have encouraged those who were abused in private life, the military, and within religious organisations to speak out. Numerous court proceedings and convictions against high-profile celebrities have demonstrated that justice is possible. Where abuse was institutional, organisations are being held to account – the Catholic Church, the BBC, and certain police forces serving as examples.

There are many ways of 'breaking the silence' concerning your experiences, and you should do what is comfortable with respect to your needs, relationships, and where you are in your recovery. For many individuals, it starts with letting someone they trust begin to know what happened to them and the way it's affected their life. You can go slowly if necessary, and then talk more when you get reassurance that the person is responding with support. Even people who care and want to help may need your advice on how you need them to respond. It can be helpful to let them know.

Society is probably more 'trauma-aware' today than ever before in history, although there is a long way to go. A trauma-aware society is one in which the general public understands that there are individuals they will come across who experienced trauma. It's not about 'walking on egg-shells', but about a reasonable sensitivity within public life and the workplace. Doctors, teachers, police, dentists, salespeople, work persons coming into your home, etc… should all be aware that on any day of the week they may be helping someone who experienced trauma. In a trauma-aware workplace, staff are provided information about the effects of trauma and how a general sensitivity (while probably a good thing for everyone) can be especially helpful for those affected by trauma. If a professional or a member of the public is not acting in a trauma-aware manner, there can be times when it makes sense to provide feedback. You are not being a 'trauma missionary' – you are just raising awareness in a way which is necessary.

Barbara experienced physical and emotional abuse throughout childhood, and her encounter with an optician is an excellent example of self-expression and how we can help society become more trauma-aware.

> **"I'd never been seen by this optometrist. He was friendly, but he spoke with this loud voice and he moved quite quickly, even when he was working very close to me. I would just 'jump' every time he spoke or moved. I said to him, *I need to mention something. You seem friendly and like you know your job, but when I was younger I had some bad experiences, and so I'm kind of sensitive when***

***people talk in louder voices or move very quickly.* He understood immediately, apologised, and changed his approach."**

Talking to a professional in this manner might seem unthinkable, but you are entitled to do it if needed. If a professional takes offence or acts defensively, you probably need to see someone else!

The idea of making allegations against a perpetrator of historical trauma can be the most challenging and complex question for some. Whether an individual comes forward with allegations to the authorities is a very personal decision. Sometimes it's not possible, such as in cases where the perpetrator is deceased. Sometimes an individual simply does not see this as a necessary part of their recovery work. However, we have worked with many individuals who brought allegations forward. Some have found this process to be an important and therapeutic part of their recovery, while others have found it to be a disappointing experience. It's such a personal decision and depends on so many factors, it's impossible for us to suggest a specific direction. If you are considering making allegations, we recommend getting professional advice. A consultation with a reputable lawyer who is experienced in this area is an option, and in some cases, there is no fee for an initial consultation. Or, if you wish, you should be able to speak to the police initially without providing the name of the perpetrator. This may help you better understand the likely local processes of investigation. If you need to speak with an officer of a particular gender, you are entitled to ask for that.

Whether beginning to tell the story with someone you trust, helping society to be that bit more 'trauma-informed', or considering bringing allegations forward, all of this can potentially support self-expression and the sense of meaning which is so important to recovery.

References

1. Dostoyevsky, Fyodor. Quote is found in multiple online sources, but the original source is unknown.
2. Frankl, V. E. (2004). *Man's search for meaning: The classic tribute to hope from the holocaust (new edition)*. London: Rider.
3. Nietzsche, F. (1998). *Twilight of the idols.* Oxford: Oxford University Press.
4. Frankl, V. E. (2004). *Man's search for meaning: The classic tribute to hope from the holocaust (new edition)*. London: Rider.
5. Windisch, S., Simi, P., Blee, K. & DeMichele, M. (2020). Measuring the Extent and Nature of Adverse Childhood Experiences (ACE) among Former White Supremacists. *Terrorism and Political Violence*, 34 (6).
6. Wolff, K. T., Cuevas, C., Intravia, J., Baglivio, M. T. & Epps, M. (2018). The Effects of Neighborhood Context on Exposure to Adverse Childhood Experiences (ACE) Among Adolescents Involved in the Juvenile Justice System: Latent Classes and Contextual Effects. *Journal of Youth and Adolescence*, 47, 2279–2300.
7. Frankl, V.E. (2010). *The doctor and the soul: From psychotherapy to logotherapy.* London: Random House.
8. Fulghum, R. (2004). *All I really need to know I learned in kindergarten: Uncommon thoughts on common things*. New York: Ballantine Books.
9. Frankl, V. E. (2004). *Man's search for meaning: The classic tribute to hope from the holocaust (new edition)*. London: Rider.
10. Harper, D. "Existence". Online Etymology Dictionary.
11. Viscott, D. (2003). *Finding Your Strength in Difficult Times: A Book of Meditations.* NY: McGraw-Hill.
12. Van Der kolk, B. (2015). *The body keeps the score: Mind, brain and body in the transformation of trauma*. London: Penguin Books.

Chapter 21

Reflecting and Looking Forward

"It's difficult to know how to think about the HTP ending.
I'm not sure whether to feel worried, sad, or relieved."
Jennifer

Every model of therapy or personal development is different. Some are gentler and ask less of the individual. While paying attention to safety and the need for participants to be well-supported, The Historical Trauma Programme is admittedly fairly intense and asks quite a lot. You have been required to explore painful memories, to work hard at developing insight, to take on board some complex psychological ideas, and sometimes to transfer what is learned into your life.

The Historical Trauma Programme thinks about *the ending* in an unusual way. While you are nearing the end of the Guidebook, you are not coming to the end of your recovery work. We hope that the HTP has helped you feel more insightful or confident in your recovery work, but the work will continue. That just seems to be the nature of childhood trauma.

Toward the outset of the Guidebook we said 'at the moment, this Guidebook is identical to every other copy. When you finish, there will be a lot of *you* between these pages.' This is true, isn't it? The Guidebook contains ideas and practices from trauma studies, the voices of others who experienced childhood trauma, and clinician observations – but your reflections, insights, and experiences are here as well. The work you have done will have at times been 'hard won' – it won't have been simple or easy. If the Guidebook helps you to face your future recovery work with a bit more insight and confidence, that will reflect what you have done here. And, if you have moments of confusion or distress (and you probably will), the Guidebook and the work you have done will be here. You own this work.

This final chapter represents an opportunity for you to pull together:

- ❖ Change which you believe you have made 'at the level of insight'.
- ❖ Change 'at the level of doing'. Some may have had moments of experimenting with change within their life, relationships, or how you relate to yourself.

- ❖ What you feel you have *not* dealt with as yet. You will realise there is more work to be done, and you can describe that as well.
- ❖ The way forward

There is a reason it can be helpful to pull together the work you have done. Past trauma is not interested in stepping aside graciously in order to make way for your on-going recovery. Despite all the work you have done, your past trauma will continue to want to run your life. Consolidating what you have learned is a good basis for the continued fight to overcome the impact of past events.

Change at the level of insight

When many people think about creating change or personal development, what comes to mind are changes which occur in their lives, like getting a new job, starting a new relationship, or taking up a new hobby. However, in respect to trauma-based therapy or personal development, being able to *see* or *think about* something from a different perspective can represent important change. We might call this *change at the level of insight*, because that's just what it is. It's important not to underestimate how important insight is and what you have had to face in order to achieve it.

However, what constitutes insight in respect to your work with the HTP programme is very individual. We can highlight what 'change at the level of insight' has meant for a handful of HTP clients to help illustrate the idea, but how insight has worked for you will be quite personal. Below represents changes at the level of insight for certain HTP clients:

"I'd heard of self-compassion, but I hadn't really thought about it. Realising how much of a problem self-compassion is for me was an eye-opener. I've seen how much work I've got to do in this area."
- Marie

"When I was little I thought my parents hurt me because I was bad. Now I can see that I just thought I was a bad kid because of the way they treated me."
-Barbara

"I'd never heard of C-PTSD. That opened my eyes because I have all of those issues. Knowing there is a name for my problems helps me think and talk about my problems differently.
- Claudine

"I've always felt like a mutant – like some sort of alien. But hearing other people's stories has made me realise that I'm not as weird as I thought."
- Reynold

"For years I've just thought I had made a mess of my life, but the Guidebook has helped me connect what happened as a child with all of the problems I've had as an adult."
- John

"I always knew that I had bad self-esteem and not much confidence, but the work on trauma-based shame sort of opened my eyes. I had just never thought of it like that. When I start to feel awful about myself, I can see it as shame and connect it to what happened to me."
- Alan

"Traumatic core beliefs were new to me, but they helped explain why I just flip into these awful thoughts and feelings when there is some trigger. I need to learn more about that when I finish the programme."
-Julie

"I've always felt everything so intensely in my body, like the way my heart pounds and I want to escape when I'm around people. A bunch of doctors have said I have an anxiety disorder, but that doesn't explain anything. The chapter on the body and that polyvagal thing helped me understand my anxiety in a completely different way."
- Mary Ann

"I've known that my relationships to men aren't good, but I've really come to see that I need to be able to set boundaries, say what I need, and not let people just keep hurting me."
-Maggy

Exercise 1: Change at the level of insight

Change at the level of insight will be personal for you. Has the programme helped you see or think about your past, yourself, or relationships differently? For some, scanning the table of contents or parts of the guidebook can help.

Change at the level of doing

Some who have engaged with the HTP will mainly have been working with 'change at the level of insight'. For these individuals, making changes in the context of one's life and relationships may take more of a 'back seat'. That's alright, and these individuals will have plenty of opportunities following their work with the HTP to transfer their insights into their lives and relationships. The severity and complexity of problems for certain individuals means that change will be slower, and everyone needs to go at a pace which they can manage.

However, some will have developed insight *and* will have been experimenting with change 'at the level of doing' (in their relationships, lives, and how they relate to themselves). Also (and this might seem odd) behavioural change can occur in your head – in the way you think. If you have been able to respond differently in how you think about situations, that's *internal behaviour* happening through your thoughts – many people forget to give themselves credit for this form of change).

There is no end to the different ways 'change at the level of doing' can happen. We have seen individuals take new risks such as joining a dating website, joining a social group, being more assertive with friends or partners, thinking differently in response to triggers, making or developing friendships, setting boundaries in relationships, ending a destructive relationship, applying for jobs or an educational programme, developing a creative project, etc… . Some will have talked about their past abuse or neglect with people in their lives rather than holding onto the secrets, which in itself is an important change.

But change at the *level of doing* does not have to be something objectively 'big' in order for it to be important to an individual. Sally experienced multiple forms of childhood abuse, and had not gone to a professional hairdresser for over twenty years. Her confidence had been so shattered and her mistrust of people so great, that she had been cutting her own hair all these years. Before the end of her therapy, she had her hair done at a solon. For Sally, that was huge change at the level of doing. Every individual is starting at a different place, and so what represents important change at the level of doing is personal.

We recall the final session of one group in which Brandon, who experienced physical and emotional abuse, appeared rather disheartened. He said, "I don't think I've made any real changes or done anything differently." Another group member then gave him some feedback, reminding him that he had previously described a long pattern of avoiding or quitting anything that caused him anxiety. In fact, he had experienced impulses to quit the therapy group on more than one occasion. The point was clear: Brandon had completed group therapy, an accomplishment which had broken a long pattern of social avoidance and disengagement.

Exercise 2: Experimenting with change at the level of doing

Can you recognise attempts you have made *to do things differently*? Don't sell yourself short. Every effort at change counts. Remember that it's not just behavioural changes happening in relationships and life, but internal change in terms of being able think differently about circumstances or yourself. What comes to mind?

Your recovery: What do you still need to work on?

The goal of this programme was never for you *to get rid of* tension or conflict. The goal was always to help you live as well as possible *with* tension or conflict. We have never had any illusions about how difficult recovering from childhood trauma can be. The exercise below offers you an opportunity to reflect on the problems you continue to struggle with.

Some will have learned that they have absorbed some very punitive messages and that they want to develop more compassionate ways of being with themselves. Some will recognise that they need healthier relationships and that they want to take some risks in making this happen. Some will have started dealing with painful post-traumatic reactions, but they have a ways to go in this respect. Some will have discovered that they really struggle with attentional problems, and approaches like mindfulness may be something they want to explore further. Some will realise that traumatic core beliefs are a significant problem, and they want to focus on this issue more. Some will appreciate that they keep being retraumatised, and it's an area needing more attention. Some will have made a start at communicating with others about what happened to them and the problems they have, but this is something they need to do further.

Exercise 3: What are the problems or issues which you continue to struggle with?
Is there something you have started working on but which you want to continue learning about or developing? Is there further personal development you want to focus on? What's your 'growing edge'?

What next?

For most, completing the Historical Trauma Programme doesn't mean they feel they are done with learning about their past and related difficulties. For some individuals, perhaps those who are newer to working on recovery, the HTP may even feel like just the beginning. Maybe after completing the HTP you feel like you need a break from thinking about your past and perhaps you just want to get on with your life for a while before picking up on further personal development work. Others may feel hungry to learn more in this area straight away. Whether you need a break from your recovery or want to dive into more work, we encourage you to keep going.

It's not unusual for participants to complete the HTP and wonder – what might I focus on next concerning my personal development? This is a very personal question and the answer will be different depending on the individual. Perhaps you will identify a way forward we haven't even considered, but below we share a few thoughts.

- ❖ There are a lot of good books to read on the subject. We highlight several at the end of this text, but web and Amazon searches can also be useful.
- ❖ If you have done the HTP as self-help, perhaps individual or group therapy is something you may wish to pursue. If you have used the HTP to support individual therapy, perhaps moving onto group therapy interests you.
- ❖ If available in your area, a community support group for people who experienced complex trauma can be very useful to some. If one doesn't exist, maybe it should. Perhaps this can be done in co-operation with mental health services in your area. At the end of this book is a section on starting a community support group.
- ❖ Perhaps your involvement with this programme has put you in touch with some creative project related to the work you have done. This might relate to writing, art, further education you wish to do, etc… . Perhaps there are social groups related to this area of interest you can consider.
- ❖ Perhaps the programme has helped you develop more confidence in yourself and a desire to develop existing relationships or create new ones.

The personalised HTP certificate of completion

The HTP is a model of self-help or can be used to support individual therapy – it's not a 'course' or training – so the idea of a personalised certificate of completion may seem odd. However, the HTP has required a great deal of time and commitment. While some do not feel the need for a certificate, in our experience many people who complete the programme wish to have one. It seems to symbolise and act as a reminder of all the work they put into it.

One person framed it and hung it on the wall of their home office. He told us he would show it to certain people who visited and joke that it was his 'sane certificate'. While a funny joke, there was something serious about the quip. He had kept his past a secret for many years, so telling people about his experience of the HTP was a way of breaking that pattern. Apparently, the certificate can also elicit some complex feelings for a few people. One person we worked with tore up a certificate and threw it in a recycling bin on the way out of a final session. Three days later she called the office, said she regretted her decision, and asked for another certificate.

If you would like a personalised certificate, one can be downloaded at the HTP website. If you have any difficulties obtaining the certificate, contact us through the website or by email (see details at the end of the Guidebook).

Finally…

You came to this programme as someone who experienced childhood trauma. What happened to you will always be a part of who you are, and so you will leave this programme as someone who experienced childhood trauma. But, as the programme has explored from many different angles, you can assert *some* control over the effects of past abuse, neglect or abandonment. Whether this means standing up to traumatic core beliefs, coping in ways in which your needs are met, avoiding retraumatisation, developing healthier relationships or creating meaning in response to your past suffering, there is always something you can work at.

If it feels like you have made substantial progress in this programme, we are pleased. But many individuals will feel there is still a long road ahead. Some will feel they are just beginning. That's okay too. Just keep going. If you have moments where you feel yourself falling into isolation, depression, or hopelessness, perhaps an idea expressed by the French-American photographer Elliott Erwitt will help: "Keep working, because as you go through the process… things begin to happen."[1]

With all of this in mind, we leave you with the words of Sam, who we quoted elsewhere. In a sense, perhaps her words say it all.

> **"I face what happened most days in my thoughts and feelings and sometimes my dreams. But what happened won't define me."**

References

1. Erwitt, E. (2014). As quoted in *Photography: The Definitive Visual History* by Tom Ang. DK Books: London.

Community Support Groups

For some people, joining a community support group can be a helpful way to receive support and stay engaged in the recovery work they are doing. Some people may join a community support group without having had therapy, but a community support group can often be a natural 'step down' from the intensity of therapy. Perhaps there is a community support group for those who experienced childhood harm you can find that may help you. If not, perhaps you can play a role in developing one. We have seen community support groups developed by experienced service users who have completed therapy and done good recovery work, often in close co-operation with mental health services.

A community support group for people who experienced childhood harm shares certain characteristics with individual or group therapy, but is also distinct. Some features are described below.

1. It's common for individual or group therapy to meet on a weekly basis. The intensity of formal therapy seems to require a greater frequency of sessions. A community support group may meet weekly, but less frequent meetings are common, e.g. monthly or fortnightly.

2. Some community support groups are facilitated by an individual or individuals who experienced childhood trauma but have done therapy and feel confident in their recovery work, and it can be helpful for them to have had some training in group facilitation and counselling. Other community support groups are facilitated by a qualified clinician, or are co-facilitated by a qualified clinician and someone who experienced trauma and has done recovery work. Either can work well, but it's usually important for the group to have a facilitator.

3. Community supports groups can be less formal than therapy, and a lot of what happens revolves around members talking, listening and offering support to one another. However, there are other ways the group can be used, e.g. occasionally having speakers join a session.

4. Safety and confidentiality are just as important in a community support group as in group therapy. For example, protecting members' identity and information, not communicating what occurs in a session on social media, and being clear about the limits concerning confidentiality.

5. In group therapy, there is often a rule against individuals socialising outside group sessions. Community support groups do not normally have such a rule.

6. The structure of what happens in a community support group session can be determined by the members and facilitator(s). However, being clear on what this structure is can add a sense of safety and stability. Some groups start with a 'check-in' where each member has an opportunity to let others know how they are, whether something important or difficult is going on for them, and whether they need any particular help. From the 'check-in', the group may decide what they want to do with the rest of the time. Perhaps certain members need particular attention in that session, or there is an important theme which is coming up that everyone can discuss together. This is only one process, and there is no 'correct' way a session must be structured.

7. Therapy groups are often limited in the number of sessions. Community support groups tend to run on an on-going basis, so there is usually no time limit concerning membership. Some members will eventually leave the group, often when they have done the work they need to, or some may move out of the area. A member may need to return if they hit a very difficult patch in life. Knowing the group is there can be reassuring. A good size for a community support group is similar to group therapy - somewhere between four and ten with 6-8 being common. If attendance gets much larger than this, a decision needs to be made. One way of resolving the issue is to start another community support group.

8. Some community support groups can create ways of communicating via social media platforms as well as in person, but if this occurs, it needs to be thought through carefully, especially concerning the issues of confidentiality or dealing with potential risk.

Recommended Reading

General books on childhood trauma

Reinventing Your Life by Jeffrey E. Young and Janet Klosko. NY; Plume. 1993.
This is an excellent personal development book which has helped many who experienced childhood harm. The book may be especially appealing if you found the chapters on retraumatisation and traumatic core beliefs useful.

The Body Keeps the Score: Mind, Brain and Body in the Transformation of Trauma by Bessel Van Der Kolk. London. Penguin.
A highly competent and comprehensive overview of the nature of traumatic experience which pays special attention to the impact of trauma on the way our brains and physiology respond. Has appeal for those affected by trauma as well as professionals.

Overcoming Childhood Trauma by Helen Kennerley. London: Robinson Press. 2000.
We've recommended this book to survivors many times over the years. It's filled with very good information about the effects of all forms of abuse and neglect, as well as practical strategies for dealing with painful psychological reactions. Highly readable and often has the effect of 'normalising' survivors experiences.

The Complex PTSD Workbook: A Mind-Body Approach to Regaining Emotional Control and Becoming Whole by Arielle Schwartz. Berkeley. Althea Press. 2017
A personal development-styled workbook with good information and practical tools. A very good introduction to complex trauma that can be used as personal development or to complement 1-1 therapy.

Anchored: How to Befriend Your Nervous System Using Polyvagal Theory by Deb Dana. Sounds True. 2021.
A compassionate and practical personal development styled book which teaches you the principles of polyvagal theory and also guides you through many exercises designed to help you reshape your nervous system. If you found Chapter 5 helpful, this book will provide more detail and depth concerning the theory and practice of polyvagal theory.

The Pocket Guide to the Polyvagal Theory: The Transformative Power of Feeling Safe by Stephen Porges. W.W Norton. 2017.
A helpful and in-depth explanation of polyvagal theory by the founder of the theory himself.

Male and female survivors of sexual abuse

Breaking Free Workbook: Practical Help for Survivors of Childhood Sexual Abuse by Carolyn Ainscough and Kay Toon. London: Sheldon Press. 2000.
This is an excellent resource for female and male survivors of sexual abuse. The workbook can be used by an individual on their own as long as they feel reasonably safe and secure. If not, the workbook is best seen as a means of supporting work you are going with a therapist, either individually or in a group.

Female survivors of sexual abuse

The Courage to Heal: A Guide for Women Survivors of Child Sexual Abuse by Ellen Bass and Laura Davies. London: Vermilion. 2002.
While several years old, this is still an excellent resource for female survivors of childhood sexual abuse.

Male survivors of sexual abuse

Victims No Longer: The Classic Guide for Men Recovering from Sexual Child Abuse by Mike Lew. NY: HarperCollins. 2004.

For people struggling with post-traumatic reactions

Overcoming Traumatic Stress by Claudia Herbert and Ann Wetmore. London: Robinson Press. 2008.
This is an excellent personal development book filled with useful theory as well as a number of strategies. Well researched but also written in an accessible and engaging style. This is perhaps the best book to get started with concerning this area.

For people who want more on emotion regulation skills

Don't Let Your Emotions Run Your Life: How Dialectical Behavior Therapy Can Put You in Control Paperback by Scott E. Spradlin. New Harbinger. 2003.
A very competent and straightforward self-help oriented book to help you learn direct skills for managing painful emotional states. Perhaps the best one to start with.

The Dialectical Behavior Therapy Skills Workbook: Practical DBT Exercises for Learning Mindfulness, Interpersonal Effectiveness, Emotion Regulation, and Distress Tolerance by Matthew McKay and Jeffrey C. Wood. New Harbinger. 2019.
Comprehensive and competent approach to emotion regulation.

Self-compassion

The Compassionate Mind Approach to Recovering from Trauma: Using Compassion Focused Therapy by Deborah Lee Sophie James. Robinson. *2012*
This book is very much self-help orientated and uses a compassion-focused approach aimed directly at adults who experienced childhood trauma. Like the HTP, there are many exercises provided for you.

The Mindful Self-Compassion Workbook: A Proven Way to Accept Yourself, Build Inner Strength, and Thrive by Kristin Neff and Christopher Germer. Guilford. 2018
This approach combines mindfulness practice with self-compassion, so if you want a resource covering both areas, this may be useful.

Mindfulness

Wherever You Go There You are: Mindfulness Meditation in Everyday Life by Jon Kabit- Zinn. Hyperion. 2005.
A beautifully written book which helps you understand the theory and practice of mindfulness.

A Mindfulness-Based Stress Reduction Workbook by Bob Stahl and Elisha Goldstein. New Harbinger. 2019.
A workbook approach designed to help you learn and use mindfulness-based stress reduction (MBSR)

Mindfulness: A practical guide to finding peace in a frantic world by Mark Williams and Danny Penman. Piatkus. 2011.
This is an 8-week course of self-help also based in the theory and practice of mindfulness-based stress reduction (MBSR).

Trauma-based shame

It Wasn't Your Fault: Freeing Yourself from the Shame of Childhood Abuse with the Power of Self-Compassion by Beverly Engel. Oakland: New Harbinger. 2015.
This is a good personal development-oriented book for male or female survivors of all forms of abuse. It is especially useful if shame is a significant issue and if you have a difficult time with self-compassion and self-soothing.

Relationship skills and social confidence

Conversationally Speaking by Alan Garner. Lowell House: Cambridge. 1997.
An excellent book for people who want to develop relationship skills and social confidence.

How To Start A Conversation And Make Friends by Don Gabor. Touchstone. Austin. 2011.
A good book for any survivors who simply lack confidence in communication and relationships. Might be seen as a bit basic for some, but for survivors who were never taught/shown how to develop and maintain good relationships, this one can be really helpful.

Overcoming Social Anxiety and Shyness: A Self-help Guide Using Cognitive Behavioural Techniques (2nd Ed.) by Gillian Butler. Robinson Press. London. 2016.
If what is getting in the way of relationship development is social anxiety, this is a good book filled with solid theory and practical strategies. If you like this book, there is a three-part workbook which acts a companion you can move onto.

For survivors currently in abusive relationships

The Emotionally Abusive Relationship: How to Stop Being Abused and How to Stop Abusing by Beverly Engel. NY: Wiley. 2003.
A good personal development book for adults who are in an abusive relationship (either as perpetrator, victim, or both).

The Verbally Abusive Relationship, Expanded Third Edition: How to recognise it and how to respond by Patricia Evans. Avon: Adam's Media. 2010.
A personal development book for those involved in verbally abusive adult relationships.

Other books

Man's Search For Meaning: The classic tribute to hope from the Holocaust (new edition) by Victor E. Frankl. London: Rider. 2013.
An autobiographical account of Frankl's experience at Auschwitz concentration camp and the psychological lessons he learned from the experience. If you found the chapter on Meaning and Self-expression important, this book may appeal to you. However, some descriptions are somewhat disturbing, so this may not be for everyone.

The Addiction Recovery Skills Workbook: Changing Addictive Behaviors Using CBT, Mindfulness, and Motivational Interviewing Techniques by Suzette Glasner-Edwards. NY: New Harbinger. 2015
A good book for any survivor who copes through addictive behaviours. A reliable and valid approach which is supportive for any form of addiction.

Further Information and Making contact

The HTP Community Website

The HTP website can be found at www.htpcommunity.org. The website allows you to connect with others, share your views, ask questions, make contact, and access further information. Free audio versions of the two HTP Guidebooks are also available for download at the website. Alternatively, you can access the audio versions on YouTube - when on YouTube, search using the words @HistoricalTraumaProgramme.

Should you wish to support the HTP

If you found the Historical Trauma Programme beneficial, we would be grateful if you could encourage others by leaving a review on Amazon. Leaving a review on the Amazon site you normally use is really helpful. And, if you have time, you can even use your normal username and password to log in separately to Amazon.co.uk, Amazon.com, Amazon.ca and Amazon.au and leave your review on all sites.

Contact

If you wish to get in touch concerning the Historical Trauma Programme to share your insights or feedback or request further information, you can do so through a link on the website (www.htpcommunity.org) or emailing **HTPcontact43@gmail.com**

However, if you are experiencing risk or need immediate clinical assistance, please do not use this email address, but instead contact your primary doctor, clinician or emergency services in your area.

www.ingramcontent.com/pod-product-compliance
Lightning Source LLC
LaVergne TN
LVHW080016210926
848481LV00011B/3041